ACCOLADES FOR
YASGUR'S HOMEOPATHIC DICTIONARY

One of our most valuable books. Jay has redone it again. Bigger, new edition and a remedy pronunciation guide, too. Everyone needs one.

Joe Lillard
Past President, NCH

We owe Jay Yasgur a debt of gratitude for a useful job well done. In these pages may be found at last the meaning of 'tetter' and 'stomacace' and a multitude of archaic terms that most of us have never heard of but can be found in our classic texts on almost every page.

Richard Moskowitz, M.D.

One of the many difficulties encountered by the persons undertaking the serious study of homeopathy is due to the fact that much of the valued literature is written in the language of another age. How often one has cried, "Why doesn't somebody make a dictionary of homeopathic terms?" Well, someone has done that, thoroughly, comprehensively and in good usable form: *Yasgur's Homeopathic Dictionary* is now revised and expanded by 400 more entries, pronounciation guide to the remedies, and in general more comprehensive. In short, here is a book which is needed in every homeopathic practitioner's library.

Maesimund B. Panos, M.D.

Yasgur's Homeopathic Dictionary belongs in the library of every homeopath and is a must for every homeopathic student. Yasgur gives clear definitions of archaic as well as modern, relevant homeopathic terms. Terminology is important—with this Dictionary we can all get it right!

Durr Elmore, D.C., N.D., C.C.H.

It is essential to be as precise as possible when practising homeopathy. A crucial part of precision is understanding the rubrics in Kent's *Repertory*. *Yasgur's Homeopathic Dictionary* is indispensible. It should be on every practitioner's desk.

Karl Robinson, M.D.

Yasgur's Homeopathic Dictionary is the Dorland of our homeopathic collection. It is invaluable to our students who often have difficulties with the meaning of the old-fashioned medical terms used in the older homeopathic literature.

Friedhelm Kirchfeld, Librarian
National College of Naturopathic Medicine

A most useful book for every homeopath.

Ellen Goldman, ND, DHANP
Chair Homeopathy Department, Bastyr University

Medical terminology is often complex because of its arid scientific nature. In the case of Homeopathy, it is even more complicated because of the obsolete character of a lot of terms used in the 19th century literature of the original authors. *Yasgur's Homeopathic Dictionary* successfully serves as a deciphering guide and a cultural bridge to help medical students in their study of classic homeopathic reference books. It represents a tremendous effort, and this useful tool should be part of every homeopathic library.

Thierry Monfort, President
Boiron-USA

This book is a necessity for the homeopathic student. Jay Yasgur has done a great service by bringing the archaic terminology together and defining those elusive terms clearly and succinctly. Aside from the over 4000 defintions there is a section on homeopathic obituaries. This is the first time this interesting information has been assembled with accuracy and completeness in one place. A pronunciation guide for over 700 remedies is also included. This book is very well done and is an essential reference for medical historian, and homeopathic practitioner and student alike.

Julian Winston
Historian and editor of *Homeopathy Today*

What a great book!   **David R. Riley, O.M.D, L.Ac., Ph.D.**

Very useful. I am glad to have it.   **Harris L. Coulter, Ph.D.**

Over the years, many homeopaths have asked me about the meaning of homeopathic terms. Non-medically trained practitioners and physicians alike can be challenged by the 19th century terminology. Jay Yasgur's dictionary can be useful for any practitioner as reflected by the following ideas expressed by two groups of homeopaths. *"I am not a medical doctor so I have been forced to look through many dictionaries to help me in my understanding of the language in both the repertory and materia medica. I have found everything I needed in this book and am thankful it has been written,"* and, *"I am a medical doctor quite familiar with medical terminology. However, homeopathic literature is riddled with terms that are no longer taught in medical school. This dictionary describes all of those words and often gives current terminology so that I can translate them into my understanding of medicine."* For these two groups of homeopaths, I like the book; it saves time!

Paul Herscu, N.D., D.H.A.N.P.

Not only a source handbook for homeopaths, but fascinating reading as well.
Irene Alleger, in *Townsend Letter for Doctors*

Yasgur's

HOMEOPATHIC DICTIONARY

and

HOLISTIC HEALTH REFERENCE
FOURTH EDITION

JAY YASGUR, R.Ph., M.Sc.

ISBN
1-886149-04-6

Publisher Cataloging-in-Publication Data

Yasgur, Jay.
    Yasgur's Homeopathic Dictionary and Holistic Health Reference/
Jay Yasgur., 4th ed.
          p. cm.
          Includes bibliography.
          ISBN 1-886149-04-6
    1. Homeopathy—Dictionaries. 2. Holistic medicine—Dictionaries.
II. Title.
RX41.Y37 1997
615.5/32/03--dc21   97-60094
                                                  CIP

Library of Congress Control Number
97-60094

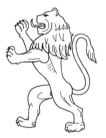

Van Hoy Publishers
P.O. Box 636 • Greenville, PA • 16125

Cover design: J. David Mata

The paper used in this publication meets the minimum requirements of the
American National Standard for Information Sciences—
Permanence of Paper for Printed Library Materials
ANSI Z39.48-1984
Printed in the United States of America

This book is dedicated to the memory of

BOAZ GOLDMAN

INEZ VAN HOY

HARRIETT YASGUR

"Still-in a way-nobody sees a flower;
really-it is so small-we haven't time,
and to see takes time,
like to have a friend takes time."

—*Georgia O'Keeffe*

CONTENTS

ACKNOWLEDGEMENTS

I would like to thank those persons who helped me, in a variety of ways, to complete this volume:

First I need to acknowledge R.P. Newstedt who has sent a number of notes detailing clarifications and suggestions for making this a better work ... thank you, R.P.

Thank you to Julian Winston and Chris Ellithorp, for this and the other contributions you've made to this dictionary. Your assistance in my times of need was greatly appreciated. I would also like to thank the members of the Homeopathic Pharmacopoeia Convention of the United States for allowing me to reprint the pronunciation guide for over 700 remedies, as found in the 8th Edition of the HPUS.

Thanks to Stella Baker, Norman Ward, DVM, S. Jubelirer, Magneto Geometric Applications (London, U.K.), The Radionic Association (Banbury, UK), William Garvin, Sherry Arrick, Durr Elmore, Karl Robinson, Maesimund Panos, L. D. Lillis, K.H. Gypser, M.D., Richard Kalin, Steven Ross *(Latin aficionado)*, Holly Pierce *(el computer wizard)*, Dorothy O'Stafy *(eagle-eye proof reader)*, Greg Bedayn, John Freedom, Thiel College, and Christine Bayuk for the special treasure which she is. Many quotes found in the text were abstracted from R.H. Langbridge's *A.B.C. of Homoeopathy*.

Thanks to the NCH and *Classical Homoeopathic Quarterly* and K-H Gypser, M.D. for their permission to use photos and text relating to Cookinham and Schmidt.

Finally, my heart-felt appreciation to editor Begabati Lennihan, whose help was greatly appreciated. Her suggestions and insights have brought this important reference to a new level.

FOREWORD

I have often told people that one way to begin to understand the language of homeopathic literature is to read 19th century literature. That was the native language of Dr. James Tyler Kent. Were Kent (or any other 19th century person) to suddenly appear today, we would have little trouble understanding them—certainly not the amount of trouble we would have understanding Shakespeare or Milton. Yet the similarity of the language is deceiving, for there are subtle shadings in the meaning of words. When the epidemic diseases of diphtheria, typhoid, malaria, and tuberculosis were such a large part of the world for the inhabitants of the 1800s, it is no wonder that they developed a whole vocabulary for talking about these things. As the diseases faded into history, so did the language to describe them. Yet it is seen every day by those who access Kent's *Repertory of the Materia Medica.*

Certainly, some of the definitions for these strange words may be found in a modern dictionary. Others can be found in medical dictionaries. But some are all but lost—to be found only in medical dictionaries that were published at the turn of the century.

Jay Yasgur has done a great service by once again bringing these definitions to our consciousness. Many of these terms are, indeed, obsolete and may refer to something that is now never seen in modern medicine. Yet others are so completely descriptive, that, as they become part of our vocabulary, our understanding of the repertory and the materia medica is enhanced.

—*Julian Winston*
Editor, *Homeopathy Today*

PREFACE

Years ago when first starting my study of homeopathy I was shocked by the number of medical terms which were not familiar to me. Even though I had taken an etymology course in pharmacy school I still found myself looking up words. It was then that the seed was planted to write this book. I did not realize how much nurturing that seed would require. In order to create this dictionary I have had to review many sources page by page, word by word...

Kent's *Repertory*

Boericke's *Materia Medica*

Julian's *Materia Medica of New Homeopathic Remedies*

Knerr's *Repertory*

Barthel's *Synthetic Repertory*

J.H. Clarke's *The Prescriber*

J.H. Clarke's *A Clinical Repertory of the Dictionary of Materia Medica*

Mathur's *Systematic Materia Medica of Homeopathic Remedies*

Boger's *Synoptic Key*

Tetau's *Clinical Homeopathic Materia Medica and Biotherapeutic Associations*

Heel's *Ordinatio Antihomotoxica and Materia Medica*

Nash's *Leaders in Homeopathic Therapeutics*

Hull's edition of Jahr's *Homeopathic Manual/Repertory*

Hull's edition of Laurie's *Homeopathic Domestic Medicine*

Hering's *The Homeopathic Domestic Physician*

Raue's *Special Pathology and Diagnostics with Therapeutic Hints*

Hahnemann's *Organon*

Obviously this has not been an easy task but it has been a task which, for the most part, I have immensely enjoyed.

Fortunately or unfortunately, the meanings associated with some terminology evolves. Words which meant one thing in the early 1800s now mean something quite different. This is the reason why you'll come across terms which have contradictory or imprecise meanings. Also, the effect that different authors had on defining terms needs to be factored in. Look at 'hemeralopia'. I've seen it defined as 'day sight' and also as 'nightblindness'. As one may imagine, this becomes more than confusing—try frustrating! In these cases one must address the context in which the term is used to obtain the exact meaning. In another example, 'orthopnea' is defined as 'difficult breathing' in an 1840 reference, *Ruoff's Repertory of Homoeopathic Medicine*. Yet in modern references it means 'labored breathing whereby the individual needs to sit up to breathe more easily'.

Or 'hypochondria'. Not only does it refer to an abdominal region, it used to mean 'of low spirits', and now the predominant definition for hypochondriasis appears to be, 'an excessive concern for one's health and well-being'. This 'low spirited' melancholic meaning has evolved into 'hypochondriac'. To see just how this term has evolved let me offer a plausible explanation. When one doesn't feel well one may feel depressed, and perhaps hold or rub the belly (hypochondria region) to provide comfort and relief. 'My stomach hurts' could be a possible way to phrase this discomfort. As medical theory was not too developed 150-200 years ago, medical reasoning might have gone something like this: 'S/he is low-spirited, and holds the belly for comfort. I'll give a medicine to affect the belly which in turn will improve the mental condition.' As time has gone by, this term evolved to mean 'sadness or depression of the spirits; gloom' and now 'obsessive worry about health, belief in imaginary ailments'. Whether or not one accepts my reasoning does not matter. The point is, elements of ambiguity are present in some definitions.

Definitions for the great variety of symptoms peculiar to homeopathy, can be found under the term *symptom*. Rather than make individual entries for particular/general/mental/new... symptoms, I decided to group them all together. This has the added benefit that all are together.

A few helpful charts are included as is an article from the early part of the 20th century. This article, by B.C. Woodbury, M.D., deals with homeopathic terminology and reflects the need which our homeopathic 'ancestors' felt for 'a dictionary of homeopathy'. I hope you enjoy this small treat.

Apparently some doubt exists about the birth/death data of Hahnemann, hence the two different astrological charts supplied by Dobereiner and by K.H. Gypser, M.D. As my astrological dexterity is virtually nil, I decided to include both! Some have criticized my decision to even remotely associate astrology with homeopathy, but I decided to include the charts, if nothing more than for interest's sake. Beware, if another chart surfaces pray tell, I'll remove myself to the environs and 'bay at the moon' (*vide* LUNATIC)!

A compilation of abbreviations and appellations (the initials after professionals' names indicating their degrees and/or licensure) and a succinct glossary of holistic health terms has been added. The obituary section contains many new characters. Yes, characters! It is just plain fascinating and inspiring to read about our 'homeopathic ancestors'.

An excellent reference has just been published, *The Mind Defined,* by L. Part and R. Preston. Like this dictionary, it is an essential book to have on one's desk while repertorizing. It defines the archaic meanings of words found in the Mind section of *Kent's Repertory.* Though many of those words can be found in my dictionary, you might consider adding this book to your library as common words which we 'know' and take for granted are defined. The compilers of that work have used older references and dictionaries just as I have done.

The *American Heritage Dictionary* defines 350,000 words; the *Oxford English Dictionary* lists 615,000; and if one adds scientific and technical terms that number rises to about two million. This dictionary has approximately 4500. There are 2,796 languages in use on this planet, and one out of seven people speaks or understands English. The German language has 185,000 words, Russian 130,000, and French less than 100,000. The average high school graduate knows about 6,000 English words, the college grad from 15,000 to 25,000. Dictionaries are important, are they not?! By the way, the first dictionary of English words was compiled in 1604 by Robert Cawdry, entitled *A Table Alphabeticall of Hard Wordes.* Samuel Johnson's (1709-1784) *Dictionary* was important because it fixed English spelling and established a standard reference for the use of modern English words. My thanks to Sherman Jubelirer for his help with this factual information.

After using the typeface Soutane for the third edition, I decided to go back to Times Roman for the fourth. It is easy to read and the standard.

Lastly, I would like to thank Begabati Lennihan who assisted me in rounding out the rough edges of this book. She came at a time when I was looking for someone to spruce up my book. It has been a meant-to-be association. She is an excellent editor and again I extend my thanks to her.

In order to make future editions more complete and error-free, I am relying on you, the user of this volume, to send me words or terms which you'd like to see included. But do not stop there; make whatever suggestions, criticisms and comments you feel necessary to improve this work. Your keen eye and diligence will aid in the production of a more educational and worthwhile book for the homeopathic community.

Be happy and smile,
Jay Yasgur

WHAT IS HOMEOPATHY?

Homeopathy is a therapeutic medical science.

All the ailments and diseases of people (and animals) can be treated with homeopathic remedies using homeopathic healing principles. This sounds like a panacea—which it is not, and yet it is. "Fantastic," you say—and that is exactly what I thought when my homeopathic studies began.

Homeopathy (from the Greek *homeo,* 'similar', and *pathos,* 'suffering'), is a scientifically proven system of healing logic which should not be confused with 'home remedies'. It uses minute doses of specially prepared substances from the plant, animal, and mineral kingdoms. Homeopathic remedies, as they are called, are non-toxic, have no known side-effects and are most commonly administered by dissolution in the mouth. The homeopathic remedy begins to work immediately, and its duration of action (which varies from remedy to remedy) can be quite prolonged. The practitioner uses his/her expertise to select the proper remedy from the nearly 2000 available. He selects the proper potency and frequency of administration depending upon the vitality of the patient and the disease being treated. During the course of treatment several remedies may be needed, yet just one is administered at a time. Because it is truly an art, the practice of homeopathy does vary from practitioner to practitioner.

As mentioned, homeopathic remedies are frequently administered in minute, incomprehensibly small doses. For example, take a 2 liter bottle of soda, empty it into the Atlantic Ocean, stir, and take one teaspoonful. That dose—and doses even far more dilute—can and do heal! Even if the ill person is incurable or organ damage has occurred, the judicious application of homeopathic remedies can palliate and ease suffering.

How do homeopathic remedies work, and if they are prepared in such tiny, tiny amounts, how could they possibly do anything in the body? There is no concrete answer to these questions. Some authorities state that the remedies stimulate or enhance the immune system of the body, or raise the opsonic index (the measure of fighting ability) of white blood cells against bacteria and infecting agents. Today much research is being conducted on the international level. To date, however, no results have been forthcoming. We really don't know how homeopathic remedies work. The point is is that they do and that fact cannot be ignored. When an ill person is given a remedy and is cured, even the most skeptical person cannot dismiss that. Probably the most validating thing about homeopathy is that it has been successfully used time and time again for the last 150 years by a huge number of practitioners in a great number of countries.

A case comes to mind of an elderly woman who had terminal cancer. Her daughter, having heard of homeopathy, approached me and asked for my advice. She explained that her mother was in great pain and injections of morphine-like pain killers provided no relief.

After 'taking her mothers case'* I suggested she give her *Arsenicum album* 30C (30C is the potency). Yes! Many remedies are made initially from poisonous substances, yet when prepared according to homeopathic principles become safe, non-toxic agents of healing. A hundred years of clinical experience has shown *Arsenicum album* to be a reliever of pain in patients stricken with cancer. The daughter administered anywhere from 2 to 6 doses per day depending upon the mother's discomfort. The remedy reduced the pain significantly. Though her condition was incurable, the homeopathic remedy allowed her mother a more restful, peaceful and dignified death.

This is but one example of the utility of homeopathy. Colds and flus, broken bones, arthritis, psoriasis, lacerations/injuries/cuts, colic, diarrhea, toothaches, and virtually anything else one might think of can be treated with homeopathy. It truly does border on being a panacea.

Do not mistake me for a medical radical or heretic, however. Certainly we cannot throw out the medicine of today. But we must integrate homeopathy as well as other holistic, alternative techniques into today's medical model. Acupuncture, massage, hydrotherapy, naturopathy, and so forth are all valuable, viable therapies which need to be incorporated into the medicine of today. It is a long and involved process, requiring inquisitive and open minds, yet for the welfare of the ill it must be done.

Explore homeopathy. It is a vast and powerful treasure chest of healing. Homeopathy is a difficult science to study and master, yet the reward is great: restored health for the patient and a deep sense of satisfaction for the healer.

---

*'Taking the case' (anamnesis) is a lengthy and involved process of gathering material (signs and symptoms, anecdotes, familial history, etc.) relevant to the patient and his/her sickness. This information is necessary in order to precisely choose the curative homeopathic remedy. Once the practitioner has enough information, he/she chooses the remedy and administers it. Treatment may involve one or more remedies or doses depending upon the case. Selection of strength (potency) also depends on many variables.

In this introductory essay, it is not my intention to go deeply into the subject. You may wish to consult basic texts in order to more fully grasp the principles and practice of this powerful healing art.

SOME NOTES ON SCIENTIFIC TERMINOLOGY
AS IT RELATES TO HOMEOPATHY

As with any body of knowledge one can distill certain truths from it with careful study. Thus in the following paragraphs I want to introduce scientific etymology simply and briefly.

Less than 5% of medical terminology is of Anglo-Saxon origin; the rest is of Greek, Latin, Arabic, Semitic, Italian and French origins. The Greek derivatives were frequently Latinized and further modified in France; we are still in the process of Anglicizing them. Therefore any effort of following Greek or Latin rules of grammar has been discarded in this volume.

Prefixes and suffixes are of great help in forming scientific terms. Without these small "bookends" we would be awash in vast amounts of cumbersome verbiage. It has been estimated that 25% of medical terms are formed with the aid of such prefixes or suffixes.

Prefixes

a-	Greek	without, lack of
ab-	Latin	from, away from
ad- (af-, an-, ap-, at-)	Latin	to
ambi-	Latin	both
amphi- (ampho-)	Greek	about, around, both sides
ana-	Greek	up, apart, across
ante-	Latin	before
anti-	Greek	against
apo-	Greek	from
bi-	Latin	twice, double, two
cata- (kata-)	Greek	down
circum-	Latin	around
co- (col-, com-, con-)	Latin	with, together
contra-	Latin	against
de-	Latin	away from
di-	Greek	twice, double
dia-	Greek	through, apart
dis- (di-)	Latin	apart from, negation
dys-	Greek	with difficulty, bad
e-	Latin	out of, out from
ec-	Greek	out from
ecto-	Greek	outer, outside
en-	Greek	in

endo-	Greek	within
epi-	Greek	on, upon
eso-	Greek	inward
eu-	Greek	good, well
exo-	Greek	outside
extra-	Latin	beyond, additional
hemi-	Greek	half
hyper-	Greek	over, above
hypo-	Greek	less, under, below
in- (im-)	Latin	in or inside; un- or not
infra-	Latin	below
inter-	Latin	between
intro-	Latin	into
meta-	Greek	beyond, after, between
ob-	Latin	inversely
para-	Greek	nearby, nearly
per-	Latin	through, super
peri-	Greek	around
post-	Latin	after, behind
pre- (prae-)	Latin	before, in front of
pro-	Greek and Latin	before, forward
retro-	Latin	backward
semi-	Latin	half
sub-	Latin	under, less than
super-	Latin	above, excessively
supra-	Latin	above, upon
syn- (sym-)	Greek	with, together
trans-	Latin	through, across, over
ultra-	Latin	beyond, in excess

SUFFIXES

A suffix is added after a word or the root to qualify meanings or indicate what part of speech is intended. The root may change its last letters to make the subsequent combination pronounceable. A few examples are as follows.

-ist, -or, -er, -ite, on a noun, express the agent or person concerned (as in doctor, psychiatrist, therapist).

-ite can also mean '-itis' or 'inflammation'.

-ia, -osis, -tion, -y, on a noun, will express action or condition (as in anemia, arteriosclerosis, ankylosis).

-osis in many instances means 'an increase'.

-y or -ity, on a noun, expresses quality (as in flabby, slimy, acidity).

-m, -ma express result of action (as in trauma.

-oma shows a neoplasm; the root attached may show the source of the neoplasm or may show what it resembles.

-ium, -olus, -olum, -culus, -culum, -cle, -cule are diminutives. They mean 'little' or 'small', as in granule ('little grain'), molecule ('little mass'), or ventricle ('little belly').

-able, -ible, added to verbs make adjectives of ability (as in flexible, digestible).

-al, -ac, -ious, -ic, express a relatedness (as in caustic, cardiac).

-id, added to verbs or nouns makes adjectives of a state or condition (as in morbid).

-ous, added to nouns make adjectives expressing material (as in mucous).

-ase, -ate, -ene, -ide, -in, -ine, -ose, are not strictly suffixes, they are endings to indicate particular kinds of chemical compounds (such as terpine, chloride, glucose, cerate, etc.).

COMPOUND WORDS

Words made up of nouns and adjectives are numerous in medical terminology and are often called compound words. Compound words may often appear to have been formed with a prefix. However, this is an error because prefixes and suffixes are prepositions or adverbs. 'Isotonic', for example, is a compound word because *isos* (meaning 'equal') is an adjective, whereas in 'hypersonic', *hyper-* is a prefix.

-algia	Greek	pain
antero-	Latin	in front of
auto-	Greek	self
bio-	Greek	life
brachy-	Greek	short
brady-	Greek	slow
-ectomy	Greek	a cutting out
iso-	Greek	equal
macro-	Greek	big
meso-	Greek	middle
micro-	Greek	small
neo-	Greek	new
-oid	Greek	resemblance
oligo-	Greek	few or scanty
ortho-	Greek	straight
pan-	Greek	all
poly-	Greek	many
postero-	Latin	behind
pseudo-	Greek	false
tachy-	Greek	fast

EPONYMS

'Eponym' comes from the Greek prefix *epi-*, 'upon', and the noun *onoma*, 'name', thus 'named after' (one's name placed upon the discovery). Therefore 'Paget's disease' is an eponym for a disease named after its discoverer, Paget. 'Bright's disease', 'Hodgkin's disease', 'Eustachian tube' and 'Addison's disease' are other examples. Strictly speaking, an eponym should be restricted to what the author originally described and shouldn't include additional features added by other observers of the condition. Later modifications or descriptions may warrant a hyphenated eponym.

Do not confuse with 'epigram'. An epigram is a pithy phrasing of a shrewd observation; a short poem, serious, witty or mocking, containing satire or eulogy and often written as an inscription. Simonides of Ceos, a Greek artist, founded this mode of expression. For example:

Treason doth never prosper;
what's the reason?
For if it prosper, none dare
call it treason.
—J. Harington's *Collection of Epigrams*
(1618)

ONOMATOPOETIC WORDS

Onomatopoeia is derived from the Greek *onoma,* 'name', and *poiein,* 'to make': a word which is intended to reproduce a certain sound and may be used as a noun to indicate sound, origin or cause. These words are echoic, i.e., they echo the sound they designate. 'Belch', 'hiccup', 'murmur', 'rale', 'retch', and 'borborygmus' are examples. 'Quackery' is another ... an echoic word imitating the sound of the duck, which is believed to reflect the boastfulness of the unethical or illegal practitioner in praising himself, his 'knowledge' and/or his methods of treatment. It is a shortened version of 'quacksalver' (Middle Dutch, *quac,* 'unguent', and *salven,* 'to salve'), which referred to physicians who merely applied ointments to skin troubles in hopes of palliating. The term evolved to 'quack' as already described.

DIPHTHONGS

A moment should be taken to discuss the diphthongs (a union of two vowels pronounced in one syllable), OE and AE. More precisely they are digraph ligatures but may also be called monophthongs as they are represented by an E or A, respectively.

OE represents the Latin OE (oesophagus, homoeopathy) or the Greek OI (oisophagos, homoiopathy), and are written in completely Anglicized words as E, as in esophagus, homeopathy, etc. In recent words derived immediately from Latin or Greek, OE is usually retained, e.g.., Oedipus, Phoebe. In scientific and technical terms (amoeba, oestrus, diarrhoea and homoeopathy) there is a tendency, stronger in America than in Great Britain, to substitute E for OE as these words pass into popular usage.

AE is a diphthong of Latin origin equivalent to the Greek AI. The AE disappeared from the language in the 13th century and was re-introduced in the 16th century in forms derived from Latin words with AE and Greek words AI. The E is now commonly substituted except in the plural termination of certain Latin words, e.g., alae.

HOMEOPATHIC ORGANIZATIONS

International Foundation for Homeopathy (IFH)
P.O. Box 7, Edmonds, WA   98020-0007   206-776-4147

National Center for Homeopathy (NCH)
801 N. Fairfax Ave., Ste. 306 • Alexandria, VA 22314   703-548-
7790

This organization coordinates a large network of study groups. Contact them to find the   closest study group to you. They also publish a directory of homeopathic practitioners.

HOMEOPATHIC PHARMACIES*

Biological Homeopathic Industries (BHI)
11600 Cochiti S.E. • Albuquerque, NM 87123   800-621-7644

Boericke and Tafel
2131 Circadian Way • Santa Rosa, CA 95407   800-876-9505

Boiron-USA
6 Campus Blvd., Bldg. A • Newtown Sq., PA 19073   800-258-8823

D. L. Thompson Homeopathic Supplies
844 Yonge St. • Toronto, 5, Ontario • Can M4W 2H1   416-922-2300

Dolisos-USA
3014 Rigel Ave. • Las Vegas, NV 89102   800-365-4767

Hahnemann Homeopathic Pharmacy
828 San Pablo Ave. • Albany, CA 94706   888-427-6422

Humphrey's Pharmacal Co.
63 Meadows Rd. • Rutherford, NJ 07070   201-933-7744

Luyties Pharmacal
4200 Laclede Ave. • St. Louis, MO 63108   800-325-8080

Standard Homeopathic
204-210 W. 131st St. • Los Angeles, CA 90061   800-624-9659

Washington Homeopathic Products
4914 Delray Avenue • Bethesda, MD 20814   800-336-1695

Weleda, Inc.
Rt. N-9W • Congers, NY 10920   914-268-8572

---

*Many pharmacies, health food stores, and individual businesses sell homeopathic remedies. This is a listing of homeopathic remedy *manufacturers*. They sell homeopathics, wholesale and retail, as well as other related products.

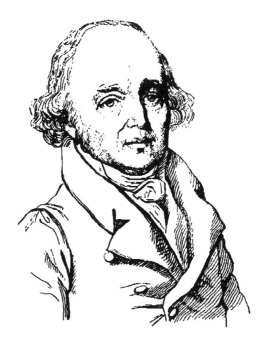

"Indolence, love of ease and obstinacy,
preclude effective service at the altar of truth."

S.C.F. Hahnemann
April 10, 1755 • July 2, 1843

a priori deduced; lit., 'from the previous causes/hypotheses'. Said of reasoning which proceeds from a known cause to a necessarily related effect.

ab usu in morbus 'from practice or use in customs'

abaissement lowering, falling, or bowing.

abasia an inability to walk even though muscular power, sensation, and coordination are unimpaired in relation to other movements of the legs.

abattoir slaughterhouse.

abaxial away from the line of the axis of the body or a body part.

abduct to draw away from the mid-line of the body or part.

aberrant deviating from the normal.

abeyance suspension; 'in abeyance', suspended or absent.

abietite a sugar found in the needles of *Abies pectinata* (the silver fir tree).

abiosis death.

abirritant a substance which eases or allays irritation.

ablactation weaning; the end of the suckling period.

ablatio retinae detachment of the retina.

ablepharia (congenital ablepharia) the absence of eyelids.

abluent detergent or soap; a cleansing or washing agent.

ablepsia blindness

ablution the process of cleansing the body.

abrosia a wasting away.

abscess a localized collection of pus in a cavity; a cavity or lump formed by the process of suppuration and disintegration of tissue.

absinthism the pathological state resulting from the excessive and habitual use of absinthe, characterized by neuritis, hyperesthesia, hallucinations, convulsions, acute mania, and even general paralysis.

abstract a preparation containing the soluble principles of a drug, evaporated and mixed with lactose.

abulia (aboulia) the loss or marked reduction in will power.

abuse of mercury the practice in the 1800s of giving large doses of mercurial purgatives to cause loose bowels in order to rid the patient of 'disease'. If repeated in large doses it can lead to a whole set of toxic symptoms, including headaches, gingivitis, nausea, dizziness, heart pain, dermatitis, excess salivation, epistaxis, keratitis, neuritis, hematological abnormalities, albuminuria, purpura, and a metallic taste in the mouth. See CALOMEL.

abyss a bottomless pit; hell. Any immeasurably profound depth or void.

acampsia inflexibility of a limb.

acanthia the spinal column. May refer to a single vertebra.

acanthesthesia a sensation of being pricked by needles.

acarophobia a morbid fear of acquiring the itch. A belief that one has scabies.

acataphasia an inability to speak a complete sentence.

acathectic unable to retain; in a state of acathexia (an abnormal loss of secretions).

acaudal without a tail.

accomodation the ability to focus ones eyes on objects at different distances.

accouchee in labor, the woman bearing the child.

accoucheur an obstetrician, one who delivers a woman in childbirth.

accoucheuse a mid-wife.

accrescent growing larger or thicker.

aceology therapeutics.

acerbity acidity in combination with sourness or astringency.

acescence the process of becoming sour.

acescent mildly sour or acidic.

acetonemia the presence of acetone in the system.

acetonuria abnormal increase in the amount of acetone in the urine (a condition found during fevers, diabetic acidosis, malignancy and intestinal disorders).

achalacia a hypo-motility.

achalybemia the lack of iron in the blood.

achlorhydria the absence of free hydrochloric acid (HCl) in the stomach, even after the administration of histamine.

achondroplasia defective development of the bones.

achor see CRUSTA LACTEA.

achylia gastrica the presence in scanty amounts or the complete absence of gastric juices.

acid mantle the slightly acid protective film produced by the skin to protect itself from bacterial and fungal infections and from excessive loss of moisture. This term was coined by Dr. Marchionini in 1923.

aciniform grape-like.

acme the height or crisis of a disease. The period of greatest intensity of a symptom.

acne a papular eruption due to inflammation, with accumulation of secretions, of the sebaceous or oil-producing glands.

acne conglobata acne in a large singular mass.

acne indurata deep-seated acne with large papules and pustules and large hypertrophic scars.

acne rosacea (acne erythematosa) acne of the cheeks and nose associated with congestion and the formation of telangiectases (stretching and dilatation of small or terminal vessels).

acne vulgaris (acne simplex, acne disseminata) common acne. Simple, uncomplicated acne.

acology the study of materia medica (remedies).

acomia alopecia or baldness.

acoria gluttony. The absence of the feeling of satiety after eating.

acousia a condition related to hearing.

acquanimitas equanimity, calmness, mental balance, evenness of temperament.

acrid harsh, caustic, sharp, biting, irritating, burning, or pungent to the senses.

acrisia uncertainty in the diagnosis and prognosis of a disease.

acrocyanosis (Crocq's disease) a circulatory disorder in which the hands (and less commonly the feet) are persistently cold, blue, and sweaty.

acromania an excessively violent mania.

acromegaly (Marie's disease) an abnormally large development of the head, thorax and extremities.

acromion that part of the scapula which forms the highest part of the shoulder.

acromion process the highest point of the shoulder.

acronarcotic a medicine which is both acrid and narcotic, e.g. *Sanguinaria, Veratrum, Aconite.*

acronyx an ingrowing of a nail.

acroparesthesia extreme paresthesia (a morbid or altered sensation). Paresthesia of the extremities. A syndrome usually seen in middle-aged women characterized by tingling or crawling sensations in the hands and fingers and coldness, pallor or cyanosis of the hands.

acrophobia an unusual fear of heights.

acroposthia the prepuce of the penis.

acrosphacelus see RAYNAUD'S DISEASE.

acrotism the absence of a pulse.

actinism the use of radiant energy or radiant heat sources to treat illness.

actinomycosis (lumpy jaw, clyers, wooden tongue) an infectious disease caused by a parasite *(Actinomyces bovis),* affecting cattle, hogs and man. The jaw is most commonly involved, being the site of slow-growing granulomatous suppurating tumors which discharge an oily pus containing yellow granules. This disease will show constitutional signs of sepsis (fever and putrefaction).

acuminate pointed, tapered or tapering to a point. To sharpen to a point. To give poignancy or keenness to.

acupuncture a therapeutic medical science which alleviates disease by stimulating points (780 of them) on the body's surface to affect physiological functions. Needles are inserted into points of the body to adjust the energy levels in the body. Acupressure is similar but uses pressure from the thumb, finger or a blunt object to stimulate the points. Auricular therapy is ear-acupuncture. There are over 200 points on the ear which reflex to the various organs and areas of the body. Acupuncture is just one aspect of Traditional Chinese Medicine (TCM); other treatments may consist of herbs, food therapy, massage and exercises. *The Web That Has No Weaver Understanding Chinese Medicine* (Ted Kaptchuk, O.M.D.) is an excellent introductory book.

acute ascending paralysis see LANDRY'S PARALYSIS.

acute condition/disease a disease state which is usually brief in duration and self-limiting, i.e. it either runs its course or the patient dies (as opposed to a chronic condition, which is usually more slowly developing and will last indefinitely).

acute intestinal catarrh (chordapsus) constriction or twisting of the intestine.

acute miasm a term used by Hahnemann to distinguish true miasmatic diseases from less deep seated ones. Scarlet fever would be considered an acute miasm as are whooping cough, mumps, chickenpox, etc. One might call the flu or cold an acute miasm. From without, the acute miasm swiftly overtakes the health of the individual and imprints itself onto the person. The person either recovers or dies in a short period of time.

acute remedy a remedy of particular use in acute conditions or situations, e.g., *Calendula* for wounds or *Bellis per.* for injuries. However, many so-called acute remedies can and are used for chronic or non-acute conditions. It is erroneous to classify remedies as either acute or chronic, for it colors one's thinking and can prevent the correct remedy from being chosen.

acyanoblepsy 'blue-blindness' (the inability to distinguish the color blue).

acyesis 1) sterility in women 2) the non-pregnant condition.

adaptogen a chemical or substance which increases the body's ability to resist stress and not suffer cumulative damage. For example, the steroidal substances in *Eleutherococcus* and ginseng support the functions of our own protective steroids. 'Adaptogenic reactions' such as fever or excessive sleepiness can shunt energy to fighting illness by forcing the ill person to slow down. Other plants with adaptogenic substances include *Schizandra chinensis, Rhodiola rosea, Acanthopanax o., Astragalus memb., Withania somni. (Ashwagandha,* or Indian ginseng). The term adaptogen was first suggested in 1957 by Russian pharmacologist I. Brekhman. According to his definition an adaptogen must have equilibrating, tonifying and anti-stress actions.

Addison's disease (adrenal cortical hypofunction, adrenal insufficency) a disease caused by the failure of the adrenal cortex (that area of the adrenal gland which produces cortisone) to function. Symptoms include ane-

nal gland which produces cortisone) to function. Symptoms include anemia, weakness, low blood pressure, hypoglycemia, feeble heart actions, small heart, and hyperpigmentation (bronzing) of the skin.

adduct to draw toward the mid-line of the body or part.

adenitis inflammation of the lymph nodes or glands.

adenoids (Luschka's glands, pharyngeal tonsils, Luschka's tonsils) the lymph nodules in the back wall of the nasopharynx (literally, 'resembling a gland').

adenoma a glandular tumor.

adenomalacia a glandular softening.

adephagia a voracious appetite, gluttony, or bulimia.

adeps (axungia porcis) lard, purified leaf lard (hog fat obtained from the omentum) used years ago in the preparation of ointments.

adhesion 1) the rejoining of parts after they have been cut (as in surgery). Pain and inflammation is often the result, and may persist for some time after the parts have healed. 2) an inflammatory band connecting serous membranes, e.g. found in the abdomen as an afteraffect of surgery.

adiposa fat.

adipose fatty or relating to fat.

adiposis an excessive accumulation (either local or general) of fat in the body.

adipositas cordis a fatty condtion of the heart.

adiposogenital dystrophy (Frohlich's syndrome, hypothalamic eunuchism) a disorder (caused by hypothalamic dysfunction) occurring in adolescent boys characterized by incomplete or underdeveloped genitals and the development of female secondary sex characteristics, including female distribution of fat. Simultaneous overeating occurs because of dysfunction of the feeding center in the hypothalamus.

adipsia the absence of thirst.

aditus an anatomical structure serving as an approach or entrance to another part.

adjuvant a medicine or therapy which assists the action of another to which it is added.

admixtion a mixture or blending of one substance into another

adnexa (annexa) appendages or parts accessory to the main organ or structure; for example, 'adnexa oculi' would mean the eyelids, lacrymal glands, etc., associated with the eyeball.

adnexitis (annexitis) inflammation of the adnexa uteri (the fallopian tubes and ovaries).

adynamia loss of vital strength or muscular powers; weakness, debility, asthenia, stagnation.

aedoitis inflammation of the labia of the female genitalia.

aerophagy the excessive swallowing of air.

aesthetic of or pertaining to the sense of the beautiful or artistic.

aestivalis pertaining to the summer season.

aet. (Latin *aetatis*), 'of age'.

afebrile without fever.

affectation a pretentious show or display. An artificial mannerism or behavior adopted to draw attention or impress others.

affected influenced by (an illness), as in 'apply to the affected area'. 'Affect' means to have an influence on, produce an effect on, effect a change in. 'Effect' means to bring about, cause, produce, or result in. 'The furlough did not affect us, so it had no effect on us when it went into effect.' 'A glass of tea may affect [alter for better or worse] his recovery.' 'A glass of tea may effect [bring about] his recovery.' 'It could seriously affect her health.' 'This will not affect [change] his purpose.' 'This will not effect [secure] his purpose.'

affection a generic term for any pathological condition of the body or mind.

afferent directed toward a central organ or section, e.g., nerves that conduct impulses from the periphery of the body to the central area or spinal cord.

afflatus 1) a form of acute erysipelas. 2) any air which strikes the body and causes disease.

after-pains pains from uterine contractions following delivery.

agalactia suppression of milk; the flow of milk is absent or scanty after childbirth.

agape wide open (mouth), expressing wonder or amazement.

ageustia (agustia) the lack or perversion of the ability to taste.

agglutinate to glue, stick or clump together.

agglutination a joining or gluing together by secretions.

aggravation (homeopathic aggravation, symbolized by <) a situation in which the patient feels worse from or symptoms are increased by a remedy. An aggravation is actually a good sign as it means the correct remedy was chosen and is working. The aggravation will soon pass and the patient will get well. See ANAMNESIS.

Some authors have suggested that neutral potencies exist (6x, 6c, 12x, 12c, 24x, 24c, 200x, 200c ...) which are gentler on the vital force and do not cause severe aggravations or aggravate at all. The author offers no opinion on this.

"Least of all, need we to be concerned when the usual customary symptoms are aggravated and show most prominently on the first days, and again on some of the following days, but gradually less and less. This so-called *homoeopathic aggravation* is a sign of an incipient cure (of the symptoms aggravated at present), which may be expected with certainty."—S.C.F. Hahnemann, *Chronic Diseases*

"An aggravation of the disease means the patient is growing weaker, the symptoms are growing stronger; but the true homoeopathic aggravation, which is the aggravation of the symptoms of the patient while the patient is growing better, is something that the physician observes after a true homoeopathic prescription. The true homoeopathic aggravation I say, is when the symptoms are worse, but the patient says, 'I feel better'."— J.T. Kent, *Lectures on Homoeopathic Philosophy*

agitans (paralysis agitans) paralysis with constant tremor of the muscles; a shaking palsy.

aglutition an inability to swallow.

agnosia absence of (or defect in) the ability to recognize persons or things.

agoraphobia fear of being in open spaces or crossing open spaces. The German neurologist C.F.O. Westphal (1833-1890) first described this state.

agranulocytosis (granulocytopenia, agranulocytic angina) a syndrome characterized by prostration, high fever, ulcerative lesions of the mucous membranes in the throat and other areas, and a marked reduction in the polymorphonuclear leukocytes (white blood cells which protect the body from invading organisms).

agremia the gouty diathesis.

agrius having an angry appearance. Often used to describe a skin disease.

agromania a morbid desire to be in open spaces or to live in solitude.

agrypnia sleeplessness, insomnia.

ague a chill; a recurrent chill or fit of shivering; an intermittent fever attended by alternating cold and hot fits (sweating, fever, and chills); the cold fit or rigor of the intermittent fever. It was often used in reference to fevers associated with malaria.

ague cake an enlargement of the spleen produced by ague.

ague-brow an intermittent neuralgia of the area just above the eye (brow area).

agustia loss of taste.

ahypnia insomnia.

ainhum (dactylolysis spontanea) the spontaneous amputation of a toe. A constricting fibrous ring develops in the digitoplantar fold (usually of the little toe) and gradually tightens, resulting in the loss of the toe. It most commonly affects black males of the tropics. The disease is symmetrical, the cause is unknown. It is pronounced 'INE-yoom'.

air castles the subject of empty theorizing, thinking, and pondering.

air of vaults underground air, as in cemetery vaults, crypts or burial chambers.

alae nasi (Latin, lit. 'wings of the nose', from *ala,* 'wing or wing-like process.') The cartilaginous flap on the outer side of each nostril.

alastrim see AMAAS.

albedo whiteness or lightness. The light reflected from a surface.

albuginea white or whitish. The layer of white fibrous tissue coating an organ or part.

albuminous resembling or containing albumin (a water soluble simple protein, whitish or clear in color, widely distributed throughout the tissues and fluids of plants and animals).

albuminuria (proteinuria) the presence of proteins (albumin, globulin) in the urine which may be caused by kidney disease.

alchemy a form of chemistry, speculative philosophy or occultism, practiced in the Middle Ages and the Renaissance, concerned with discovering methods for transmuting metals of a lesser value into gold or silver. 'Alchemists' searched for a precious substance (a catalyst, tincture, elixir, or 'philosopher's stone') to initiate the transformation. Alchemical work has three stages: separation, purification, and recombination ('chymical wedding').

Alchemy may have its basis in depletion gilding, the process used to make the 2000-year-old 'Corinthian Bronze'. Depletion gilding was developed by the Hellenistic Greeks and independently by the Quechua of pre-Hispanic Peru. A copper alloy ingot containing 5% silver and 12% or more of gold is heated in air to produce an ingot coated with black oxide. This is then marinated in a warm solution of salt and copiapite (basic iron sulfate, which is gold in color), which dissolves the surface copper and silver leaving a spongy gold surface which, when burnished, becomes bright gold in color. It seems this was the secret alchemical process shrouded in occultism and astrology by which base metals were turned into gold!

"The intrinsic meaning is of the transformation of the lower nature of man into the highest form, metaphorically into that of gold: sun, heart, and feeling."—E. Whitmont, M.D. *(The American Homeopath,* 1: p. 23. 1994). "As nature is extremely subtle and penetrating in her manifestation, she cannot be used without the Art. Indeed, she does not produce anything that is perfect in itself, but man must make it perfect, and this perfecting is called alchemy."—Paracelsus. See SPAGYRIC.

Alcottism a system of diet and health maintenance devised by William Alcott. See GRAHAMISM.

alexia an inability to read; word-blindness.

alexipharmic a medicine which neutralises a poison.

alexipyretic an agent which lowers a fever.

algid chilly or cold.

algomenorrhea (dysmenorrhea) painful menstruation.

algorithm a recipe or set of steps which can be taken to solve a particular problem. The 'lather, rinse, and repeat' instructions on the back of a shampoo bottle make up an algorithm.

alible nutritious; capable of nourishing.

alienatio mentis loss of reason; lunacy. A term applied to insanity as distinguished from other forms of derangement such as delirium.

alienist a popular term for psychologist in the late 19th century, so termed because mentally ill persons were considered alienated from their true nature and society. An expert in mental pathology.

alimentary pertaining to the intestine; also nourishing, nutritious, related to the diet.

alkaloid any of various physiologically active nitrogen-containing organic bases derived usually from plants, e.g., nicotine, quinine, cocaine, atropine. They are generally bitter in taste, alkaline, and unite with acids to form salts. Their common names usually end in '-ine'.

alkalometry (dosimetrics) a popular method of dosing in the mid to late 1800s. It sought a middle ground between homeopathy and allopathy by advocating the administration of small doses of potent drugs given at short intervals. These drugs were not potentized.

W.C. Abbott, M.D., editor of the *American Journal of Clinical Medicine,* provided this definition: "Use the smallest possible quantity of the best obtainable means to produce a desired therapeutic result." Alkalometry emphasized drug purity in stabilized amounts in the form of soluble granules or tablets. For example, the alkaloid aconitine in doses of 1/500 grain would be given every 30 minutes for fevers or inflammation.

allergic contact dermatitis an acquired, or non-atopic, allergic skin reaction resulting from contact with an allergen to which the person has been sensitized by previous exposure. Sometimes it is called eczematous contact dermatitis (which is inaccurate, since the condition is not always oozing or eczematous).

alliaceous garlic-like. Having the quality of garlic.

Alnaschar a daydreamer; one given to imaginings, as in 'Alnaschar visions'. One who plans great works and yet never carries them out. From a character in the *Arabian Nights.*

allopathy (heteropathy, antipathic, enantiopathic, palliative) the treatment of disease using medicines whose effects are different from those of the disease being treated and which have no relationship to the disease symptoms. Allopathy is based on the principle of *contraria contrariis,* or the Law of Opposites, as opposed to homeopathy, which is based on *similia similibus curentur,* or 'like cures like'. See HOMEOPATHY.

"The failure of allopathy was that it treated disease, or a part of an organ, or tried to do so, whereas the only means of cure was to treat the whole patient."—Fergie Woods

allosteatodes an alteration in the quality of the sebaceous or oily secretions of the skin.

alogia the inability to speak due to nerve damage or lesion.

alopecia (morbus vulpis) loss of hair. 'Alopecia areata' is loss of hair in patches.

alphaism a women's reformist movement mildly popular, especially in Washington, D.C., in the second half of the 19th century. It advocated women's rights, the education of women about their bodies and health concerns, and in particular the reservation of sexual intercourse for procreative purposes only.

alterative a medicine which alters the course of disease, modifying the nutritive processes while promoting waste, and thus indirectly curing some chronic diseases. An alterative acts to correct disordered metabolism and promote repair.

alternation "the successive administration of two or more remedies which recur in turn in a regular order and at intervals sufficiently approximated so that the duration of the action of the one drug may not be quite exhausted before another succeeds it."—Martiny & Bernard *(Trans. of the International Homeopathic Convention, London, 1881,* and *Medical Counselor, 8/1881, #5, Vol. #5).*

"As a shot gun maims where the rifle would kill, so alternation may change and modify and maim the disease, but it never does nor can effect the clean, direct and perfect cure that a single remedy, exactly homoeopathic, will accomplish."—C. Dunham, *Homoeopathy: The Science of Therapeutics.*

"Alternation or rotation of remedies is reprehensible since it leads away from accurate and definite knowledge of drug effects and sooner or later to poly-pharmacy which is the most slovenly of all practice."—G. Boericke, *Principles of Homoeopathy.*

R. Hughes in *The Principles and Practice of Homeopathy* (p. 506) says: "The Piles accompanying it [abdominal plethora] are of the 'Blind' character; they bleed little, but are very annoying for their fulness. It is here that *Sulphur* and *Nux vomica* display their great Anti-haemorrhoidal virtues. They seem to act better conjointly (i.e., in alternation) than when either is given separately."

alternative medicine see COMPLEMENTARY MEDICINE.

alveolar pertaining to or shaped like a small cell or cavity. May refer to the alveoli of the lungs or to the tooth-socket.

alvine relating to the abdomen or intestines; the belly.

alvine flux diarrhea.

Alzheimer's disease (dementia presenilis, senile dementia-Alzheimer type, SDAT) a presenile syndrome characterized by confusion, memory failure, disorientation, hallucinosis, speech disturbances, restlessness, agnosia, etc. From the German neurologist Alois Alzheimer (1864-1915). 'Presenile dementia with cerebral atrophy'.—O.A. Julian, *Materia Medica of New Homeopathic Remedies.*

amaas (milk-pox, alastrim) a non-fatal disease especially prevalent in Brazil and the West Indies resembling smallpox but without a secondary rise of temperature and the pustules are not raised as much. Vaccination does not seem to afford permanent immunity.

amara a drug used for its bitter taste, primarily to increase the appetite. Bitters.

amasesis the inability to chew.

amative inclined to love; sexually passionate.

amanuensis one who takes dictation or copies manuscripts.

amaurosis partial or total blindness, usually without an apparent lesion or injury of the eye.

ambergris a grey, waxy material with a marbled appearance, formed in the intestines of sperm whales. The source of the homeopathic remedy *Ambra grisea*.

ambient surrounding or encircling.

amblosis an abortion or miscarriage. Some authors use the term 'abortion' to signify premature deliveries before the fourth month, with deliveries between the third and seventh months termed 'miscarriages'. Today the meaning of 'abortion' is very different, meaning the forcible removal of the developing fetus. Cf. EFFLUXION.

amblyopia dimness of vision without apparent physical defect or disease of the eye. Blurred or weak vision.

amblyopia potatorum dimness of vision caused by excessive drinking of alcoholic beverages.

ambulatory shifting or walking about. Having the ability to walk or move.

ambustion a burn or scald.

amenia (amenorrhea) the absence of menstruation.

amebiasis (amoebiasis) infestation with *Endamoeba histolytica* and the subsequent production of dysentery.

amebic (amoebic) referring to parasites found in the digestive tract. Infestation of the colon with these parasites leads to dysentery.

amelioration (symbolized by >) an improvement of the patient or decrease in symptoms. See AGGRAVATION.

"Immediate amelioration often indicates the absence of deep-seated disease."—J.T. Kent, *New Remedies*.

Concerning the analysis of a case, H.A. Roberts, in his *Principles and Art of Cure by Homoeopathy*, had this to say: "In analysing the case, very valuable symptoms are those pertaining to the aggravations and ameliorations, because the aggravations and ameliorations are the natural modifiers of diseased states and are the definite reaction of the man himself."

amenorrhea (suppressio mensium) the absence or abnormal cessation of menstruation.

ametropia the inability of the eye to focus images clearly on the retina.

Amicus Plato, amicus Socrates, sed magis amica veritas "Dear is Plato, dear is Socrates, but truth is dearer."

ammoniacal like or combined with ammonia.

ammotherapy the therapeutic application of sand-baths.

amok see AMUCK.

amomum Indian spice plant. A genus of plants of the *Zingiberaceae. A. cardamomum* refers to cardamom. *A. granum paradisi* ('grains of paradise') possesses diuretic properties (see GRAIN). Also a generic term for any spice.

amorous loving, affectionate, inclined to love.

amorphous shapeless, formless, lacking definite form.

amphemerous (quotidian) recurring daily, as a fever. Recurring every 24 hours.

amuck (amok) a condition of mania first observed in Malaysia. The individual becomes acutely maniacal and exhibits wild and uncontrollable behavior, threatening to do injury to others. 'To run amuck' is a common expression which means 'to go wild or go crazy' in a damaging or destructive way.

amygdalae the tonsils; also a small lobe of the cerebellum (lit. 'almond-shaped', from the Latin *amygdalus*, almond).

amygdalitis (tonsillitis) inflammation of the tonsils.

amylaceous starchy or starch-like in nature.

amylocardia weakness of the heart muscle.

amyloid a starch-like substance. A protein deposit resulting from degeneration of tissues.

amyostasia difficulty in standing due to muscular incoordination or tremor.

amyotrophia the atrophy (wasting away) of muscular tissue.

amyotrophic lateral sclerosis (Charcot's disease) the deterioration of spinal nerve pathways which in turn causes muscle deterioration and wasting. From J.M. Charcot (1825-1893), a French physician and one of the greatest neurological researchers in medical history.

anabolism constructive metabolism; the process by which simple substances are synthesized into the complex materials of living tissue. For example, anabolic steroids cause a building up of the bodily tissues.

anacatharsis severe and long-continued vomiting.

anakusis (anacusia) complete deafness.

analepsis the restoration of health.

analeptic an agent which restores health after illness.

analgesia an insensibility to pain. Usually the relief of pain without the loss of consciousness.

analgesic an agent such as aspirin which causes analgesia (relieves pain).

anamnesis lit., 'the act of remembering.' The medical history of a patient previous to his present illness.

C. Rousson once said, "[You must] look at, listen to, question, examine, and above all understand [your patient]." And Pierre Schmidt, who wrote *The Art of Interrogation,* commented, "You don't have a good consultation unless your patient cries and smiles." Three mistakes are often made in examining the case: interrupting the patient, asking direct questions, and making answers conform to some remedy which you might have in mind.

anapeiratic resulting from overuse, as in writer's cramp.

anaphalantiasis the loss or absence of eyebrows.

anaphia a defective or absent sense of touch.

anaphoresis diminished activity of the sweat glands.

anaphrodisia impairment of the sexual appetite. Reduced libido.

anaphylaxis an acute, often explosive, systemic reaction occurring in a previously sensitized person after receiving foreign serum, certain drugs or diagnostic agents, desensitizing injections, or insect stings. The person might be agitated and flushed, complaining of a sense of uneasiness. Palpitations, paresthesias, pruritus, throbbing in the ears, coughing, sneezing and difficult breathing are typical signs. Signs of shock may develop shortly thereafter, with the patient becoming incontinent, convulsive, and unresponsive; death may ensue.

anasarca (hyposarca) a general dropsical condition. A generalized, systemic edema. A general infiltration of clear watery fluid into the subcutaneous connective tissue.

anastasis convalescence or recovery.

anatripic a remedy to be applied by friction or rubbing (as an ointment).

anchilops a swelling or inflammation at the inner corner of the eye and nose.

anchylosis (ankylosis) an abnormal immobility and unusual stiffness of a joint.

ancipital two-headed or two-edged.

andromania nymphomania.

androphobia an irrational or insane fear of men or of the male sex.

anemia hypoglobular (hypocytosis, cytopenia, oligocythemia) the lack of cellular elements in the blood.

anemia (anaemia) a deficiency in the constituents of blood which may result in shortness of breath (dyspnea), pallor, palpitation of the heart and a general weakness. There are many kinds of anemia including a reduction in the amount of blood, a deficiency in red blood cells, and a deficiency in hemoglobin.

Gabriel Andral's (1797-1876) *Essai d'Hematologie Pathologique* (1843) was the first monograph on hematology establishing exact knowledge of the blood components. He coined the terms 'anemia' and 'hyperemia' and described numerous blood diseases including septicemia, lead poisoning, and polycythemia. He was the first to urge the clinical examination of blood in disease states.

anergic lethargic, inactive.

anesis the remission of a disease.

anesthesia loss of sensation, especially of tactile sensibility. A state of insensibility. In the late 1800s words such as narcotism, stupefaction, sopor, etherization, anodyne process, letheonization, hebetization, and apathisation were used instead of anestheia to describe that state. Bailey's English dictionary (1724) defined anesthesia as 'a defect in sensation'.

aneurysm an abnormal dilatation of an artery, generally producing a sac as a result of the arterial wall stretching. The resultant sac is thin, weak and prone to rupture.

Paul Broca, the great French physician and anthropologist, wrote the classic work on aneurysms, *Des Aneurysmes et de Leur Traitement* (1856).

angiectasis dilation of lymphatic or blood vessels.

angina 1) sore throat from any cause. Inflammation of the throat. 2) A severe cramp-like, constricting pain; commonly used in the term 'angina pectoris'.

angina faucium a sore throat, particularly of the fauces (the walls of the rear portion of the throat and pharynx).

angina gangrenosa a malignant sore throat.

angina granulosa (granular pharyngitis) see CLERGYMAN'S SORE THROAT.

angina ludovici (Ludwig's angina) an acute streptococcal infection of the floor of the mouth. It begins suddenly with marked swelling under the jaw, rapidly extending into the neck. The floor of the mouth becomes swollen and indurated and the tongue is pushed upward. Speech and swallowing are impeded, and the disease is frequently fatal.

angina parotidea see MUMPS.

angina pharyngea an inflammation of the mucous membranes of the throat.

angina pectoris paroxysmal pain characterized by a sense of suffocation and oppression and severe constriction about the chest. The pain radiates from the precordium to the left shoulder and down the arm along the ulnar nerve. The pain is caused by myocardial ischemia (lack of oxygen due to a lack of blood). This syndrome was first described by Wm. Heberden, M.D. in 1768 in a lecture he gave before the Royal College of Physicians.

angina tonsillaris (quinsy, angina vera) see QUINSY.

angina vera (quinsy, angina tonsillaris) see QUINSY.

angioglioma a blood-tumor of the spinal cord.

angioma a tumor with a tendency to consist primarily of blood vessels.

angioneurotic edema (urticaria, hives) an edema, currently termed 'angio-edema', caused by a disturbance of the vasomotor system either through injury, spasms, or paralysis of blood vessels. Whereas urticaria is local blisters/bullae and redness, a. edema is a similar eruption but with larger edematous areas that involve subcutaneous tissues as well as the skin.

angiosclerosis the induration and thickening of the walls of the blood vessels. See ARTERIOSCLEROSIS.

angitis (angiitis) inflammation of a blood vessel.

angor restlessness.

anhaphia see ANAPHIA.

ani referring to the anus.

anidrosis (anhidrosis) deficiency or absence of sweat.

animal economy all matters relating to animal life; physiology. In the 18th century this term was often used to refer to the ability of an individual to carry out basic physiological processes.

John Gardiner's *Observations on the Animal Oeconomy, and on the causes and cure of diseases* (1784) was a very early treatise on this subject.

animal heat the body's inherent heat or energy.

animal magnetism (animalism) see MESMERISM.

aniridia the absence of the iris of the eye.

ankylosis (anchylosis) an abnormal immobility and unusual stiffness of a joint.

ankylostomiasis (hookworm disease, uncinariasis, tropical chlorosis, mountain anemia, brickmaker's anemia, miner's anemia, dochmiasis, tunnel disease) infestation of the intestine with *Ancylostoma duodenale* (a hookworm), resulting in anemia, emaciation, dyspepsia and swelling of the abdomen with mental and physical inertia.

anlage a fundamental principle or foundation.

annular ring-shaped.

anodyne quieting pain. An agent which has the power to relieve pain.

anomia inability to name familiar objects due to failure to recognize them.

anon time after time; now and then, as in 'ever and anon'.

anorexia absence or loss of appetite. 'Anorexia nervosa' is an abnormal or hysterical aversion to food which can lead to serious malnutrition. Bigarexia is the opposite.

Anorexia nervosa was first described by R. Morton (1637-1698) in his book on pulmonary tuberculosis, *Phthisiologia seu exercitationes de phthisi* (1689).

anosmia the loss of the sense of smell.

antalgic (anodyne) an agent which has the power to relieve pain.

antagonistic remedies see INIMICAL.

antecedent preceding, former, prior. That which precedes.

antepartum before birth (usually considered to refer to the last four months of pregnancy).

antephialtic that which acts to prevent a nightmare.

anterior situated before or in front of; toward the ventral (front) aspect of the body; denoting the forward/front part of an organ.

anteversion a turning forward or bending forward. Inclining forward as a whole without bending. 'Anteversion uteri' refers to a malposition of the uterus.

anthelmintic (vermifuge) having the power to destroy or expel intestinal worms.

anthrax (charbon, wool-sorter's disease, tanner's disease, splenic fever) from the Greek, 'a live coal'. An acute infectious disease of cattle and sheep transmissible to man, caused by *Bacillus anthracis*, and producing carbuncles.

"This is a species of malignant tumor. It commences as a livid red swelling, attended with a burning, itching, smarting pain, which gradually grows worse as the disease progresses. After 5 or 6 days, softening and suppuration takes place, and when it bursts, instead of having a central opening as a boil, it is flat on top with several openings which discharge a thin, acrid fluid. These openings gradually widen, coalesce, and large pieces of decayed cellular tissue are thrown off by sloughing."—*I.D. Johnson's Therapeutic Key.*

anthropophobia the abnormal fear of people or of society.

anthroposophical medicine as defined by the Anthroposophical Society in America, anthroposophical medicine "does not regard illness as a chance occurrence or mechanical breakdown, but rather as something intimately connected to the biography of the human being. Handled appropriately, it represents opportunities for new balance and maturity. The patient is treated holistically as a being of body, soul and spirit. This approach integrates conventional practice with new and alternative remedies, dietary and nutritional therapy, massage, hydrotherapy, art therapy and counseling." See ANTHROPOSOPHY.

anthroposophy 'the science of the knowledge of man'. This vast body of knowledge, mainly attributed to the work of Rudolf Steiner (1861-1925), touches virtually every realm: philosophy, medicine, architecture, spirituality, food production, nature awareness, etc.

In medicine, the anthroposophical view is that man is a threefold being. He has nerve/sensory functions (nervous system and brain which support the mind and the thinking process), rhythmic functions (the physical processes of a rhythmic/periodic nature-pulse, breathing, intestinal rhythmswhich support the emotional or feeling processes), and metabolic functions (digestion, elimination, energetic metabolism and voluntary movement processes which supports the aspects of human behavior that express the will). The rhythmic aspect mediates the other two.

From an understanding of this concept comes a deeper understanding physical therapies, homeopathic and anthroposophical remedies, rhythmical massage, hydrotherapy, compresses and external applications, movement therapy (curative eurythmy), counseling, painting, sculpture, and music and speech therapy.

For more information you may wish to contact: Physicians' Association for Anthroposophical Medicine (PAAM), PO Box 269, Kimberton, PA 19442, or Weleda Inc., Rt. N-9W, Congers, NY 10920. 'Weleda' ('Velledas' is the Celtic spelling) refers to a Celtic wise woman or healer-priestess who provided understanding of nature to her followers. Consult Francis X. King's *Rudolf Steiner and Holistic Medicine* for a lucid and interesting introduction to anthroposophy.

antidote an agent which neutralizes a poison or counteracts its effects. In relation to remedies, some remedies act to neutralize other remedies. For example, *Bell.* is antidoted by *Coffea, Aconite* and *Opium* and *Chamo.* is antidoted by *Nux v.* and *Puls.* This antidotal effect can be complete, partial, or merely a modification of action. In relation to taking homeopathic remedies their effects are antidoted or nullifed by coffee, strong mints and odors, extreme stresses to the patient, etc. With few exceptions *Camphora* antidotes most remedies.

"It is often as important to be able to arrest a medicinal action as it is to start it. A prescriber who cannot antidote a drug effect is like the driver of a motor who cannot put on the brake."—J.H. Clarke, *Clinical Repertory*

"An interesting and little-understood phase of antidotal relationship is the power of a higher potency to modify the action of the same drug in a lower potency."—R.H. Langbridge, *A.B.C. of Homoeopathy.*

"The following general rule holds here: Practically any agent which can exert a medicinal effect on the human being is capable of serving as an antidote to a homeopathic remedy. By the same token, any influence which can induce a hyperactive, nervous state, or which can artificially bring about a state of sedation or sleep, can interfere with the action of a homeopathic remedy."—George Vithoulkas, *(Biological Therapy,* 14:1, January 1996, p. 167-68).

antidysuric a remedy to relieve painful or difficult urination.

antefebrin (antifebrin salicylate, salifebrin) acetanilide (an aspirin-type product employed years ago to bring down a fever or allay pain).

antihomotoxic therapy see HOMOTOXICOLOGY.

antikamnia a no-longer-in-use proprietary product having antipyretic, analgesic and hypnotic qualities. It contains acetanilide, acetophenetidin, caffeine, and sodium bicarbonate. Recommended dosage was 300-600 mgs.

antimiasmatic against or countering a miasm. *Sulphur* is an antimiasmatic, specifically an antipsoric, for it works against the psoric miasm. *Medorrhinum* is an antimiasmatic, specifically an antisycotic, for it works against the sycotic miasm, etc.

antimony a metallic element (symbol Sb) often used in a variety of alloys. In homeopathy, often refers to *Antimonium crudum.*

antipathic (allopathic, enantiopathic) averse, contrary or opposed to. See ALLOPATHIC.

antiperiodic a remedy that prevents or lessens the severity of the seizures associated with a periodic febrile disease, e.g. *China.* Herbal antiperiodics include senna, rue, and skullcap.

antiphlogistic a term applied to medicines, diets and/or other measures (venesection, rest, cold packs, counterirritation) which tend to oppose or decrease inflammation. These measures often work by weakening the system by diminishing the activity of the vital power.

18th century chemists believed that a substance burns as a result of 'phlogiston' escaping from it. Thus an inflamed part or feverish person would have been given drugs thought to counteract phlogiston. Even after evidence proved there to be no such substance, the remedies used to treat inflammations and fever continued to be called antiphlogistic. Bleedings and blisterings became popular because 19th century physicians considered them antiphlogistic. Today there is still an ointment available with the trade name 'Antiphlogistine'!

antipilus an agent which removes hair.

antipones to place before, set before, prefer.

antipsoric a homeopathic remedy which acts to treat, nullify or rid the body of the psoric miasm. *Psorinum, Calc. carb., Arsenicum*, and *Sulphur* are examples. 'Antipsorica' means a remedy which is curative of the itch or psora. In some early references the terms *Psoricum* and *Antipsorinum* were used for the nosode. These are synonymous with today's *Psorinum.*

antipyretic lowering the body temperature, or a substance which has this effect.

antipyrine (antipyrina, phenazone) an antipyretic and pain reliever no longer used today, as its side-effects can be quite toxic.

antipyrotic an agent which heals burns.

antiscorbutic an agent which cures scurvy.

antiseptic tending to inhibit the growth and/or reproduction of microorganisms, especially pathogenic ones. Also an agent used to inhibit that growth.

antisycotic a homeopathic remedy which acts to treat, nullify or rid the body of the sycotic miasm. *Medorrhinum, Nat. sulph., Sepia, Thuja, Acidum Nitricum,* and the *Argentums* are examples of remedies which have antisycotic qualities.

antisyphilitic a homeopathic remedy which acts to treat, nullify or rid the body of the syphilitic miasm. *Syphilinum, Acidum Nitricum, Aurum, Ars. i.,* and the *Mercuries* are examples of remedies which have antisyphilitic qualities.

antitragus a projection of the ear opposite and superior to the tragus (the small prominence of cartilage projecting over the meatus of the external ear).

antivivisection against or opposed to vivisection. See VIVISECTION.

antrum any nearly closed cavity, or hollow space, particularly one with bony walls.

antrum of Highmore (sinus maxillaris) an air cavity (sinus) above the upper jaw (maxilla), connecting with the middle meatus of the nose.

anuria total suppression or lack of urine.

aortic pertaining to the aorta.

aorta the large artery arising from the heart sending fresh, oxygenated blood to the body.

aortitis inflammation of the aorta.

aperient a mild laxative or medicine, especially one which is effervescent, which opens the bowels gently.

apex the summit or extremity of anything. The extremity of a conical or pyramidal structure, such as the heart or the lung.

aphasia the loss of the power of speech. A defect in the ability to talk. The French physician Paul Broca did seminal work in *aphemie* as he called it. From this work, the first on cerebral location, he concluded that articulate speech was localized in the third frontal convolution of the brain.

aphonia loss of voice. 'Aphonia clericorum' is clergyman's sore-throat.

aphoria sterility in women (Gr. *a-,* 'not', and *phorein,* 'to bear') .

aphrodisiac (aphrodiasiacum) anything which arouses or increases sexual desire (from *Aphrodite,* the Greek goddess of love).

aphrodisiae a morbid or immoderate sexual desire.

aphthae small whitish ulcers of the mouth; canker sores. May also refer to thrush or sprue. See THRUSH.

aphthous ulcer (aphthous stomatitis, canker sore) a superficial ulcer usually occurring on a mucous membrane, for example the mouth. See CANKER SORE.

apices the upper portion of the lungs (plural of 'apex').

apitherapy the use of injected bee venom and/or actual stings of bees to cure or alleviate a variety of illnesses, especially arthritis and multiple sclerosis.

aplastic anemia a form of anemia in which the formative processes of the bone marrow are lacking or nil.

apocenosis a discharge or evacuation.

aponeurosis a fibrinous extension of a tendon. The passage of muscle into tendon. A fibrous sheet or expanded tendon, giving attachment to muscular fibers and serving as the means of origin or insertion of a flat muscle.

apoplectic referring to a sudden loss of consciousness followed by paralysis.

apoplexy (stroke, cerebral hemorrhage, cerebral thrombosis) sudden loss of

apoplexy (stroke, cerebral hemorrhage, cerebral thrombosis) sudden loss of muscular control with a lessening or loss of sensation and consciousness due to a blood clot in the brain. It is seldom instantly fatal but may cause paralysis or other mental affections. Commonly referred to as a stroke (technically, a stroke can occur anywhere in the body).

aposia (adipsia) absence of thirst or of the feeling of thirst.

apostacy the act of forsaking what one professed or believed in.

apostems an abscess.

appendicitis (typhlitis, perityphlitis, apophysitis, scolecoiditis) inflammation of the appendix. See PERITYPHLITIS.

Charles McBurney, a New York physician, was the first to describe (1889) where the area of greatest pain could be found in the appendicitis patient, thence called McBurney's point. "The seat of greatest pain, *determined by the pressure of one finger*; has been very exactly between an inch and a half and two inches from the anterior spinous process of the ilium on a straight line drawn from that process to the umbilicus."—*New York Medical Journal* 50:676-84, 1889.

appetite a desire for food, as opposed to hunger (which has discomfort, weakness, or pain, caused by the need for or lack of food).

approbation praise, commendation, approval.

apraxia the inability to perform skilled or learned movements, such as typing or opening a glove compartment.

aprosexia the inability to concentrate or fix the attention.

apyrexia lack of fever.

arachnitis (arachnoiditis) inflammation of the arachnoid membrane (the middle layer of membranes covering the brain and spinal cord).

arachnoid resembling a cobweb or spider web. The arachnoid membrane is the middle layer of the membranes which cover the brain and spinal cord.

archetype the original pattern or model from which all other things of the same kind are made; a prototype.

archoptosis prolapsed anus.

arcus senilis (gerontoxon) the whitish or greyish ring of fatty degeneration seen around the cornea in older persons.

areola a colored or darkened ring surrounding some central point or space, such as a nipple or pustule.

argillaceous clay-like or composed of clay.

argyria (argyriasis, argyrism) a slate-grey discoloration of the skin, deeper tissues and organs due to insoluble deposits of silver-protein (albuminate of silver). It usually occurs as a result of prolonged ingestion or exposure to silver salts.

armamentarium all the means (books, medicines, instruments, etc.) at the doctor's disposal to help him practice his profession, namely, to heal the

Arndt-Schulz Law (hormesis, biphasal response/effect, Type-Effect Hypothesis, Time-Response Curve, biphasal-paradoxical effect, Bier-Huchard Rule) the law stating that a small stimulus enhances growth, a medium stimulus impedes it or maintains normality and a strong stimulus inhibits, or destroys activity. This law of Western medicine supports the fundamental concept of homeopathy in that a substance which has harmful effects in large doses can have beneficial effects in minute ones. After Rudolph Arndt (1835-1900) and Hugo Schulz (1853-1932).

This law or postulate was first put forth in 1880, as Schulz conducted experiments using chemicals to stimulate growth and respiration in yeast. Schulz presented his premise formally in 1888: 'Uber Hefegifte' in *Pflugers Archiv Gesammte Physiologie* (Vol. 42, p. 517).

More precise versions were formulated by Karl Koetschau in the 1920s and Joseph Wilder in the 1930s. See KOETSCHAU'S HYPOTHESIS, WILDER'S LAW.

'Hormesis' is a modern term given to the growth-stimulating effect of minute quantities of toxic substances in living organisms, as demonstrated by experimental data. See HORMESIS.

aromatherapy the use of plant essences either inhaled or applied/massaged to the skin to effect therapeutic changes. Their effects are said to be psyche-related, due to the ethereal nature of the oils. A whole range of correspondences can be established with other modalities (e.g.., cinnamon with the color orange, the planet Sun, the element fire, and yang activity in Traditional Chinese Medicine). The practitioner's intuitive powers no doubt play a large role in the therapeutic setting. For more information: American Aromatherapy Assoc., PO Box 1222, Fair Oaks, CA. 95628.

arrhythmia a lack of rhythm, as in an arrhythmic heart.

arsenical yellow in color. Of, pertaining to, or containing arsenic.

arsphenamine see SALVARSAN.

arteriole a very small artery.

arteriosclerosis hardening and thickening of arterial walls which interferes with blood circulation. 'Angiosclerosis' is a general term used to describe hardening of the walls of blood vessels; 'arteriosclerosis' is a general term for a disease characterized by thickening and loss of elasticity of arterial walls. 'Atherosclerosis' is a type of arteriosclerosis in which deposits of yellow plaque containing lipid material and cholesterol are formed within the lining of medium and large arteries.

arteritis inflammation of an artery.

arthragra gout of the joints.

arthritis chronica chronic gout.

arthritis vaga wandering gout. Now it commonly means inflammation of the joints.

arthrocace caries or wasting of bone tissue, especially in a joint.

arthrolithiasis gout.

arthrophlogosis an inflammation of the joints.

articular referring to the joints.

articulation joint. Any connection allowing motion between the parts.

artificial phlyctenular autotherapy see PHLYCTENULAR AUTOTHERAPY.

aryenoids 'ladle-like' (referring to cartilage and muscle of the larynx).

ascariasis an intestinal infestation with worms *(Ascaris lumbricoides)*; worms may also be found in the stomach, liver and lungs.

ascarides (sing. ascaris) roundworms. "A genus of intestinal round worms."— E.A. Neatby, *A Manual of Homeopathic Therapeutics*. There are two types of ascaris: 1) *Ascaris lumbricoides*, long round worms, like the earthworm, and 2) *Ascaris vermicularis (Oxyuris vermicularis)*, the thread worm or maw worm. See OXYURIS.

ascites (hydroperitoneum, abdominal dropsy) accumulation of fluid in a cavity, usually the abdomen.

asepsis the absence of harmful bacteria. The removal or destruction of infected material or organisms causing disease.

aseptic without germs, disease or infection. It is possible to have an 'aseptic fever' or a fever unassociated with infection. Mechanical injury (a blow, fall or crushing trauma) may cause fever even though no pathogens are present.

asphyxia unconsciousness due to suffocation or interference of any kind with oxygenation of the blood.

asphyxiation (suffocation) lack of oxygen.

assuage to ease or make less severe or burdensome. To satisfy or appease.

asteatosis any skin disease characterized by scantiness or lack of sebaceous secretions, the skin becoming dry, scaly, and often fissured.

asteroid star shaped.

asthenia weakness or debility.

asthenopia weakness of the ocular muscles or of visual power. Eyestrain with spasm of accommodation.

asthma a disease characterized by difficult breathing, coughing, wheezing, mucoid sputum and constriction of the chest. Spasms of the bronchioles may occur and edema may be present.

asthma humidum 'spitting asthma'.

asthma thymica (asthma thymicum kopii, thymic asthma of Kopp) asthma erroneously thought to be due to an enlargement of the thymus gland. It is synonymous with LARYNGISMUS STRIDULUS *(vide)*. Another source says "an asthma reflexively produced by the irritation of an enlarged thymus, usually seen in infants."

astigmatism a condition of unequal curvature of one or more of the refractive surfaces (cornea, lens, or eyeball) of the eye whereby images are not focused onto a single point of the retina but spread out in a line and are blurry.

astragalus 1) the ankle bone (also called 'talus') 2) a Chinese herb.

astraphobia the morbid fear of thunderstorms.

astringent causing contraction of tissues. An agent which causes contraction of the tissues, arrests secretions, or controls bleeding.

asynesia stupidity or dementia..

asystolia (asystole) lack of heart action.

ataraxia muscular coordination.

ataxia muscularis see THOMSEN'S DISEASE.

atelectasis imperfect expansion of the lungs. A collapsed or airless state of the lungs.

atelia (ateliosis) incomplete development of the mind or the body or any of its parts; infantilism.

athelia absence of the nipples.

atheroma (steatoma) a fatty cyst. Fatty infiltration of the walls of the arteries in arteriosclerosis.

atheromatous having a hard quality.

atherosclerosis see ARTERIOSCLEROSIS.

athetosis (Hammond's disease) a condition characterized by recurrent, slow, and continual change of position of the fingers, toes, hands, feet and other parts of the body.

First described by W.A. Hammond (1828-1900), an American neurologist (who also, by the way, founded the Army Medical Museum).

atonic relaxed; without normal tone or tension.

atopic eczema (atopic dermatitis) an inflammatory skin reaction that occurs when an atopic (genetically allergic) person is exposed to an allergen. Although contact with an allergen can be a factor, atopic eczema is a distinct clinical entity not to be confused with acquired allergic dermatitis or contact dermatitis.

atresia failure of a cavity or duct to develop or open up completely to the connecting organ.

atrichia the absence of hair, whether congenital or acquired.

atrophic wasting away, withered; relating to atrophy.

atrophic rhinitis inflammation of the nasal mucous membrane with subsequent wasting away of those membranes.

atrophy a shriveling or wasting of the tissues of a part or of the entire body.

attenuantia remedies that penetrate and divide the humors (see HUMORS) into smaller parts.

attenuation potency, or dilution. Some homeopaths say, "I gave the 30th attenuation," which is just like saying, "I gave the 30th potency" or "I gave the 30th dilution." 'Attenuation' would actually mean the process of potentizing. "I attenuated the substance" would be the same as "I potentized the substance." But in the literature of old (or even today) you may come across statements such as "I gave the 30th attenuation," which is perfectly acceptable. See POTENCY.

attrition wearing away by friction or rubbing.

audacity boldness or daring. Unrestrained impudence, insolence, or presumption.

aude sapere a Latin expression which can be loosely translated as 'dare to be better', 'dare to understand', 'dare to go higher', 'dare to know', etc. Hahnemann's epigram for his *Organon*.

audiatur et altera pars 'let another part be heard' (Latin).

aura 1) a subtle, invisible (perhaps visible to some) emanation from a substance. 2) The peculiar sensation, as of a light vapor, or cold air, which rises from the trunk or limbs towards the head, and serves as a premonitory symptom of epilepsy (aura epileptica) or hysterics. Some migraine sufferers and epileptics say they see aura-like disturbances in their visual field before their respective attacks.

aural referring to the ear.

aural polypi polyps in the ear canal.

auricle (pinna) the external ear.

auricular/atrial fibrillation a cardiac arrhythmia due to abnormal excitation of the upper heart (atrium) muscle which causes an irregular and rapid ventricular heart rate, the end result being a rapid and irregular heart rate.

aurigo/auriginous (aurugo) jaundice or icteric.

auscultation physical examination by listening to the sounds made by the organs of the body, the contracting muscles, the blood in the vessels, the fetus, etc., in order to diagnose potential diseases or assess the functioning of the body.

autohemic therapy/autohemotherapy (plasmapheresis) a variation of isotherapy in which a very small amount of the patient's blood is withdrawn, treated with homeopathic remedies, ozone, etc., then either potentized or not potentized, and then re-injected into the patient.

L.D. Rogers, in the early 1900s, modified this procedure by using multiples of five drops of blood added to nineteen times as much water. She exposed this solution to varying degrees of heat and made further dilutions as dictated by the condition and patient being treated. See AUTO-SANGUIS THERAPY.

autointoxication a poisoning of the body by accumulation and subsequent absorption of waste products.

autoisopathics remedies prepared from secretions or excretions from the patient, such as urine, serous discharges, blood or plasma.

autolysates the disintegration or dissolution products of dead bacteria.

autophony the phenomenon by which a person's voice seems more resonant to himself.

auto-sanguis therapy/cure a method of mixing the patient's blood with homeopathic remedies, potentizing the mixture, then injecting this newly prepared remedy back into the patient. Specifically this term applies to the method as taught by the late Dr. H.H. Reckeweg (1905-1985) and other homotoxicologists. Vannier did seminal work in this area, as espoused in his paper 'Sanguineous Autotherapy' (1936). J. Roy and J.M. Munoz conducted research as well. It differs from merely making a blood-nosode or blood-isode from the ill person, since it involves mixing remedies with the patient's blood. Also see AUTOHEMIC THERAPY, HOMOTOXICOLOGY.

autumn the fall; that particular season of the year which is characterized by hot days and cold nights.

autumnal catarrh hay fever.

auxiliary symptom see entry under SYMPTOMS.

avarice greed. An excessive desire to amass wealth.

avaunt a command to 'go away' or 'go forward'.

aversion not merely a dislike for something, such as a food, but an intense dislike, a loathing.

Avogadro's number (6.023×10^{23}) the number of molecules contained in one mole of a substance. One molecule of a remedy substance in a mole is approximately equivalent to the 24x (12c, Q3) dilution level. In other words, mathematical calculations show that not one molecule of the original substance or material can be found in a homeopathic remedy of the 24x or 12c dilution level. Amadeo Avogadro (1776-1856), the physicist for whom this principle was named, stated his observation in 1811. It was not officially recognized as a mathematical or physical constant until 1865 when J. Loschmidt (1821-1895) calculated the exact number which Avogadro had proposed. Loschmidt's number, which some confuse with Avogadro's number, is the number of molecules in 1 cc of gas at standard temperature and pressure, 2.67×10^{19}. It is because Loschmidt did the calculations to come up with 6.023×10^{23} that his name is associated with that figure.

avulsion a forcible separation or setting loose from where something was previously.

awn a slender, bristlelike terminal process, like an asparagus tip.

axilla armpit.

Ayurveda 'the knowledge or science of life'. The traditional medicine of India, developed over more than 4000 years and first recorded in the Vedas, the sacred scriptures of Hinduism. Traditional Chinese Medicine and Ayurveda are thought to have developed together and then split at some point. They have many common aspects: energy points, pulse diagnosis and herbal remedies. The Chinese divide the world into yin and yang, the Ayurvedics into vata (air and ether), pitta (fire), and kapha (water and earth). Tibet, at the crossroads of India and China, blended both, to create a unique and esoteric system—Tibetan medicine. Consult Svoboda and Lade's *Tao and Dharma*.

azoturia an increase in the nitrogenous substances in the urine. Excess urea in the urine.

BBBB**B**BB

Bach flower remedies the 38 flower essences of Dr. Edward Bach (1886-1936), a British bacteriologist and homeopath, who along with Dr. F.J. Wheeler identified and classified eight bowel organisms in the first quarter of the 20th century. (Bowel nosodes were subsequently made of these organisms.) Dr. Bach abandoned his successful medical practice in 1930 to 'retire' to the countryside to seek out herbs which would heal the sick. He felt that the basis of disease was found in the disharmony between the spiritual and mental aspects of the human being. Dr. Bach theorized that conflicting moods lowered the body's vitality and allowed disease to occur. Therefore the remedies which he intuitively developed were for the mood and temperament of the patient, not necessarily for the physical illness. As the patient's emotional sphere became more balanced or healthy, he reasoned, the accompanying physical illness would dissipate. He said, "The mind being the most delicate and sensitive part of the body shows the onset and the course of disease much more definitely than the body, so that the outlook of mind is chosen as the guide to which remedy or remedies are necessary. "

Many believe that Bach remedies are homeopathic. This is incorrect as they have arisen from a different philosophical premise in addition to not being potentized in the homeopathic manner. Also, Bach remedies have not been proven in the homeopathic sense. They can not only be taken orally or used topically but can be added to bath water. They are often used in conjunction with positive affirmations.

Dr. Bach originally developed twelve flower essences (described in his book *The Twelve Healers*) which corresponded to the twelve mental states he felt were responsible for illness: fear, terror, mental torture or worry, indecision, indifference or boredom, doubt or discouragement, over-concern, weakness, over-enthusiasm, pride or aloofness, self-distrust, and impatience.

For example, Bach said that the essence for worry was Agrimony, for over-concern Chicory, and for over-enthusiasm, Vervain. Later he added 26 more to make a total of 38 (Agrimony, Aspen, Beech, Centaury, Certo, Cherry Plum, Chestnut Bud, Chicory, Clematis, Crab Apple, Elm, Gentian, Gorse, Heather, Holly, Honeysuckle, Hornbeam, Impatiens, Larch, Mimulus, Mustard, Oak, Olive, Pine, Red Chestnut, Rock Rose, Rock Water, Scleranthus, Star of Bethlehem or Ornithogalum, Sweet Chestnut, Vervain, Vine Walnut, Water Violet, White Chestnut, Wild Oat, Wild Rose, and Willow). Consult *Bach Flower Therapy* (M. Scheffer) and *The Medical Discoveries of Edward Bach, Physician* (Nora Weeks).

Baelz's disease (chilitis glandularis, myxadenitis labialis) a chronic painless ulceration of the mucous glands of the lips, after the German physician E.B. von Baelz (1845-1913), who lived for many years in Tokyo.

bakers' eczema (bakers' itch) eczema caused by the irritation from handling yeast.

balanitis inflammation of the head (glans) of the penis or the head of the clitoris.

balanoblennorrhoea gonorrhea of the glans penis.

balanoposthitis inflammation of the glans penis and the prepuce.

balbuties stuttering, stammering.

bandyleg bow-legged. See GENU VARUM.

Banquo's ghost simply means 'a ghost'. Generically, something which comes back to haunt a wrongdoer. Banquo was a Scottish general (c. 1066) who figures in Shakespeare's play *Macbeth*. Upon Macbeth's orders, Banquo is murdered, after which his ghost terrifies Macbeth at a royal feast.

Banti's disease (Banti's syndrome) idiopathic (meaning 'of unknown origin') enlargement of the spleen characterized by anemia, leukopenia, hemorrhage, and cirrhosis of the liver.

Bantingism a dietary method of treating obesity by eating chiefly lean meat, avoiding fats and carbohydrates. After Wm. Banting (1797-1878), a London undertaker.

barber's itch (sycosis coccygenica, sycosis vulgaris, ringworm of the beard, Jackson's itch, sycosis, tinea sycosis) a pustular folliculitis of the hairy areas of the face, and neck and nape of neck. Pustules form around hair follicles after which they may break and form hard brown crusts. These crusts slough off in a few days, leaving purple pimples which gradually disappear.

Barlow's disease (Moller's disease, Cheadle's disease) infantile scurvy. A wasting condition resulting from feeding infants improper foods; symptoms include pallor, foul breath, coated tongue, and diarrhea.

Bartholinitis inflammation of a vulvovaginal gland (Bartholin's gland). After Thomas Bartholin (1616-1680), a Danish physician.

baruria an increase in the solid constituents of the urine which results in a high urinary specific gravity.

Basedow's disease see GRAVE'S DISEASE.

basso profundo deepest bass voice; having a range below the ordinary bass staff.

bastinado beating of the soles of the feet, a form of punishment used in Turkey and China. During the late 1800s it was used to revive patients who had passed out or had received too much anesthesia.

Batavian fever an intermittent fever which originated from what is now Holland.

bat's wing disease see LUPUS.

baunscheidismus (baunscheidtism) a form of therapy based on the use of a mechanical instrument (lebenswecker) containing twenty or more one-inch-long slender needles arranged in a series of circles, used to produce counter-irritation. All the needles are introduced into the tissue of the patient at once. Then croton oil or another irritant is rubbed in, in order to increase and maintain the irritation, thus assuring a good counter-irritant effect.

It was invented by Carl Baunscheidt, a 19th century German businessman and inventor, to blend acupuncture and counter-irritant effects. He called it Lebenswecker ('great resuscitator' or 'life-reviver'). Baunscheidt attributed the alleviation of arthritic pains in his hand to gnat bites and thus invented his instrument. Perhaps he should have looked into a proving of gnat.

In 1911, John Linden (a non-homeopath) wrote *Manual of the Exanthematic Method of Cure also Known as Baunscheidtism*. See BLEEDING.

Bazin's disease (tuberculosis cutis indurativa, buccal psoriasis, leukoplakia buccalis) white or bluish white patches on the surface of the tongue or the mucous membrane of the cheeks, due to excessive growth of the oral mucosa. Also the formation of hard nodules below the skin which break down, forming ulcers. This phenomenon usually occurs on the calves, occasionally on the thighs or arms, and is generally associated with tuberculosis. From the Paris dermatologist Bazin (1807-1878).

beal pustule or boil. To suppurate. Also (not commonly used) 'bealed ear' or 'to have a bealing hand lanced' are former uses for 'beal'.

Beard's disease neurasthenia or nervous exhaustion. The chief symptoms are insomnia, headache, feelings of constriction around the head, back pain, exhaustion after slight mental or physical exertion, increased sensitivity to noises, irregular heart actions, vertigo, dyspepsia, visual disturbances, and loss of memory. In general, the individual has an intensely nervous irritability and weakness. Named after the American physician G.M. Beard (1839-1883).

Bechterew's disease chronic arthritis of unknown origin with progressive deformity, stiffness, and bony fusion of the vertebrae. From the Russian neurologist V.M. Bekhterev (1856-1927).

beclouded covered, made obscure or gloomy.

Bell's palsy (prosopoplegia, peripheral facial paralysis) peripheral paralysis of the facial nerve. Dr. Sir Charles Bell (1774-1842), a Scottish surgeon and anatomist, demonstrated the sensory motor function of the seventh cranial nerve and the cause of facial palsy or Bell's palsy ('On the Nerves', 1821). It is a unilateral paralysis of the facial muscles causing pain, weakness, and paresthesias (abnormal sensations) of that area. As nerve function is interrupted, normal muscular tone is decreased and the face may look deformed and droopy.

Bell was one of the greatest scientists in medical history. All his discoveries were, in his own words, "deductions from anatomy." He was an anatomist, physiologist, neurologist, and surgeon and an accomplished artist. All the drawings for the illustrations in his books were made by him, and they stand unrivaled for their facility, elegance, and accuracy.

bellwether any leader of a blindly following crowd.

beri-beri (kakke, Singhalese, endemic neuritis) polyneuritis occurring especially in tropical and mild temperate regions. The muscles are stiff and atrophied with accompanying nerve pains and paresis. Dyspnea is frequent and in certain forms (e.g., wet beri beri) edema is a prominent symptom. This term comes from the Singhalese meaning 'extreme weakness'. It is a deficiency disease due to a lack of vitamin B1 (thiamine) in the diet. In the Far East it is largely due to the almost exclusive use of polished rice.

Berkeley's elements the elements or fundamental aspects of the universe in Chinese Medicine (fire, earth, air, water, and ether) as related by Berkeley Digby to homeopathic remedies. An awareness of the predominance of these elements or energies allows one to better select a homeopathic remedy for the patient. For example, "If the person appears to be splenic/psoric in their thinking and feeling, and there is difficulty in deciding between *Phosphorus* and *Sepia*, then *Sepia* will likely be the best choice [because Sepia is a splenic or earth-element remedy]" or "The lungs tend to create armoring in response to being hurt, thus they are associated with the element 'metal' in Chinese medicine [and thus 'metal' remedies will be most efficacious for lung problems]." "Remedies demonstrating these qualities are *Tuberculinum, Ignatia, Natrum mur., Stramonium, Phosphorus, Coca, Platina*, etc."—B. Digby (in Kent Homeopathic Associates brochure).

Bernard's canal (Santorini's duct, ductus pancreaticus accessorius) the excretory duct of the head of the pancreas.

besotted having a muddled or stupefied expression, especially after drinking liquor, as in "he was besotted with liquor."

BEV (bio-electronic Vincent) an electronic instrumentation method which uses pH, reduction-oxidation (redox) potential, and resistance of bodily fluids (namely, blood, saliva, and urine), in order to diagnose disease, to suggest methods of treatment and to show bio-compatibility of medications and drinking water. One of the main thrusts of BEV (and EAV) is to improve the 'soil' or terrain of the individual, thus improving the overall health. This technique was originated by French researcher Louis-Claude Vincent. See EAV.

Bibron's antidote an antidote to the rattlesnake bite, consisting of 2.5 drams of bromine, 2 grains of potassium iodide, and one grain of corrosive chloride of mercury, diluted with 30 oz. of dilute alcohol. A teaspoonful of this mixture was given in wine or brandy as necessary.

bibulous 1) absorbent. Having the ability to absorb water. 2) tending to festive and social drinking.

Bier-Huchard Rule see ARNDT-SCHULZ LAW.

Biermer's anaemia (pernicious anemia, Addisonian anemia) see PERNICIOUS ANEMIA.

bifida forked, divided in two, as in spina bifida (rachischisis), a birth defect resulting from the absence of the vertebral arches. Spinal membranes and/or nervous tissue can thus protrude out of the spinal cord, generally in the lumbosacral region.

bifurcation division into two branches. A forking.

bigarexia a constant appetite for food (opposite of anorexia).

bilharziasis (schistosomiasis, swimmers' itch, swamp itch) a papular and pustular dermatitis occurring on the skin of persons wading or swimming in freshwater lakes of the northern U.S. and Canada.

bilious 1) pertaining to bile, or disorders arising from an excess of bile. 2) bitter, ill-humored, resentful, discontented, as in a bilious temperament.

bilious fever fever with digestive disturbances (vomiting, copious clayey stools)

"It is still more difficult to confound the so-called bilious fevers with typhus; for in their case the bilious vomiting and stools, the jaundiced complexion and the dark-brown urine with a greenish tint, together with the violent inflammatory fever might induce a belief that we have to deal with hepatitis or acute jaundice; but the slight painfulness of the liver which is in no proportion to the febrile heat, together with the marked sensation of pressure and fullness in the region of the stomach, and more particularly the copious evacuations by the mouth and rectum, exclude the idea of jaundice and hepatitis insofar as in both these conditions we have constipation or a discharge of hard, gray, clayey stools with retching rather than, as in bilious fever, copious yellow, green and brown stools; whence it is evident that in this case the symptoms point to a functional derangement of the digestive process rather than to a local affection of some definite organ."—Jahr,*Therapeutic Guide: Forty Years Practice*.

Binet test a series of graded tests which compares the mental age of the individual with his chronological age. The individual is asked a series of questions graded according to the intelligence of normal children at different ages; according to the answers given, the individual is graded as normal, backward, a moron, an imbecile, or an idiot. After Alfred Binet (1857-1911), a French psychologist. This test, though once popular, has since been modified to become the Stanford-Binet test. Now the Wechsler Scales have become quite popular and are frequently used to measure the intelligence of adults and children. The terms 'idiot', 'moron' and 'imbecile' are no longer used.

biochemics (celloids, biochemic salts, cell salts) see SCHUESSLER.

biocybernetics the science of communication and control within a living organism.

biological terrain assessment (BTA) the evaluation of the blood, urine, and saliva to determine the health of the 'terrain' or 'soil' of the person.

Louis Claude Vincent conducted much research in this area and in the assessment of an individuals 'interior' environment. He found that the key to healing was not just in drugs but rather in bodily biochemistry. He used the information (ph, redox potential, resistivity, etc.) from the building blocks of life (amino acids, enzymes, biochemicals found in blood, urine, and saliva) to gain information on how the body was functioning. This information can then be used to chose treatments designed to alter abnormal biochemistry in order to make the terrain more healthy and thus the person more healthy. See TERRAIN.

bio-oxidative therapy the medical use of oxygen, ozone and peroxide to cure disease or balance health. This is a vast subject and far too broad to discuss here. For example, the naturopath Eugene Blass developed a method of oxygen therapy in the early 1920s to cleanse the blood and vital organs by oxidizing the toxins. He created products (Calozone, Magozone, etc.) which delivered nascent oxygen to the body. Since then many others have done research in this area. Perhaps one of the earliest was Wm. F.

Koch, who invented a product called Glyoxylide which, he claimed, restored proper oxidation in body cells and converted toxins to antitoxins in a chain-like reaction "where dehydrogenation [removal of a hydrogen atom] initiates oxidation in the cell and destroys the pathogens integrated with the cell." Koch felt that insufficient oxidation due to the accumulation of toxins in the body is a factor in the development of cancer and other diseases.

There are many books on the subject, including two comprehensive texts: R. Viebahn, *The Use of Ozone in Medicine* (1987), and H.E. Satori, *Ozone: The Eternal Purifier of the Earth and Cleanser of All Living Beings* (1994).

There are instruments which generate ionized oxygen for inhalation and drinking. Some of the effects of ionized oxygen include improvement of the microcirculation, stabilization of cell membrane potentials, correction of side effects from radiation and chemotherapy, regeneration of the organism, and reduction of pain and inflammation.

bioresonance and multiresonance therapy (BRT) a method of therapy which, along with resonance homeopathy, maintains that electromagnetic processes are functionally superordinate to biochemical processes. Thus via the use of specific frequencies (all matter has a specific frequency) normal physiological processes can be enhanced. Likewise, specific frequencies can be applied to kill pathogens or inhibit pathological processes. See RESONANCE HOMEOPATHY, MORA-THERAPY.

biotherapic see NOSODE and BIOTHERAPY.

biotherapy the general term describing the use of homeopathic preparations from living tissue or discharges (tissues, nosodes, sarcodes, serums, etc.) to treat illness and disease. See NOSODE.

biphasal effect (biphasal paradoxical effect) see ARNDT-SCHULZ LAW.

bistoury a type of scalpel.

bitters (amara) a bitter, usually alcoholic liquid made with herbs or roots and used in cocktails or as a stimulant tonic for the stomach. Bitters promote the flow of digestive juices, stimulate the appetite, increase the flow of bile and aid the liver in detoxification. Angostura bitters, which you may be familiar with, is made from the bark of a tree, *Galipea cusparia,* and is named after the Venezuelan town, Angostura. Swedish bitters is made from a combination of herbs following a traditional recipe dating back to the medieval physician Paracelsus.

Blackmore's celloids mineral remedies based on the theories of Australian homeopath M. Blackmore (1906-1977) and described in his *Celloids: A Text Book for Physicians.* He claimed to have refined Schuessler's theories, stating that Schuessler's tissue salts are too minutely prepared to have any therapeutic effect on the body. Blackmore's products have substantial amounts of salts and no sodium chloride. For example, his Silica compound contains 25mg Silica and 200mg of Sodium phosphate.

blacksickness see KALA-AZAR.

blackwater fever (hemolytic malaria, malarial hemoglobinuria) a fatal and contagious malarial disease of the tropics, with fever, chills, vomiting and dyspnea.

blebs a bulla; a soft blister approximately 1cm in diameter.

bleeding the 'therapeutic' technique to relieve fevers or plethoric conditions in the body, in vogue during the 18th and 19th centuries. Lancing veins, scarring tissues, and leeching (leaving leeches on to suck blood until they dropped off) were the methods employed; cupping and blistering (using fly pastes) were related techniques.

Bloodletting was thought to be one way to correct the imbalance in the humors (see HUMORS). Bleeding usually involved opening a vein (at the bend of the elbow, on the bottom of the foot, or even under the tongue) and allowing 10-12 ounces of blood to escape. This was done repeatedly at the discretion of the physician. One reference reported nearly five gallons of blood were drained from a woman patient over a period of six weeks.

According to the eminent Scottish physician Wm. Cullen, "bloodletting is a powerful means of diminishing the activity of the body and is thus the most effective way to quell feverish reactions." (This was the same doctor whom Hahnemann translated and then disagreed with concerning the action of quinine.)

The appearance of Pierre C.A. Louis' *Recherches sur les effets de la Saignee dans quelques maladies inflammatoires* (1835) marked the beginning of the decline of bloodletting. He offered statistical evidence proving that the barbaric practice was of little use in pneumonia as well as other diseases. Furthermore, he showed that statistics can be used as an instrument of precision in cases where proper clinical methods are wanting. Louis is considered the father of medical statistics.

blennorrhea (blennorrhagia, urethrorrhea) gonorrhea, gonorrheal urethritis. Also a copious mucous discharge from the vagina or urethra.

blepharitis inflammation of the eyelids.

blepharitis marginalis (b. ciliaris) inflammation of the hair follicles and sebaceous glands along the margins of the eyelids.

blepharophthalmia inflammation of the eyeball and lids.

blepharoplegia paralysis of an eyelid.

blepharoptosis drooping of the upper eyelid.

blepharospasm (nictitation) excessive winking or an involuntary, forceful spasmodic winking.

blind not visible, as in 'blind piles' (hemorrhoids which are present within the rectum and do not protrude through the anus or occur outside of it).

bloody-flux see DYSENTERY.

blue skin disease (cyanosis, morbus coeruleus) see CYANOSIS.

bodkin a small thin instrument with a sharp point used for making holes in cloth or leather.

Boeck's sarcoid (sarcoidosis, Besnier-Boeck-Schaumann syndrome) a connective tissue tumor, usually highly malignant, and of unknown origin, which involves the lungs, lymph nodes, skin, liver, spleen, eyes, bones of the fingers and toes, and parotid glands. These tissues gradually become fibrous (harden). Named after P.M. Boeck (1845-1917), a Norwegian dermatologist. 'Sarcoid' means 'resembling flesh'.

Boenninghausen Clemens Maria Franz von Boenninghausen (1785-1864) was a lawyer and physician who wrote *Therapeutic Pocket Book* (1847), the first repertory. Ill with pulmonary tuberculosis and with no cure in sight, Boenninghausen began writing farewell letters. One letter was to August Weihe (the elder), who responded, advising Boenninghausen to give homeopathy a chance. (It was August Weihe's grandson, August Weihe III, who developed the 'points of Weihe', which blended the use of acupuncture and homeopathic remedies.) Boenninghausen sent his symptoms to Dr. Weihe, which indicated *Pulsatilla* to be the curative remedy. *Pulsatilla* did in fact cure him in 1828. Boenninghausen then studied homeopathy, wrote, treated the ill and eventually became one of Hahnemann's best friends.

Hahnemann said of Boenninghausen, "If I were ill and could not help myself, I would not entrust myself to any physician in the world except him." Also, "Not one of my students in the profession has thus far done even half as much as you have done to further our Beautiful Art." Boenninghausen is considered to have had the largest homeopathic practice of any homeopathic physician.

One of Boenninghausen's significant contributions was the concept that a person expresses parts of a grand symptomatology. See BOENNINGHAUSEN CONCORDANCES.

Boenninghausen concordances (Boenninghausen's relationships of remedies) the section on remedy relationships in Boenninghausen's *Therapeutic Pocket Book* (a concordance is an alphabetical index of subjects or topics). It was the first repertory and its arrangement is based on a practical analysis of symptoms into their component elements of location, sensation and conditions. He felt that many allied remedies could be grouped together which, in turn, would allow one to easily find an alternate remedy if the previously given remedy(s) failed, or acted partially.

"Suppose you have given *Aconite* to someone, it worked well but the patient is left with some symptoms that you have to translate to rubrics to find the follow-up remedy. What Boenninghausen did was to divide these symptoms into groups. For example, if the main symptoms left over after *Aconite* was given are mind symptoms, he found out which specific follow-up remedies come forward for mind symptoms after *Aconite.* He has found out which remedies come out more when they have extremity symptoms, and digestive tract symptoms, circulation symptoms, or sleep symptoms, etc."—R. van Zandvoort, *The American Homeopath,* 1:1, p. 58, 1994.

boggy like a bog, swampy or mushy.

borborygmi intestinal rumblings or gurglings; the rumbling noises caused by gas in the intestines.

bougie a slender cylindrical instrument used for dilating then exploring the urethra and other canals.

bowel nosodes nosodes made from cultures of the bowel intestinal flora as found in human fecal material. They were originally introduced into homeopathic practice in the 1930s as seminal research was carried out by Edward Bach (a bacteriologist and formulator of the Bach Flower Remedies), and Dr. John Paterson with his wife, Elizabeth. These researchers noticed that certain diseases and certain homeopathic remedies produced an abundance of specific bacilli in the stool of patients. "The potentized bowel nosode can therefore be considered as a complex biochemical substance having the characteristics of the disturbed metabolism and thus be similar to the disease, and by the Law of Similars, to have the power to restore the balance."—W.J. Diamond, *Biological Therapy,* 13:3, p. 128.

Bach and Paterson saw relationships between the symptomatology of certain homeopathic remedies and a corresponding bowel nosode. For example, the bowel nosode *Sycotic Co.* seems to cover a totality of symptoms associated with three remedies, *Rhus tox., Nitric ac.,* and *Arg. nit. Morgan Pure* is associated with *Sulphur, Graphites,* and *Calc. carb.* Usually one of the associated remedies represents the bowel nosode quite closely and is called the Prototype Remedy. Other bowel nosodes are *Morgan gaertner, Proteus, Mutabile, Bacillus No. 7, Gaertner, Dysentery col.,* and *Faecalis.* Bowel nosodes are often employed when a case is not proceeding to cure even though carefully selected remedies or antimiasmatics have been administered.

Treatise on Bowel Nosodes (Y.R. Agarwal), *A Repertory of Bowel Nosodes* (Murray Feldman), *Bowel Nosodes* (J. Paterson), and *Intestinal Nosodes of Bach-Paterson* (O.A. Julian) are just a few resources available on this subject.

Boyd's drug groups/classification a classification of remedies according to their electrophysical properties, by Wm. Ernest Boyd (1891-1955), a British homeopath. Boyd developed 12 groups and felt that specific relationships exist between the individual remedies within the group. He believed that constitutionally a person tends to remain in a particular group for his entire life and that if one remedy in that group doesn't seem to act curatively then another item within that same group will fill that void or complete the cure. Like many, he believed that the remedies emanate resonant energies and developed a diagnostic instrument called the Emanometer. He measured energies from the patient's lachrymal fluid (tears) and maintained that improperly chosen remedies could further imbalance the patient and do harm. He rarely prescribed above the 30C potency. Dr. Boyd died before completing his research.

brachial plexus a network of nerves located in the neck and armpit composed of the lower four cervical and first thoracic nerves.

brachialgia severe pain in the arm or in the neck and armpit areas.

bradycardia a slow heart rate, usually less than 60 beats per minute.

bradyspepsia slow digestion.

Braidism hypnosis. See MESMERISM.

brain fag (brain-tire, cerebral asthenia, encephalasthenia) exhaustion of the mental faculties through overwork of an intellectual character.

Interestingly enough, a paper appeared in *Society, Science and Medicine*, 21:2, p.197-203 (1985) by Raymond Prince entitled 'The Concept of Culture-Bound Syndromes: Anorexia nervosa and Brain-Fog'. Brain fog (f-o-g) was first described in Nigeria in 1982. According to this essay half of all students suffered from a 'painful burning or crawling sensation' in their heads. Perhaps this is somehow related to brain fag?

brain fever inflammation of the brain. See ENCEPHALITIS.

brandy nose (whiskey nose, spider nevus, spider cancer, telangiectasis faciei) see ACNE ROSACEA.

brash (water-brash, pyrosis) acidity of the stomach with belching of sour, burning fluid.

breakbone fever see DENGUE.

breast-pang see ANGINA PECTORIS.

bregma the upper part of the skull/head.

Bright's disease (chronic nephritis, parenchymatous nephritis) a chronic, inflammatory disease of the kidneys.

"A morbid condition of the kidneys; the term is 'generic' and includes several forms of acute and chronic disease of the kidney, usually associated with albumin in the urine, and frequently with Dropsy, and with various secondary symptoms."—Ruddock's *Vade Mecum*, p. 570. "Bright's disease is a generic term embracing the various forms of organic kidney disease of inflammatory origin, with resulting albuminuria and dropsy."—Raue, *Special Pathology*, p. 589. "In the more acute cases the disease hastens, with uniform rapidity, onward towards a fatal termination. If the disease runs a more chronic course, its intensity varies; remissions . . . are observed."—Baehr, *The Science of Therapeutics I,* p. 602.

brimstone sulphur; especially sublimed sulphur remelted and then cast into cones. In the Bible, the stuff of which Hell is made; hence 'fire and brimstone'. "One does not wonder that hell is represented as being heated by this substance [*Sulphur*], for it seems by its pathogenesis as though it were *eternally burning.*"—E.B. Nash, *Leaders in Homoeopathic Therapeutics.*

bromidrosis (osmidrosis, bromhidrosis) secretion of sweat with an unpleasant odor. Hexenoic acid has been isolated as the substance which causes the odor.

brominism a disease or poisoned state caused by the prolonged administration of bromides (bromides were at one time used therapeutically as hypnotic and sleep-inducing agents and as anti-epileptics). It is characterized by headaches, sleepiness, apathy, cold extremities, bad breath, and an acneform eruption. A loss of strength and sexual desire, associated with testicular or breast atrophy, may occur.

bromo-chloralum a mixture of solutions of the bromide and chloride of aluminum, used as a disinfectant.

bromomenorrhea an excessive menstrual flow with a foul odor.

bronchiectasis dilatation of bronchi due to an inflammatory or degenerative process, usually associated with chronic suppuration.

bronchocele goiter, especially cystic goiter.

bronchorrhagia hemoptysis (the spitting or coughing up of blood). Bleeding from the lungs or bronchial tubes.

bronchorrhea excessive secretion from the bronchial mucous membrane.

brow ague (brow ache, brow pang) migraine, supraorbital nerve pain.

brucellosis see MEDITERRANEAN FEVER.

Brunonian school/healing a theory developed by John Brown in the late 18th century stating that life depends on stimulation and lack of it results in death. Thus stimulants (such as laudanum and whiskey) were advocated in the treatment of illness.

Brunner's glands small branched and coiled tubular glands in the submucosa of the first part of the duodenum. They were discovered by the Swiss anatomist J.C. Brunner (1653-1727) who did pioneering research on the pancreas.

bubo an inflammation and swelling, often very tender, of the lymphatic glands (nodes) of the groin or armpit; e.g., venereal bubo. An abscess.

bubonic plague (pest, black death) an acute infectious disease caused by *Yersinia pestis* and marked clinically by high fever, toxemia, prostration, and a petechial eruption. Glandular swellings (lymphatic buboes of the armpits and groin), pneumonia, and hemorrhage from the mucous membranes are also often present. It is primarily a disease of rodents and is transmitted to man by fleas which have bitten infected animals.

The Black Death of 1348 and two later plagues, *pestis secunda* (1362) and *pestis tertia* (1369) killed one quarter of the world's population, some 60 million people. "Europe did not attain its thirteenth-century population levels again until the sixteenth century." Asia and Africa were devastated as well.—A. Nikiforuk, *The Fourth Horseman,* p. 50.

buccal referring to the cheek.

buccula the fatty puffing under the chin; a double chin.

Buerger's disease (Winiwater's disease, Winiwater-Buerger disease) see THROMBOANGITIS OBLITERANS.

buffoonery clowning around. A buffoon is a witless person who makes coarse jokes.

bugantia see CHILBLAIN.

bulbar paralysis a progressive atrophy and paralysis of the muscles of the tongue, lips, palate, pharynx, and larynx, occurring in later life and due to atrophic degeneration of nervous tissue of the medulla oblongata.

bulimia (bulimy) insatiable, ravenous appetite. Excessive, morbid hunger. The contemporary meaning is an insatiable craving for food, with episodes of continuous eating and often followed by self-induced vomiting or purging, depression and then self-deprivation.

bulla (bleb) a large skin blister/vesicle (> 1cm. in diameter) filled with serum. 'Bullae' is the plural.

bung hole the hole on the side of a barrel where the cork is inserted.

bunion a chronic low-grade inflammation of the first joint of the big toe associated with swelling, pain, redness, and a painful thickening of that area.

Burgi's principle a principle of synergism formulated by Emil Burgi of Switzerland in 1910: If two pharmacological agents with similar actions are given in combination, the resultant effect is not merely additive but super-additive (synergistic). For example, *Berberis, Colocynthis* and *Veratrum* more than likely have different mechanisms of action (MOA), even different sites of action, yet are more useful in combination than separately for irritation/inflammation in the urogenital and biliary region. Or *Belladonna* in combination with *Echinacea* proves very efficacious for localized inflammations (boils, carbuncles, etc.), more so than either agent given singly.

Burn's amaurosis postmarital amaurosis. A blindness or impaired vision following sexual excesses.

bursa a saclike bodily cavity (generally filled with fluid), especially one located between joints or at points of friction between moving structures.

bursitis inflammation of a bursa.

byssus lint, cotton.

CcCCCCc

CC   another way of indicating the 200C potency.

cf. to compare (Lat. *confer*, imperative of *conferre*, to compare).

CR an abbreviation for van Zandvoort's *Complete Repertory*, e.g. CR-47 means the symptom may be found on page 47 of the *Complete Repertory*.

cacesthesia any disorder of the senses. A morbid or unusual sensation. Malaise.

cachectic/cachexia a general lack of nutrition and wasting occurring in the course of a chronic disease or emotional disturbance. Weakness and wasting caused by some serious disease. A devitalized constitution; bad habits.

According to C. G. Puhlmann (*Handbook of Homoeopathic Practice*, p.12), "Dyscrasia is known in medicine as the chronic impoverishment in old age of the normal composition of the blood, with the consequent development of alterations in the tissues. By cachexia is meant a long continued general dyscrasia through which the nutrition of the body has already become undermined, so that in the whole outward appearance the condition of the patient is discernible. In the cachectic state, the derangements of nutrition which have set in are generally considered incurable."

cachexia ex nimio usu hydrargyri (cachexia mercurialis) cachexia from the abuse of mercury. See ABUSE OF MERCURY.

cachexia malaria (quinine cachexia, malarial cachexia, chronic malaria) a condition developing after repeated attacks of malaria, yet the patients may have had no distinct paroxysms of chills and fever. They are anemic, emaciated, with sallow complexions. Ankle edema, feeble digestion, enlarged spleen, muscular weakness, and mental depression may also be found.

cacoplastic relating to or causing morbid or abnormal growth.

caduca (decidua, tunica decidua, membrana decidua) the mucous membrane of the uterus, especially that part specially modified in preparation for pregnancy and which is first cast off during parturition.

caecal (cecal) referring to the region of the right side of the large intestine. The area where the small intestine meets the large intestine.

caecum (cecum, typhlon, blind gut) the cul-de-sac, about 2 ½ inches in depth, lying below the ileocecal valve, forming the first part of the large intestine.

calcaneus the heel bone.

calcar a spur or spur-like process.

calcareous having the nature of chalk or lime. Referring to deposits of calcium in a part.

calculi stones. The plural of 'calculus', as in urinary calculi/us.

callosity (callus) an area of thickened skin caused by irritation, friction or pressure. Also new growth of incompletely solidified bony tissue surrounding the bone ends in fractures; a part of the reparative process.

calmant a sedative.

calomel (hydrargyrus) mild mercuric chloride used as a laxative. Mercurius dulcis is dulcified mercury; 'dulcify' means 'to sweeten' which is exactly what happens during the preparation of calomel. The bitterness of mercurous sulfate is removed when sodium chloride is added, and the 'sweeter' mercurous chloride produced.

Though not used today, calomel certainly had a long reign as 'king-laxative', having been discovered by Sir Theodore Turquet de Mayerne in the early 17th century. Around the turn of the 20th century it was used in approximately 2 grain (130 mg) doses to produce bowel movements, which were often of a green color. This promulgated the belief that calomel stimulated bile secretion. This is not the case, but rather it indicates the failure of biliverdin (a green bile salt) to be converted to bilirubin. This conversion is inhibited by mercury. The mercury content in calomel inhibits the absorption of water by the intestine, thus causing diarrhea or loose stools. Calomel has some action as a diuretic but is no longer used for that purpose either. Calomel ointment was used as a prophylactic to prevent syphilitic infection. Members of the armed forces (WWI and II) received 'pro' kits which contained calomel ointment. They were instructed to use such ointment after coitus as a local antibacterial agent.

calor heat. One of the four classical signs of inflammation, as assigned by Celsius (*calor, rubor, tumor,* and *dolor,* or heat, redness, swelling and pain, respectively).

calor mordax a biting or caustic heat. 'Mordacious' means biting or caustic.

calumniate to slander or falsely accuse.

calvarium the uppermost portion of the skull above the eyes and ears. The top of the skull.

camp diarrhea a diarrhea of soldiers in their encampments. "Camp diarrhea of the European and American soldiers—the result of continued heat on the one hand, of bad diet, exposure and foetid exhalations on the other."—R. Hughes, *Principles and Practice of Homeopathy,* p. 495,6. A "chronic diarrhea contracted in Southern camps."—H.C. Allen, *Materia Medica of Nosodes, p. 175.*

camp fever (typhus fever) see TYPHUS.

cancer 1) a disease characterized by malignant growths (neoplasms) which invade and destroy other tissues and have a tendency to spread, ultimately ending in death. 2) A pernicious and proliferative evil.

cancrum gangrenous ulceration; a rapidly progressive ulcer. 'Cancrum oris' is canker sores or ulceration of the mouth. See NOMA.

canine hunger ravenous hunger.

canities greyness of the hair.

canker sore a small, painful, soft ulcerous lesion of the mucous membrane of the mouth. These occur inside the mouth, as opposed to cold sores which occur outside the mouth (lips or near lips). Canker sores are not contagious and are usually caused by streptococcus bacteria.

cannonade sounds as if from cannons or artillery.

cannula a tube inserted into a bodily cavity to drain fluid or insert medication.

canthus (pl. canthi) The corner at either side of the eye, formed by the meeting of the upper and lower eyelids. The palpebral angle.

capricious fickle or impulsive. Characterized by or subject to whim; unpredictable.

caput gallinaginis (snipe's head, colliculus seminalis, verumontanum) 'woodcock's head' (Latin). The longitudinal fold of the lining membrane in the prostatic portion of the urethra. An acute inflammation of this fold is most commonly induced by an extension of gonorrheal inflammation.

carbo-nitrogenoid one of the three constitutions of Edward von Grauvogl (1811-1877). It is characterized by an excess of carbon and nitrogen in the system, caused by an insufficient oxygenation of the blood. It corresponds to the psoric miasm of Hahnemann. The two other Grauvogl constitutions are HYDROGENOID (sycotic) and OXYGENOID (syphilitic).

carbuncle (furunculus malignans, whelk) a large and usually deep infection, more extensive and serious than an abscess. Since it is a more severe infection, systemic effects may be present such as malaise, fever, and depression. Cf. ANTHRAX.

carcinoma ventriculi cancer of a ventricle (a small belly-shaped cavity).

cardiac asthma asthma that occurs when the left heart is weak or fails, causing blood to dam up or congest the lungs. It usually comes on at night and wheezing is the primary symptom.

cardiac dropsy edema caused by diminished heart functioning.

cardiac dyspnea difficult or labored breathing due to cardiac failure.

cardiac uremia uremia (a toxic condition of the blood from an accumulation of urea) as a result of poor or compromised heart action.

cardiagra gout affecting the heart.

cardialgia heartburn; pain in the region of the stomach or a non-specific term for heart pain. A gnawing pain in the stomach. This pain may extend to the back, cause faintness, nausea and vomiting, cold extremities, and anxiety. It is usually due to eating foods which disagree.

cardiogmus disease of the heart.

cardiopalmus heart palpitations.

carditis inflammation of the heart.

careworn showing the effect of grief and anxiety, and thus 'worn' out.

caries usually refers to decay of bone. An ulcerous inflammation of bone, whereby bone becomes fragile, thinned, and breaks down with the formation of pus. Years ago it was often associated with tuberculosis. May also refer to tooth decay, i.e., dental caries.

carminative an agent which relieves flatulence (gas). Preventing the formation or causing the expulsion of flatus.

carotid referring to the heart or associated with the heart, e.g. carotid arteries (those vessels running from the heart to the head along the lateral sides of the neck).

carphologia (floccillation) an aimless, semiconscious picking or plucking at the bed clothes, as if one were picking off threads or pieces of lint. Often occurs in the delirium of a fever or stuporous condition. Reaching out or grasping with hands.

carphopedal referring to the wrists and feet, or the fingers and toes.

carriage sickness the seasick feeling caused by riding in a carriage (horse-drawn or motor powered).

carrion dead and decaying flesh.

carriwitchet conundrum, pun or tricky question. A piece of jocularity or facetiousness.

caruncle (caruncula) a small fleshy mass or growth usually occurring at the meatus of the female urethra (caruncula myrtiformes). Or caruncula lachrymales, the small fleshy bodies found in the inner angle of the eye.

caseation a form of tissue death (necrosis) whereby there is loss of cellular outline and the tissue resembles crumbled cheese/cottage cheese. Cheese-like necrosis.

caseous cheese-like.

castile soap a hard, white odorless and gentle soap made with olive oil. It can also be found as a liquid as in castile shampoo.

casts plastic looking, often cylindrical coagulated proteins found in urine. There are many types (blood c., fatty c., pus c., renal c., waxy c., granular c.) which can be indicative of various urinary tract diseases.

catabolism destructive metabolism; the breakdown of living matter into simpler chemical compounds. Cf. ANABOLISM.

catalepsy a lack of responsiveness or awareness of the environment. A trance-like state with rigidity of the limbs. The limbs can be placed in various positions and stay there for quite some time. Catatonia. A sustained immobility.

catamenia menstruation. The menstrual period.

cataplasm a poultice. A soft magma or mush prepared by wetting various powders or other absorbent substances with oily or watery fluids, sometimes medicated, and usually applied hot to the surface. It exerts an emollient, relaxing, or stimulant counter-irritant effect upon the skin and underlying tissues.

catarrh an increased mucus discharge from mucous membranes which have been inflamed by any variety of irritants. An increased secretion of mucus from the membranes of the nose, fauces, and bronchia with fever and attended sneezing, cough, thirst, lassitude and want of appetite. Two types: *catarrhus a frigore* (cold in the head), and *catarrhus a contagione* (the flu).

catarrhal increasing the flow of mucus.

catarrhal fever an archaic term for the common cold.

cathartic laxative. An agent which causes a bowel movement.

catheter fever (urinary fever) a sharp elevation of bodily temperature sometimes following the introduction of a catheter into the urethra.

causa morbi morbid cause; cause of disease or death.

causalgia (RSDS, Sympathetic Reflex Dystrophy Syndrome, Sudeck's atrophy) the burning pain which sometimes accompanies injuries of the nerves, especially those nerves supplying the palms and soles of the feet. It may also affect the knee, shoulder, and hip. With time, weakness and wasting of the tissues in the affected areas develops.

causal chains a term coined by acupuncturist and bio-energetic physician Helmut W. Schimmel to help describe the meaning of disease symptoms. "Symptoms do not exist in isolation, but are part of a constellation of causes and effects usually triggered by a maximally disturbed organ." This thought is shared by practitioners of TCM (Traditional Chinese Medicine).

causal therapy therapy directed against the cause of disease (e.g. using antibiotics to kill pathogenic bacteria).

causam tolle 'remove the cause' (Latin. One of the three methods of cure outlined by Hahnemann, and the one he called 'the most sublime'. The other two were based on the Law of Contraries (allopathy) and the Law of Similars (homeopathy) .

caustic burning, corroding, or dissolving. Biting or cutting ('caustic wit').

cauterize to burn, sear or seal flesh in order to stop blood flow or destroy a growth such as a wart or tumor, using either heat, extreme cold, or a caustic agent.

cautery destruction of tissue by the application of a cauterizing agent.

caveat emptor 'let the buyer beware' (Latin). *Caveat vendor* means 'let the seller beware' and first applied to physicians, as mentioned in the Code of Hammurabi (2250 B.C.). This code protected patients by setting fees and establishing punishment for physicians who harmed their patients.

cecitis (typhlitis) appendicitis. Inflammation of the CAECUM *(vide)*.

celialgia colic, abdominal pain.

cell salts, celloids see SCHUESSLER.

cellular pathology the theory (as opposed to the humoral theory of pathology), first formulated by Virchow in 1858, that the cause of disease is the result of damage or improper functioning of individual cells or tissues (*omnis cellula a cellula,* 'everything cell by cell'). See MOLECULAR PATHOLOGY.

cellulitis a diseased condition with inflammation of cellular or connective tissue.

celonychia see SPOON-NAIL.

cenestopathy a derangement or inability of the individual to sense bodily stimuli in a normal fashion. 'Cenesthesia' refers to one's sense of existence as derived from all the various stimuli and reactions throughout the body at any specific moment to produce or register a feeling of health or illness.

censorious critical.

centesimal (1 to 100 dilution ratio) the most widely-known and used potency scale, the one originally developed by Hahnemann. See POTENCY.

centrifugal moving away from the center. Moving outward.

centripetal moving towards the center. Moving inward.

cephalalgia (cephalea) pain in the head.

cephalagra gout affecting the head.

cephalea (cephalalgia) head pain.

cephalhematoma a bloody cyst or tumor of the scalp in a newborn infant.

cerebrospinal fever meningitis.

cerebro-spinalis referring to the head and spine area. More specifically perhaps to the occiput (the back of the head) and spinal muscles which run on either side of the spinal cord from the occiput to the sacrum (tail-bone area).

cerous wax-like.

cerumen earwax.

cervical referring to the neck.

cervix the neck, particularly the back part. More commonly means any neck-like structure, especially the lower cylindrical portion of the uterus (the neck of the womb).

cessat effectus cessat causa 'when the effect stops, the cause stops' (Latin).

cessatio mensium discontinuance of the menstrual flux/flow.

ceteris paribus 'all else being equal' (Latin).

Chagres fever a malignant form of malarial fever, named after Panama's Chagres River.

chagrin a feeling of embarrassment or humiliation caused by failure or disappointment.

chalazion a stye. A tumor, cyst or lump on the border of the eyelid due to inflammation of the Meibomian gland.

chalazoe (Meibomian cyst) a tumor of the eyelid from the blocked secretion of the Meibomian gland.

chalybeate relating to or containing iron. A therapeutic agent containing iron.

chancre the lesion, usually an ulcer, formed at the site of primary inoculation or infection. Generally refers to the initial lesion of syphilis.

chaos an imperceptible state of order.

characteristic symptom see entry under SYMPTOM.

charbon a malignant pustule. See ANTHRAX.

charpie lint, scraped linen.

Charcot's disease see AMYOTROPHIC LATERAL SCLEROSIS.

chasma (pandiculation) yawning.

cheilocace (lip evil) an induration or swelling of the lower lip. See CHEILOSIS.

cheilosis symptoms of riboflavin deficiency, in which the corners of the lips turn pale, followed by a softening and breakdown of the lips. Fissures may develop, becoming deep and extending into the cheek.

cheiritis inflammation of the hand.

chelate (in the non-scientific sense) to grasp or hold firmly.

cheloid (keloid) a raised, irregularly shaped scar.

chemosis edema of the conjunctiva, forming a bulging around the cornea.

Cheyne-Stokes respiration an irregular, intermittent breathing. A pattern of heavy breathing followed by apnea (lack of or very shallow breathing) lasting 10-60 seconds followed by increased respirations. The respiration rate returns to normal for a varying brief period of time before the cycle recommences. It is often seen in patients with cerebral arteriosclerosis, senility, brain damage, chronic hypoxia, and heart disease, especially left heart failure and severe congestive heart failure (CHF).

After the Scottish physician John Cheyne (1777-1836) and Irish physician Wm. Stokes (1804-1878). Dr. Cheyne (pronounced 'Cheen'), one of the founders of the 'Dublin school', first described this type of respiration in 1818, but did not attach any great importance to it. Stokes, a contemporary of R.J. Graves (the discoverer of Grave's disease), showed the diagnostic significance of this breathing pattern.

chiasma a crosswise intersection of nerve trunks, as of optic nerve fibers at the base of the brain.

chickenpox (variola spuria) see VARICELLA.

chilblains (pernio) redness of the hands and feet, with burning and itching, sometimes with chapping and ulceration, caused by damp cold. An inflammation of the extremities from the application of cold, attended by violent itching and, if prolonged, the formation of a gangrenous ulcer. In order to conserve heat the blood vessels of the affected part constrict. However, the body over-reacts by over constricting, which produces the symptoms of redness, inflammation, throbbing, pain, etc. This excessive reaction of the body can be expressed in three degrees, much the same way burns are categorized: first degree, red skin in patches, and slightly swollen; second degree, vesicles appear with the adjacent skin being blue/purple; this may further degenerate into the third degree, formation of superficial ulcers. Chilblains differs from frostbite, in which severe cold (at least 10 degrees below freezing) quick-freezes the part, producing numbness and stiffness. The part is pale with a bluish tint and the circulation is severely restricted. If very severe, gangrene and tissue death occur from frostbite.

child-bed fever see PUERPERAL FEVER.

chimney sweeper's cancer cancer of the scrotum of chimney sweeps, supposedly due to continual contact with soot.

chiragra gout in the hand.

chiropractic a method of treating disease, invented in 1895 by D.D. Palmer (1845-1913), which relies on manipulations of the spine and other joints of the body. The term 'chiropractic' was suggested to Dr. Palmer by a clergyman, Rev. Samuel Seed.

Chiropractors (D.C.s) believe, in contrast with the osteopathic theories, that when subluxations or misalignments of the joints and/or spinal vertebrae are corrected, nerve functioning is improved and thus overall health improves. For a good historical treatment read J. Stuart Moore's *Chiropractic In America* (1993). See OSTEOPATHY.

chlamydia a generic term referring to the bacterial genus *Chlamydia,* a genus of microorganisms (rickettsiae) which cause a wide variety of disease in man and animals, e.g., trachoma, proctitis, inclusion conjunctivitis, nonspecific urethritis, ornithosis, and a venereal disease called lymphogranuloma venereum. There are two species, *C. trachomatis* and *C. psittaci.* Usually 'chlamydia' refers to the infectious venereal disease, which evolves in the following way: 7-12 days after contact with a chlamydia carrier a herpes-like vesicle appears on the genitals. It ruptures and heals with no pain. Then after 1-8 weeks the regional lymph nodes become inflamed, tender and suppurative. These inflamed lymph nodes or buboes gradually heal, leaving scars which obstruct lymphatic flow. Allopathic treatment consists of tetracycline administration.

chloasma (liver spots, moth patches, melasma, melanoderma) deposit of pigment in the skin, occurring in patches of various sizes and shapes and of a yellow, brown, or black color. In the repertory see 'discoloration, spots'.

chloro-anemia see CHLOROSIS.

chloroform an organic solvent used medicinally at one time as an anesthetic, anodyne, and antispasmodic. In the 1800s it was administered chiefly by inhalation as a general anesthetic and is more potent and more rapid acting than ether, as well as more dangerous. Internally it was used as a carminative and anodyne. It is no longer used internally or as an anesthetic because of its severe liver toxicity. Topically it is still used in liniments for its counter-irritant effects.

chloroformism the state produced when toxic doses of chloroform are ingested. Prostration, protracted nausea and vomiting, jaundice, and coma are produced. Hypotension, cardiac arrest, and arrhythmias are common. Chloroform came into vogue in the mid-1800s and was no doubt abused by pleasure seekers, causing many needless deaths due to autointoxication.

chlorosis (green sickness, morbus virgineus, emansio mensium) a form of anemia most commonly seen in young women, marked by a greenish pale color of the skin and menstrual disturbances. One source says that chlorosis can occur after a young woman's first menses but menses fail to occur for several months after. It is characterized by a reduction of hemoglobin in the blood, out of proportion to the diminution of red blood cells. A disease which affects young women, characterized by depraved appetite, headaches, anemia, disturbed sleep, nervousness, bad digestion, livid paleness, great debility, painful menses or suppression of the menses. The tongue may become white.

chlorotic relating to CHLOROSIS *(vide).*

choanae posterior nares; the rear opening of the nose into the nasopharynx.

cholagogue stimulating the flow or secretion of bile.

cholangitis (angiocholitis) inflammation of the bile duct.

cholecystitis inflammation of the gallbladder.

cholelithiasis (gallstone, biliary calculus) a condition in which concretions (stones, hardened deposits) are present in the gall bladder or bile duct.

cholera (c. indica, epidemic c., virulent c., c. vera, classic c., asiatic c.) an acute infection caused by *Vibrio cholerae* (isolated by Koch in 1883), a short, aerobic rod bacteria. It involves the entire bowel, producing profuse, painless watery diarrhea, vomiting, muscular cramps, dehydration, oliguria, acidosis, and collapse.

This form of enteritis is prevalent or endemic in India and southeast Asia, with outbreaks occurring in other regions of the world. The bacteria produce an enterotoxin which is responsible for the tremendous purging of bodily fluids. Cholera is spread by feces-contaminated food and water. In the literature of the early to mid 1800s the term 'cholera' was used as a nonspecific term for a variety of gastrointestinal disturbances.

"In all that has preceded it will be understood that I have been speaking of true Cholera, i.e., where in addition to rice-water vomiting and purging, cramps, and suppression of urine, there is some amount of algidity and cyanosis."— R. Hughes, *Principles and Practice of Homeopathy,* p.

267. "Where the cholera first appears, it usually comes on in the commencement in its first stage ... the face bluish and icy cold, as also the hands, with coldness of the rest of the body."—R.E. Dudgeon, ed., *The Lesser Writings of Samuel Hahnemann*, p. 773.

cholera infantum (infantile cholera, acute milk infection, summer complaint) an acute intestinal poisoning of bacterial origin in infants and young children. It starts with severe vomiting and diarrhea, and may be followed by fever, shock and collapse. C. infantum and c. morbus may be one and the same because their symptomatology is much the same. The disease is related to cholera only in similarity of symptoms. *Vibrio* are not found. It is possible that this milder form is caused by *Escherichia coli.*

cholera mitis mild cholera. See CHOLERA INFANTUM.

cholera morbus (summer cholera, cholera nostras, cholera europea, summer complaint) acute gastroenteritis characterized by diarrhea and vomiting usually occurring in the summer. Nearly all references consider c. infantum and c. morbus to have the same symptoms and thus to be virtually the same disease, with the only difference being in name: c. infantum is used when referring to infants and young children.

cholera nostras same as cholera infantum and cholera morbus, or cholerine.

cholera sicca 'dry cholera', cholera without the diarrhea. Upon autopsy the bowel is often found filled with rice water material. "The most dangerous of all forms of the disease. The full incidence of the disease is on the internal vital organs, with no relief either in vomiting or purging, which do not appear at all. There are merely great anxiety and terrific pain in the chest; the patients are speechless, suffocated, and gasping for breath. Death follows in two or three hours unless relief is obtained."—J.H. Clarke, *Cholera, Diarrhea and Dysentery*, p. 37.

choleraic/choleric quick-tempered, bilious, ill tempered, easily angered, touchy. Also, pertaining to the highly infectious and acute bacterial disease cholera, whose characteristic symptoms include stomach pains, vomiting, acute diarrhea which could be so severe as to cause death because of the sudden loss of fluids and cramping.

cholerine (English c., bilious cholera, choleraic diarrhea, sporadic cholera) a mild form of cholera common during epidemics of Asiatic cholera, but it is not determined whether it is simple cholera morbus, or the true epidemic disease in mild form.

cholesterolaemia elevated cholesterol levels in the blood.

cholelithiasis gall stones present in the gall bladder or bile-duct.

chololith gallstone, biliary calculus.

choluria bile in the urine.

chondralgia pain in the cartilage.

chondroma a benign bone tumor located within the marrow cavity.

chorda a collection of fibers which form a cord.

chordapsus constriction or twisting of the intestines. Acute intestinal catarrh.

chordee a painful downward curved erection of the penis usually caused by gonorrheal inflammation of the corpus spongiosum.

chorea (Sydenham's chorea, St. Vitus's dance, choromania, dancing chorea, chorea Sti. Viti, morbus saltatorius, chorea minor) a disorder, usually of childhood, characterized by irregular, spasmodic, involuntary movements of the limbs or facial muscles; when used without qualification the term usually refers to Sydenham's c. or St. Vitus's dance.

Chorea was first described in the Middle Ages, but Sydenham first accurately described it in 1686 and the first book published on the subject was written by E.M. Bouteille in 1810, *Traite de la Choree, ou Danse de Saint-Guy.*

choreic relating to chorea. See CHOREA.

choroiditis inflammation of the choroid coat of the eye (the sheath surrounding the eye carrying the blood supply, via a capillary network, to the eyeball).

chromatopsia see CHROMOPSIA.

chromidrosis the secretion of colored sweat.

chromophytosis see TINEA VERSICOLOR.

chromopsia (chromatopsia) colored vision. A condition in which all objects appear abnormally colored.

chronic remedy a homeopathic remedy especially indicated and useful in chronic, long seated diseases, e.g., *Sulphur* in Psoriasis, *Arsenicum* in diabetes. However, 'chronic remedy' may be a misnomer and wrongly influence one's thinking in regards to choosing the correct remedy. To be sure, so-called acute remedies can be the simillimum in chronic conditions and visa versa.

"It is a *fundamental rule* in the treatment of chronic diseases: *to let the action of the remedy, selected in a mode homoeopathically appropriate to the case of disease which has been carefully investigated as to its symptoms, come to an undisturbed conclusion, so long as it visibly advances the cure and while improvement still perceptibly progresses.* This method forbids any new prescription, any interruption by another medicine as well as the immediate repetition of the same remedy." *and* "The cure of great chronic diseases of ten, twenty, thirty, and more years' standing may be said to be quickly annihilated, if this is done in one or two years. Only an ordinary ignorant practitioner can lightly promise to cure severe inveterate disease in four to six weeks."—S.C.F. Hahnemann, *Chronic Diseases.*

"Only chronic diseases can be complicated with each other. The acute is never complicated with the chronic; the acute suppresses the chronic and they never become complex."—J.T. Kent, *Lectures on Homoeopathic*

Philosophy.

chyle a milk-white emulsion of fat globules in lymph formed in the small intestine during digestion. This chyle is absorbed via the lacteals (lymphatic vessels) which carry the chyle away and into the general circulation ultimately to be utilized by the body for energy.

chyluria the presence of lymph (chyle) fluids in the urine.

chyme the partly digested food mass created by emulsification in the stomach and passed in semiliquid form to the small intestine.

chymification the first stage of food digestion occurring in the stomach.

cicatrice (cicatrix) scar; the fibrous tissue replacing the normal tissues destroyed by injury or disease.

cicatrization the process of forming a scar.

ciliary 'hairlike', referring to the eyelash (e.g., the ciliary muscle is the eyelash muscle).

ciliary neuralgia nerve pain in the eyelash area.

cinchona (Peruvian bark) the dried bark of any of the trees of the genus Cinchona. It was the first medicine proved by Hahnemann. As a homeopathic remedy, it is better known as *China*. Cinchona is named for the countess who introduced it into Europe in the 17th century.

cinchonism the systemic effect of cinchona (Peruvian bark, which contains quinine) when given in large doses; symptoms produced are tinnitus, deafness, headache, giddiness, dimness of sight and a weakened heart action.

cinesia (kinetosis) the symptom-complex caused by unwanted motion, i.e., vertigo, nausea, vomiting and prostration. Sea-sickness, car-sickness, swing-sickness, etc.

cinnabar (HgS, red mercuric sulfide, cinnabarite, native vermilion, Chinese vermilion) the basic ore from which mercury is obtained, usually by sublimation. Heated to 835⁰F, cinnabar sublimes. Oxygen combines with the sulfur vapor passing off as sulfur dioxide, leaving the pure mercury behind. Cinnabar is also called red sulphide of mercury, because mercury and sulfur are found in combination. Cinnabar is formed when black mercuric sulfide is heated. Most deposits of cinnabar are red or brown granular masses found near hot springs and volcanos.

cipher (cypher) The figure zero, or any figure. Also, a message in code, or a secret system in which letters are arbitrarily substituted according to a predetermined key. 'To decipher' would mean 'to solve the message by figuring out the predetermined key'.

circinatus having a well-defined round edge (referring to ringworm).

circle group "a unique method of organizing one's thoughts in order to develop accurate leads for rubric choices based on the patient's story. It is a simple, non-linear system of recording ideas for clarity and reference. As the patient tells his/her story, the practitioner writes down and circles each of their expressions that refer to their experience. Then lines are drawn between the circles, linking them into groups and sequences relating to their reported or observed intensity, clarity and peculiarity. At the center of the cluster are the symptoms which the case pivots or rests upon— moving outward from particular to general. Arranging the case in such a way gives the practitioner a visual image of the patient's spoken record that can be organized and changed into varying orders of interest."—Greg Bedayn, RSHom (NA). These thoughts are not unique to homeopathy. Consult *Writing the Natural Way* (G. Lusser Rico) and *Use Both Sides of the Brain* (T. Buzan).

circumcision the removal of the foreskin of the penis; excision of a circular piece of the prepuce.

circumduction the continuous circular movement of a limb.

circumspection prudent, carefully considering all circumstances and consequences.

cirrhosis (hob-nailed liver, granulated liver, hepar adiposum) a chronic disease of the liver marked by progressive destruction and regeneration of liver cells and increased connective tissue formation, ultimately resulting in blockage of portal circulation, portal hypertension, liver failure, and death.

cirsocele see VARIOCELE.

cirsophthalmia dilatation of the conjunctival blood-vessels.

cito, tuto et jucunde 'quickly, safely, and pleasantly' (Latin).

CK centesimal Korsakovian. See POTENCY.

clairaudient able to hear that which is not discernible by ordinary means; a type of ESP (extrasensory perception).

clairvoyance the supposed ability to perceive things that are out of the natural range of human senses. ESP.

clap gonorrhea.

classic fever see TYPHUS.

claudicatio intermittens (intermittent claudication) cramp-like pains and weakness in the legs (especially calves) induced by walking and relieved by rest; associated with excessive smoking, vascular spasms and arteriosclerosis.

claudicatio spontanea a sudden or spontaneous limping or lameness.

claustrophobia a morbid fear of being in a small, enclosed or confined place.

clavicle collar bone

clavus (clavus pedis; pl. clavi pedis) corn, a small conical callosity caused by pressure over a bony prominence, usually on a toe.

clavus hystericus sensation as if a nail is being driven into the head.

cleptomania see KLEPTOMANIA.

clergyman's sore throat (angina granulosa, granular pharyngitis) inflammation of the mucous membrane and underlying parts of the pharynx whereby the lymph follicles are enlarged, studding the surface and forming minute nodules or granules.

climacteric (climaxis, menopause) a period of life at which the body undergoes marked changes, specifically as it relates to women. Some older references equate it with the 63rd year. "The premenopausal period which culminates in the stoppage of menses." —T. P. Chatterjee, *Highlights of Homeopathic Practice.*

clinker a hard, dried mass of mucus in the nasal cavity.

clonic marked by alternate contraction and relaxation of a muscle, as in a clonic spasm.

club foot see TALIPES.

clubbed fingers (clubbed digits, Hippocratic digits) fingers with knob-like terminations, often indicative of heart disease or tuberculosis.

clyers see ACTINOMYCOSIS.

clyster (enema) an injection into the bowels for promoting an evacuation and relieving constipation.

coal oil kerosene.

coaptation the joining together of two surfaces, e.g., the ends of a bone fracture or edges of a wound.

coccygodinia neuralgic or rheumatic pain in the coccyx region.

coccyx the 'tail bone'.

coction digestion or the process of digestion.

codex a code of laws or statutes. For example, Jahr's *Symptom Codex* is an authoritative compendium of symptoms and associated remedies.

coelialgia stomach pains.

coition coitus; sexual intercourse.

coitus copulation, coition, sexual union/intercourse.

cold sore (fever blister) a small, painful, hard or crusty ulcer which often breaks open and oozes, caused by Herpes simplex virus Type I and occurring outside the mouth on the lips or nearby tissue. Cold sores are contagious (*cf.* CANKER SORE), spreading via saliva and skin contact.

coleocele (colpocele, elytrocele) a hernia or any tumor which projects into the vagina.

Coley's toxins a mixture of *Streptococcus pyogenes* and *Serratia marcescens* which, when injected into a patient ill with cancer, causes a high fever and mobilizes the patient's immune system to fight the cancer cells.

Wm. B. Coley was a bone surgeon who lived at the turn of the twentieth century. He was an early pioneer of immunotherapy. Coley's toxins are no longer available for use in the United States.

colic (gripe) acute paroxysmal pain in the abdomen, usually resulting from gas, spasms, or obstructions in the digestive system. Commonly refers to abdominal pain in infants. However, this term could be used to describe effects on other viscera, i.e., renal colic.

colica pictorum see PAINTER'S COLIC.

colica plumbae (lead colic) colic caused by ingestion of high amounts of lead.

colicodynia pain in the large intestine.

colitis inflammation of the colon.

colliquative progressively wasting or melting away the body, generally by excretion of liquids (as a c. diarrhea or a c. sweat). Characterized by excess discharge of any secretion.

colliquitine to reduce, to melt away or to melt together.

collodium, collodion a liquid prepared from gun-cotton (pyroxylin), ether, and alcohol. When applied to wounds it evaporates and leaves a glossy contractile film protecting the area. It may also be used as a vehicle for the local application of medicinal substances. Pyroxylin or gun-cotton is obtained by the action of nitric and sulphuric acids on cotton.

colloma a cyst containing colloidal matter.

collous gluey.

collum the neck. The constricted or neck-like portion of any organ or structure.

collyrium an eyewash. A medicinal lotion for the eyes.

collutorium a mouth-wash or gargle.

colonic 1) relating to the colon. 2) a procedure designed to cleanse the colon (lower bowel, large intestine). It involves the insertion of a tube into the rectum and the introduction of water to loosen and remove waste and putrefying fecal material. The water is then allowed to flow out, and fresh water instilled again. This process is repeated over and over to cleanse the colon. Generally a series of colonics carried out with regularity is necessary to cleanse the colon.

colostrum the first milk from the mother's breasts after the birth of the child. It is laxative, and assists in the expulsion of the meconium. It contains greater quantities of lactalbumin and lactoprotein than later milk, and also the friendly flora necessary for the baby's digestive and immune systems.

colpitis (erosio portionis, fluor albus) inflammation of the vaginal mucous membranes.

coma an abnormally deep sleep; stupor; drowsiness. A state of profound unconsciousness from which one cannot be aroused.

coma vigil a state of muttering delirium in which the person is lethargic and partly conscious, yet never actually sleeping or completely comatose. Delirious lethargy with open eyes.

combination remedies (complex remedies) 1) homeopathic products containing more than one remedy. In the 1800s the term 'poly-pharmacy' was used to mean the practice of giving many remedies at the same time. 2) The combination of two remedies into one, the new substance exhibiting properties of both constituents. For example, *Ars.* is restless and *Iodine* is restless therefore *Ars. iod.* has extreme restlessness. *Mag.* is not refreshed after sleeping, but *Phos.* is, therefore *Mag. phos.* is no better or worse by sleep. And yet there is nothing about *Calc.* or *Phos.* which would allow one to imagine that *Calc. phos.* would crave smoked foods. Two elements in combination may yield predictable symptoms as well as unique, unpredictable ones.

Though different, see SYNTHETIC REMEDIES.

combustiones burns or scalds.

comedo (pl. comedones) a blackhead; a collection of sebaceous (oily) material and dead cells retained in the hair follicle and excretory duct of the sebaceous gland, the surface covered with a dark crust. It is the primary lesion of acne vulgaris.

commissure the point of union of the lips, eyelids, or labia majora.

common symptoms see entry under SYMPTOMS.

commotio cerebri concussion of the brain/head either by a blow or violent shaking. Symptoms are nausea and vertigo followed by coma with slow respiration and a weak pulse. Acute cerebral concussion. ('Commotio': a concussion or shock).

compatible remedies remedies which follow each other well, acting better if given in a series. They are not of the same family and are dissimilar, e.g., *Lyco.-Sulphur-Calc. c.* in chronic cases; *Bell.* and *Merc.*, *Puls.* and *Sepia* follow each other well.

complementary remedies (concordant remedy) a remedy which assists or reinforces another remedy in its actions. For example, *Sulphur* and *Nux vomica* are complements because if *Nux* is given and seems to help the case but not in a complete way, the practitioner may choose *Sulphur* in order to finish what *Nux* started. Or work begun by *Apis* is finished by *Nat. mur.; Aconite* is best followed with *Sulphur,* with the second remedy in each case being a deeper-working, more chronic version of the first.

complementary medicine (alternative medicine) according to a definition adopted by the British Medical Association, "those forms of treatment which are not widely used by the orthodox health care professions and the skills of which are not taught as part of the undergraduate curriculum of orthodox medical and paramedical health care courses." Another definition might be: Complementary medicine encompasses all health systems/modalities/practices which are not a part of the dominant health care system of the society or culture. "Complementary and alternative medicine is defined through a social process as those practices that do not form part of the dominant system for managing health and disease."—Office of Alternative Medicine, National Institutes of Health.

complete symptom see entry under SYMPTOMS.

complex disease two or more chronic dissimilar diseases present in the patient at the same time. See DISSIMILAR DISEASE.

complex remedies/homeopathy see COMBINATION REMEDIES.

complicated disease see DISSIMILAR DISEASE.

concha the outer ear.

concomitant existing or occurring concurrently. An accompanying state, circumstance or thing. In describing symptoms, symptoms that occur in conjunction with the chief complaint or illness.

concordant remedy see COMPLEMENTARY REMEDY.

concubitus sexual intercourse.

concussive like a blow or shock, e.g., a 'concussive cough' is a cough which comes on suddenly, like a blow to the body, and shakes the whole body.

condyle a rounded articular surface at the extremity of a bone.

condyloma (pl. condylomata) a wart or wart-like growth or tumor, usually near the anus or pudendum. A typical expression of the sycotic miasm.

condyloma acuminata (HPV, human papillomavirus) venereal warts. Ten percent of sexually active adults have HPV and HSV (herpes simplex virus) and lesions will develop in > 50% of those adults.

confrere a fellow member or associate.

confluent joining or running together, as in certain skin lesions which become merged, forming a patch.

congestio ad caput (cerebral congestion) a congestion of blood in the head.

congestio ad pectus a congestion of blood in the chest.

congestive fever a fever due to an excessive accumulation of blood in a vessel, an organ or area of the body.

conglobata a 'single mass', usually referring to lymph glands/tissues.

conglobate glands an archaic term for the lymphatic glands, or glands resembling them (of a globular form, with no excretory duct, composed of a texture like lymphatic vessels).

conjugal relating to marriage.

conjugal onanismus the act of withdrawing the penis prior to ejaculation during sexual intercourse.

conjunctiva the mucous membrane covering the anterior surface of the eyeball and lining the eyelids.

conjunctival pertaining to the mucous membrane which lines the inner surface of the eyelid and the exposed surface of the eyeball.

conjunctivitis inflammation of the CONJUNCTIVA *(vide)*.

consanguinity pertaining to or descended from a common ancestor. Blood relationship, affinity.

consociatio (consociation) union, association, or connection.

constipation (costiveness) a condition in which bowel movements are absent or infrequent, or the bowels are evacuated only with great difficulty.

constitution 1) the overall mental, emotional and physical makeup of the person, including temperament, appearance and behavior, corresponding to one of the major homeopathic remedy types. 2) The physical makeup of the body, including the mode of performance of its functions, temperament, appearance, behavior characteristics, the activity of its metabolic processes, the manner and degree of its reactions to stimuli, and its power of resistance to the attack of disease-causing organisms. "He has an excellent constitution" would mean the person in question rarely gets sick and if he does get ill he has such a good vitality that he 'throws' the sickness off easily.

Much has been written about constitutions, constitutional medicine and typology in homeopathy. Von Grauvogl in the late 1800s developed his three constitutions: hydrogenoid (corresponding to sycosis) carbonitrogenoid (psora) and oxygenoid (syphilis); later A. Nebel theorized three others: carbonic ($CaCO_3$, psora/sycosis), phosphoric ($CaPO_4$, tubercular) and fluoric (CaF, syphilitic). Still later H. Bernard in his approach emphasized an embryological facet: in the individual if the endodermic layer predominates the person is carbonic; if mesodermic, the person is sulfuric; if ectodermic, the person is phosphoric; and persons who are mixed or dystrophic are fluoric. Thus fundamental and deep-acting remedies effect the person's constitution, improving the person's health in all aspects. *Ammonium carb., Ars. alb., Bryonia, Calc. carb., Calc. fluor., Calc. phos., Chamo., China, Ignatia, Kali c., Lachesis, Lyco., Nat. sulph., Nux v., Phosphorus, Puls., Rhus tox., Sepia, Silicea, Sulphur,* and *Thuja* are examples of constitutional remedies.

Just as with many aspects of life, we study constitutional medicine because we want to know man and disease in a more intimate fashion. For more information you may wish to consult: L. Vannier, M.D., *Typology in Homeopathy*, C.R. Coulter, *Portraits of Homeopathic Medicines*, E.C. Whitmont, *Psyche and Substance: Essays on Homeopathy in the Light of Jungian Psychology*, and J.H. Clarke's *Constitutional Medicine*. See TYPOLOGY, CONSTITUTIONAL REMEDY.

constitutional remedy a remedy of fundamental importance to the health of an individual during his entire lifetime. The constitutional remedy for a person is determined by the homeopath who uncovers certain fundamental truths about the person and then repertorizes that symptomatology or examines that typology in order to uncover the patient's nature or constitution, and the corresponding constitutional remedy.

For example, the *Sulphur* constitution or type is primarily a male falling into one of two personality types, the philosopher or practical idealist. Some of the more notable characteristics of the *Sulphur* type are laziness, anxiety, egotism, an overly critical nature, and slovenliness.

"The philosophical type has great intellectual interest but poor connection with friends and family. He is a truly deep thinker, looking long at profound questions in a detached manner. His intelligence tends to set him apart from others and he becomes egotistical concerning his mind and accomplishments. His greatest desire would be to discover some truth or knowledge which will make him famous. He is ambitious, intellectual, detached. This gives him a cynical and condescending attitude. He may even feel disgust for others. His self-confidence is unshakable." -R. Morrison (*Desktop Guide to Keynotes and Confirmatory Symptoms,* p. 368).

This method of classification has good and bad points. Bad because it can lead to keynote prescribing not based on the simillimum and good because it does allow one to more deeply understand the person. For a partial listing of constitutional types/remedies, see CONSTITUTION.

constringing shrinking.

consumption (phthisis) a generic term for wasting away or atrophy, usually referring to tuberculosis, especially of the lungs or intestine.

contact dermatitis (dermatitis venenata) the general term for inflammatory skin reactions resulting from contact with an allergen or a primary irritant. These reactions comprise the two main types of contact dermatitis: allergic contact dermatitis and irritant contact dermatitis.

contagion 1) transmission of an infectious disease by contact with the sick. The process whereby disease spreads from one person to another, by direct or indirect human contact or by an intermediate agency. "The term 'contagion' is used when disease transmission may or may not involve microbes or definitely does not, such as the dynamic action of a disgusting sight upon one's imagination which results in nausea."—*Organon of the Medical Art* (Brewster-O'Reilly, p. 297). 2) The germ or virus which causes a communicable disease (contagium).

It was Athanasius Kircher (1602-1680) who first explicitly stated the theory of 'contagion by animalculae' as the cause of infectious disease (*Scrutinium Physico-Medicum Contagiosae Luis, quae Pestis dicitur...* , 1658). If not the first, he was probably one of the first to use the microscope to do his investigations: "a countless brood of worms not perceptible to the naked eye, but to be seen in all putrefying matter through the microscope." He could not have seen the plague virus but no doubt described microorganisms.

contemporary homeopathy the use of homeopathic remedies not necessarily in accordance with the classical homeopathic method. This method almost exclusively employs large numbers of remedies in one product in an attempt to carry out cellular detoxification or enhance metabolic and biochemical pathways in the body.

continence a voluntary restraint or temperance in regards to sexual activity.

contorted twisted.

contradictory symptom see entry under SYMPTOMS.

contraria contrariis curentur curing by opposites. See ALLOPATHY.

contre-coup fracture due to a counter-stroke. A fracture or injury in an area which did not receive the blow.

contuse to bruise.

contused wound a bruised wound, generally produced by a blunt object.

contusion a bruise or bruised wound.

convulsions see these particular varieties: CLONIC, TONIC, TETANIC.

cophosis a loss of hearing or deafness.

copiopia a tired condition of the eyes.

copious abundant. Large in quantity or amount.

coprophagia eating of feces.

cor pulmonale (Ayerza's ds., Ayerza-Arrillaga syndrome) dilation and failure of the right side of the heart, secondary to (due to) lung dysfunction. It is a syndrome of chronic cyanosis, dyspnea, erythremia, and sclerosis of the pulmonary artery. It was first described by Corvisart in 1806.

coram publico 'before the public/people' (Latin).

corneitis inflammation of the cornea.

corona crown. Usually refers to the head of the penis (c. glandis).

coronaritis inflammation of the vessels which encircle the heart.

corporeal having a material body or substance. A 'corporealist' is one who denies the reality of spiritual existences. A materialist.

corpulent excessively fat, obese.

corroborant an invigorating remedy. A tonic.

corrosive sublimate *Mercurius corrosivus.* See MERCURY.

corrugator a muscle which draws the skin together causing it to wrinkle.

corybantism a wild delirium with hallucinations.

coryza (common cold, gravedo, rhinitis, nasal catarrh, cold in the head) an acute, mild upper respiratory infection which leads to invasion of the respiratory tract by pathogenic bacteria. It is usually short-lived yet highly contagious. The onset is marked by a chilly sensation followed by sneezing, watering of the eyes, nasal discharge, cough and a mild fever. It may simply refer to an increased discharge of mucus from the nose.

coryza, annual hayfever.

cosmoline (vaseline, petrolatum) a trade name for petroleum jelly as is Vaseline. It is a jelly-like preparation obtained from residues of the petroleum distillation process. It was introduced as an emollient and ointment base by A.W. Miller, M.D. in 1873.

costal referring to the ribs or rib area.

costive congested, constipated. 'Costiveness' is being in a congested state.

counter-irritant an agent producing an irritation of a part of the body to produce a stimulant effect on another, perhaps far removed, diseased part. An agent which causes irritation or a mild inflammation of the skin with the purpose of relieving a deep-seated inflammatory process, a sort of 'like cures like'!

coup-de-soleil (solis ictus) sunstroke.

cowperitis inflammation of the bulbourethral glands (Glands of Cowper), usually gonorrheal in origin.

Cowper's glands (bulbourethral glands, antiprostate) two small glands, situated near the prostate, which provide some of the fluid in the ejaculate. After Wm. Cowper (1666-1709), a London anatomist.

cowpox (vaccina) a contagious disease of cows marked by pustular eruption on the teats and udder and communicable to man. A disease, usually local and limited to the site of inoculation, induced in man by inoculation with the virus of cowpox (vaccination), and conferring immunity against smallpox.

coxagra inflammation of the hip joint. 'Cox' is the hip or haunch.

coxalgia (luxatio spontanea femoris) pain in the hip or hip joint.

coxarthritis arthritis of the hip joint.

coxarthrocace inflammation or disease of the hip joint.

coxarum morbus (coxarius morbus) hip joint disease. Scrofulous disease of the hip.

coxitis inflammation of the hip.

Coxsackie virus a very small, round virus first isolated in Coxsackie, N.Y., which causes inflammation of the muscles and muscular paralysis.

CR an acronym for van Zandvoort's *Complete Repertory*, e.g.., CR-440 would mean that symptom may be found on page 440 of the *Complete Repertory*.

cradle cap eczema of the infant's scalp.

craniotabes (circumscribed craniomalacia) a disease marked by areas of thinning and softening in the bones of the skull, usually of a syphilitic or rachitic origin.

crasis constitution or temperament.

craurosis vulvae atrophy of the skin of the female genitalia.

craving a pronounced longing for something, usually a food; more than just a liking for it.

crepitant making a crackling, grating sound, closely resembling the sound produced by rubbing hair between the fingers close to the ear.

crepitus a crackling or grating sound.

crepuscular hazy or dim. Resembling twilight.

crescendo becoming louder.

cretinism a condition occurring in young children due to a lack of thyroid secretion resulting in retardation of mental and physical development.

cri a chirping, crying, or shouting sound.

cribriform sieve-like; containing many perforations.

cri encephalique (crie cerebrale, encephalitic cry, brain cry) the characteristic crying sound made by infants or children suffering from encephalitis or meningitis, or other intracranial pathology of some severity.

crisis the turning point or height of symptoms of a disease.

crissum movement of the buttocks during intercourse.

critical in crisis, e.g., a disease in a 'critical' stage can go in two directions: either resolve favorably or unfavorably.

Crohn's disease (terminal ileitus, regional ileitis, regional enteritis) intestinal inflammation characterized by patchy, deep ulcers that may cause fistulas, and narrowing and thickening of the bowel by fibrosis. First described by B. Crohn, a New York physician, in 1932.

croup (cynanche trachealis) an inflammation of the trachea usually seen in children. A condition of the larynx characterized by a harsh brassy cough, crowing, and difficult respiration. Any affection of the larynx in children characterized by difficult and noisy respiration and a hoarse cough, sometimes marked anatomically by the formation of a pseudomembrane. Croup can be further broken down into two general divisions, membranous (laryngitis with fibrinous exudation) and spasmodic (see LARYNGISMUS STRIDULUS).

cruels see HERPES ZOSTER.

cruor clotted blood.

crural relating to the leg or thigh; a leg-like structure.

crus the leg, especially the segment between the knee and the ankle.

cruro-genital referring to the upper thigh or leg close to the groin area or genitals.

crusta lactea (favus, milk scab, scald-head, milk crust) seborrhea of the scalp in an infant, similar to cradle cap.

crusta serpiginosa (serpentine scall) a crust which resembles or is indicative of ringworm. A round crust.

crusts (scabs) plates of dried serum, blood, pus or sebum, perhaps mixed with epidermal debris, that form upon the surface of a vesicular, bullous or pustular lesion when it ruptures, e.g., impetigo and infected contact dermatitis.

cryptogamia a division of flowerless plants (never having true stamens and pistils) which propagate themselves via spores; the source of a family of remedies.

cryptorchism see KRYPTORCHISM.

crypt a small sac or follicle. A glandular cavity.

cui bono 'whose good? who benefits?' (Latin) (the concept that the one responsible for an act is most likely to be the one who benefits the most from it).

cupellation the process of assaying, refining, or separating. The purifying of perfect metals by means of an addition of lead.

cupping the process of drawing fluids (primarily blood) from the body by creating a vacuum at a point on the skin. A glass cup (bellshaped and capable of holding approximately 3-4 ounces) is applied to the skin and a vacuum is created within the cup, which in turn draws the fluid out. See BLEEDING.

curare cito, tuto et jucunde 'to cure quickly, safely, and pleasantly' (Latin).

curettage scraping of the interior of a cavity, such as the uterus.

Cushing's syndrome/disease (adrenal cortical hyperfunction) a disorder which results from increased secretion of corticosteroids (cortisol, cortisone) from the adrenal glands. It can have many causes and its characteristics include facial and torso obesity, high blood pressure, osteoporosis, plethora of the face, muscular weakness, menstrual dysfunction, hyperglycemia, psychiatric disturbances, moon face, acne, and virilism in females. From the discoverer, Harvey W. Cushing (1869-1939), who wrote the much acclaimed work *The Life of Sir William Osler*.

cutaneous referring to the skin.

cuticle the epidermis, the skin; specifically, the skin surrounding the fingernail.

cutis anserina (gooseskin, horripilation) gooseflesh, goosebumps.

cutis skin

cyanosis (blue-skin disease, morbus coeruleus) a bluish or purplish discoloration of the skin and mucous membranes due to deficient oxygenation of the blood.

cybernetic the philosophical approach which attempts to explain how complex feedback-dependent systems work. Usually such systems (man, computers) contain feedback mechanisms and controls which in turn effect the system, constantly changing it. Thus, explanations and ways to impact such systems are difficult, requiring many approaches. This applies to medicine in that the clinician must realize that the ill person can be helped by number of different techniques chosen at a variety of appropriate times and in a variety of settings.

cyclothymic (manic depressive) according to the current official definition, a 'chronic mood disturbance of at least two years' duration involving numerous periods of depression and hypomania that are not of sufficient severity to meet the criteria for a depressive or manic episode'.

cyesis pregnancy.

cynanche any inflammatory disease of the throat. 'Cynanche cellularis' would mean a sore throat accompanied by excessive cellular growth (hyperplasia). 'Cynanche' was an archaic term for any acute disease of the throat in which the patient struggles for breath, e.g., c. tonsillaris (quinsy), c. trachealis (croup), c. parotidea (mumps), or c. maligna (as in the putrid sore throat associated with scarlatina).

cypher see CIPHER.

cyphosis see KYPHOSIS.

cyst an abnormal sac containing gas, fluid or semi-solid material.

cystalgia pain in the urinary bladder.

cystitis with chorda inflammation of the bladder which when palpated (felt) feels as though cords are stretched across it.

cystitis strangury; inflammation of the bladder. ('Strangury' actually means a painful urination in drops.)

cystocele prolapse of the bladder into the vagina. Hernia of the bladder.

cystodynia bladder pain.

cystoplegia paralysis of the bladder.

cystopyelitis inflammation of both the urinary bladder and the pelvis of the kidney.

cystospasm spasm of the bladder.

D D D D D D D

DAB unripe coconut milk/juice.

dacryadenitis (dacryoadenitis) inflammation of the lacrimal gland.

dacryocystitis inflammation of the lacrimal sac of the eye.

dacryolithiasis the formation and presence of concretions (calculi, stones) in the lacrymal or nasal duct.

dacrosyrinx (lacrymal fistula) abnormal opening of the tear duct.

dactylitis inflammation of one or more fingers.

daft mad, crazy, foolish or stupid.

dainties snacks, especially sweet snacks such as cakes, pies, ice creams, jams and jellies.

damp houses may not strictly mean damp houses but may simply refer to places which are heavily laden with moisture or humidity. Thus individuals living in such an environment may feel as though their tissues are soaked, dense and heavy, under the pressure of a lot of moisture in the tissues. This state corresponds to the sycotic miasm. Depending upon the degree to which a person has the sycotic miasm their tissues may be waterlogged, they may not have the ability to handle water, or they may be unable to live comfortably in moist, humid places. See SEWER GAS.

dandy fever see DENGUE FEVER.

DD see DIFFERENTIAL DIAGNOSIS.

death-rattle the gurgling of mucus in the throat of a dying individual.

debauch an act of debauchery. Also to corrupt morally, seduce, pervert.

debauchery extreme indulgence in sensual pleasures; intemperance.

debile low, feeble, weak

debility feebleness, fragility, the state of abnormal bodily weakness.

decalvant removing the hair, making bald.

decidua the mucous membrane of the pregnant uterus which forms an envelope for the fetus.

decillionth (X^0) the 30th centesimal level of dilution.

decimal (1 to 10 ratio, X, D) a scale of potency developed in the 1830s by Samuel Dubs which allows for 'intermediary' potencies between the centesimal levels (5x is mid-way between the 2C and 3C in dilution, although not always in succussions, depending on the pharmacy). It is indicated by an X or D after the number. Interestingly enough, this scale was developed at just about the same time by a German physician, Vehsemeyer. See POTENCY.

decoction the process of boiling down in order to concentrate a mixture (as opposed to an infusion, where the medicinal substance steeps in hot water or liquid.

decrescendo becoming softer in sound.

decubitus bedsore.

deductive logic a process of reasoning in which a conclusion follows from stated premises. Reasoning is from the general to the specific.

deerfly fever/malady (tularemia, rabbit fever) a disease caused by *Pasteurella tularensis,* which is transmitted to man from rodents through the deer fly *(Chrysops discalis)* or other insect bites. It can be transmitted by animal bites as well or from an infected carcass. Symptoms are akin to undulant fever or plague and consist of a lengthy fever, lymph node swelling, etc. From Tulare, a county in California, where it was discovered.

defervescence the falling of an elevated temperature.

deflorescence the disappearance of the eruption in scarlet fever or other exanthemata.

deglutition the act of swallowing.

delirium animi fainting fits.

delirium a condition of mental excitement, confusion and clouded sensorium, usually with hallucinations, illusions, and delusions.

delirium furibundum delirium plus tetanic spasms, with stiffness of the whole body.

delirium tremens (DT's) a delirious state marked by distressing delusions, illusions, hallucinations, constant tremor, fumbling movements of the hands, insomnia and great exhaustion. Usually associated with alcohol poisoning but may appear in arteriosclerosis, in schizophrenia or manic-depressive psychoses. See MANIA-A-POTU.

deltoid referring to the shoulder muscle or that area of the shoulder.

delusion a representation of the patient's innermost feelings which in the broad sense involves holding onto a false belief in spite of evidence to the contrary. A wrong perception of reality. Consult R. Sankaran's *The Substance of Homeopathy* (1995).

dementia a deterioration of intellectual faculties with concomitant emotional disturbance resulting from organic brain disorder.

dementia praecox a term first coined by Benedict Morel (1809-1873) which refers to a syndrome very much like schizophrenia yet different in that its course is chronic and deteriorating and includes hallucinations and delusions. See SCHIZOPHRENIA.

demulcent a mild, viscid fluid which protects tender surfaces (such as a sore throat) from the action of irritating substances.

dengue fever (dandy fever, breakbone fever) an acute, infectious tropical and subtropical epidemic disease characterized by paroxysmal fever, rash, and severe pains in the bones and joints. Transmitted by mosquitoes, it has an incubation period of 3-5 days, the onset being sudden with high fever (over 104^0 F). This fever lasts approximately 3-4 days and subsides only to reappear again in 2-4 days. The recovery is slow.

dentagra tooth-ache.

dentition teething. The cutting of the teeth.

dentoid tooth-like.

denudation the removal or lack of a protective covering or layer.

deobstruent an agent or drug which removes an obstruction or obstructive material.

depilatio the loss of hair.

depravity moral corruption; a wicked or perverse act.

depurative an agent or process which removes waste products or promotes the excretion and removal of waste.

Dercum's disease (lipomatosis dolorosa, adiposis dolorosa) a condition characterized by the deposit of symmetrical nodular or pendulous masses of fat in various areas of the body which, as a result of being so massive, cause pain and discomfort. After the 19th century neurologist F.X. Dercum.

dermatalgia pain, burning and other sensations of the skin, unaccompanied by any structural change.

dermatomycosis a general term for any fungus infection of the skin.

dermatitis venenata (contact dermatitis) a skin inflammation produced by local irritation by irritant substances, usually plants.

dermatostomatitis a severe form of erythema multiforme which may involve the conjunctiva of the eye, causing blindness.

dermoid skin-like, resembling the skin.

descemetitis (keratitis punctata, serous cyclitis) inflammation of the membrane on the posterior surface of the cornea. This membrane is named after its discoverer, Jean Descemet (1732-1810), a French physician.

desiccative 1) dry; lacking moisture. 2) uninteresting; lacking spirit, animation, or spontaneity.

desquamation shedding; a peeling and casting off, particularly of the skin in scales or shreds.

diabetes insipidus (neuropituitary syndrome) a disease characterized by the passage of large quantities of urine, intense thirst and dehydration, due to an inadequate output of pituitary antidiuretic hormone (ADH). "It is the condition in which polyuria occurs without glycosuria or hyperglycemia. The specific gravity of urine is low."—K.N. Mathur, *Diabetes Mellitus: Its Diagnosis and Treatment.*

diabetes commonly refers to diabetes mellitus.

diabetes mellitus (diabetes, sugar diabetes, melituria,'sweet urine') the disease generally referred to as diabetes, characterized by the inability of the body to metabolize carbohydrates normally. Generally it is a result of an inadequate secretion of insulin and/or a resistance of the body's cells to insulin. It manifests itself with excessive blood sugar, sugar in the urine, excessive urination, acidosis, intense thirst and hunger, weakness and a loss of weight. As the disease progresses degenerative changes take place (arteriosclerosis, cataract formation, and neuropathies occur). "A constitutional disease, characterized by an excessive discharge of pale, sweet and heavy urine, containing grape-sugar (glucose)... Diabetic urine is of a pale straw-color, has a faint smell of apple, hay or milk, is of high specific gravity and is passed in large quantities."—E. H. Ruddock, *Vade Mecum,* p. 286-7.

diabrotic corroding or a corrosive agent.

diaphoresis sweating, perspiration.

diaphoretic causing the body to sweat.

diaphragmitis inflammation of the diaphragm.

diaphysis the shaft of a long bone.

diarrhea (flux) (Greek, 'a flowing through') an increased frequency of watery bowel movements. "Diarrhea is, in fact, a catarrh of the intestinal mucous membrane, just as an ordinary cold is a catarrh of the mucous membrane of the nose."—J.H. Clarke, *Cholera, Diarrhoea and Dysentery,* p. 42.

diastole the period when the heart is relaxed and full of blood. 'Systole' is when the heart is contracting, pushing out the blood.

diathermy (transthermia, thermopenetration) a special form of high-frequency current which when applied to affected tissue causes an increase in temperature of that tissue, inducing a healing response.

Karl Franz Nagelschmidt is considered the Father of Diathermy ('Ueber Diathermie', *Muenchener med. Woschr.,* 56:50, pp. 2575-76, 1909). He employed high-frequency currents in treatment after the suggestions of Tesla and Nernst. The current is usually applied via two pads, one placed on the affected part and the other underneath. A sensation of warmth or tingling may occur during the 10-12 minute treatment. Sinusoidal current, fulguration, and the Morse Wave Generator are other methods of applying electricity in the treatment of disease. See GALVANIC and FARADIC.

diathesis natural predisposition to a disease. A constitutional or hereditary influence. A state or condition of the body or a combination of attributes in an individual causing a susceptibility to disease. For example: sycosis or the sycotic diathesis is a tendency to retain water in the tissues, to produce small cutaneous fig-like tumors, chronic catarrh of the mucous membranes, and the slow, insidious progressive development of these and other symptoms.

dichrotism having two qualities at the same time.

dicrotic having a secondary beat, as the pulse.

differential diagnosis differentiation between two or more similar remedies under consideration for a patient.

Often a patient's symptoms are so similar to those of a number of remedies that selection becomes very difficult. For example, *Cuprum* and *Arsenicum* have enormous anxiety, caution, fear of death, restlessness, etc. *Sepia* as well as the metals *Aurum, Ferrum* and *Plumbum* have these symptoms. Points which can direct one to choose *Cuprum* include the appearance of the patient:

"The combination of blue sclera, protruding eyes and swelling around the eyes is a very strong indication. Secondly, there is TENSION from anxiety plus anticipation, overworking, fear of failure and mental, emotional or physical suppression. They try to control everything in a rigid manner, are fastidious and have to respect the rules. They plan everything and have difficulty to adapt. They are serious and don't like to take risks. *Cuprum* patients feel better (less anxious) when occupied. Their anxiety for others, especially family members, has been verified many times. On the physical level there is always some form of cramp or tension: migraine, epilepsy, asthma, hypertension, angina pectoris, tension in the neck and shoulders and cramps in the muscles, especially the toes. With all this there is often an exhaustion and prostration—'burnt-out'."—'A Compilation of Links', *Homeopathic Links,* 1992, vol. 5 p. 12.

diffident 1) lacking self-confidence, timid, reserved or modest. 2) suspicious or distrustful of others.

diffusa scattered or spread out.

dilate to broaden or make wider.

dilation (dilatation) the act of enlarging an opening or cavity.

dilution the process of diluting a substance; also, the final alcoholic solution (87% alcohol) which is used to impregnate blank pellets. You may also see it as 'I gave the 30th dilution', which is the same as 'I gave the 30th potency' or 'I gave the 30th attenuation'. See POTENCY.

Dioscorides a Greek scholar and herbalist who lived during the 1st century ACE. He wrote on medical botany as an applied science and was the first to write a materia medica. He recognized family relationships between plants 17 centuries before Linnaeus. His works formed the foundation of scientific botany and pharmacy and were regarded as the ultimate authority on materia medica for 1600 years! He described over 600 plants and was the first to recognize the analgesia provided by opium and the medicinal usefulness of aloes, ammoniac, aconite and ginger. Wrote *De Materia Medica*.

diphtheria (diphtheritis, garotilla) an acute and highly contagious disease caused by *Corynebacterium diphtheriae* usually affecting the mucous membranes of the throat (occasionally the nose) wherein a fibrinous exudate is formed and the patient is depressed and toxic. It is characterized by the formation of a false membrane adhering to the pharynx, larynx, and trachea (occasionally of the vagina and conjunctiva). It produces pain, swelling and obstruction, and the toxin may produce such systemic effects as fever, prostration, heart damage, paralysis, and rarely, death. It is caused by a Kleb-Loeffler type bacillus which distinguishes it from false diphtheria or croupous tonsillitis.

diphtheritic referring to DIPHTHERIA.

diplegia paralysis of similar parts on the two sides of the body.

diplocoria the presence of a double pupil in the eye.

diplopia double vision.

dipsomania an uncontrollable craving for alcohol; alcoholism.

dischromotopsia a disorder of vision in which color impressions just appear.

discutient an agent which disperses a tumor or pathological accumulation of material.

disease 'dis-ease', a lack of ease. Simply, an illness or sickness; a disturbance in structure or function of an organ, organ system, or part of the body. An abnormal condition of an organism or part thereof as a consequence of stress, infection, inherent weakness or environmental stressors which impairs the normal functioning of the organism. A state of disease is present if two of the following are present: consistent anatomical alterations, a recognizable etiological agent, or the identification of signs and symptoms.

According to Hahnemann, disease is a derangement of the vital force (that spiritual/dynamic force or quality which enlivens us). Though vague, he does acknowledge the energetic and psychic level of disease.

Disease, however, is a vast limitless concept to explore. To look at disease with a philosophical eye provides much insight. For example, the chief proponent of the notion of disease as illusion is Sankaran. He terms it a 'central delusion' in that a disease has a central theme (something which the patient does not perceive correctly). Sankaran recommends prescribing the remedy based on finding that central delusion, then finding the remedy that describes that delusion. Often we hear a symbolic complaint like 'I can't stomach that', which is often indicative of psychological problems, maladjustments, and/or stresses within relationships.

Disease can also be viewed as a myth which has central recurring themes. What is often helpful is when the patient recognizes him or herself in the myth. Then healing can begin, albeit on a much deeper level. A brief yet adequate compendium of the meanings of 'disease', for initial reference, may be found in Jan Scholten's interesting work, *Homoeopathy and Minerals* (1993).

"In all diseases and especially in chronic diseases, the discovery of the true and complete disease-picture and of its individualities demands particular insight, scepticism, knowledge of human nature, wariness in enquiry, and patience of the profoundest kind."—S.C. F. Hahnemann, *Organon*.

"Disease itself is impossible of observation; we only see and record the effects of disease; we can only record the symptoms ... the inner expressions are dynamic in nature, their outward expression is functional."—H.A. Roberts, *Principles and Art of Cure by Homoeopathy*.

"There are no such things as 'diseases' in the abstract to treat, only diseased persons; and each case must be individualized and treated on its merits, and not according to the name of the disease, by some drug that has been named the 'anti-' to it. Every case of disease is a problem in itself

—presenting a new combination of morbid phenomena."—J.H. Clarke, *Homoeopathy Explained.*

dispensatory a reference book where the preparation, uses, and contents of medicines are described. 'Dispensatory' and 'pharmacopoeia' may be considered synonymous but at one time they were not. Before the 18th century, pharmacopoeias were a compilation of standardized recipes for making drug preparations from plants, whereas a dispensatory included chemicals as well.

The pharmacopoeia had its origins in Italy in the 1490s. Slowly its predecessors, the 'herbals', were being replaced by pharmacopoeia. At that time, pharmacopoeia were written by physicians for use by pharmacists so that the same drug compounded by different pharmacist/apothecaries would be identical. Often districts had their own pharmacopoeia, thus assuring correct prescriptions no matter which pharmacist compounded the physician's order.

Today 'pharmacopoeia' implies an official, standard compendium such as the HPUS (Homoeopathic Pharmacopoeia of the United States) or the USP (United States Pharmacopoeia). "It is the object of a pharmacopoeia to select from among substances which possess medicinal power, those, the utility of which is most fully established and best understood; and to form from them preparations and compositions, in which their powers may be exerted to the greatest advantage."—USP, 1820 (1st ed.)

dissecting wounds cuts or wounds which should be healing yet are splitting or pulling apart.

disseminated spread about, scattered.

disseminated sclerosis see MULTIPLE SCLEROSIS.

dissimilar disease this as well as concepts of 'similar disease' and 'complicated (complex) disease' are very involved. Detailed explanations may be found in Para. 35-49 of Hahnemann's *Organon,* 6th ed.:

"If two *dissimilar* diseases meet together in the human being and they are either of equal strength, or the *older* one happens to be *stronger,* then the older one will keep the new one away from the body." Para. 36, Brewster-O'Reilly ed., p. 81.

"Or the *new dissimilar disease is stronger.* In this case, the weaker disease that the patient already has is postponed and suspended by the stronger supervening disease until the new one has run its course or been cured, and then the old one comes forth again *uncured."* Para. 38, p. 82.

"It can also happen that the *new disease,* after impinging for a long time on the organism, *joins the old one that is dissimilar to it,* and they form a *complicated* disease. Each disease takes on its own region in the organism, that is, it takes the organs especially appropriate to it. As it were, it takes only the peculiar place that is proper to it, leaving the rest of the organism to the dissimilar disease." Para. 40, p. 86.

"Two [similar] diseases, differing as to mode but very similar in their manifestations and actions, in the sufferings and symptoms they cause, always and everywhere annihilate one another as soon as they meet in the organism; that is, the stronger disease annihilates the weaker one. It is not difficult to guess the cause of this: Due to its active similarity, the stronger additional disease potence claims, by preference, *precisely* the *same* parts in the organism that were, until then, affected by the weaker disease irritant. Consequently, the weaker disease can no longer impinge upon those parts, and it expires."

distention bloated or swollen as if from internal pressure. Dilitation. Stretched out in all directions.

distichiasis (distichia) an extra row of cilia (eyelashes) at the border of the inner eyelid, which in turn rubs on the cornea.

diuresis an abnormally increased excretion of urine.

diuretic tending to increase the discharge of urine.

diurnal enuresis an incontinence of the bladder during the day or on a daily basis. Nocturnal enuresis (bedwetting at night) is just the opposite. 'Diurnal' refers to the day or daily.

diverticulum a pouch or sac which opens from a tubular organ, e.g., the colon.

diverticulitis an inflammation of the diverticula particularly of the large intestine, in which these pockets become filled with stagnant fecal material and become inflamed.

diverticulosis the presence of many diverticula (usually referring to the large intestine).

doctrine of signatures a postulate first proposed in the Middle Ages which says that external characteristics (including color) of a substance serve to indicate possible therapeutic effects, e.g., *Euphrasia* is a good remedy for the eyes, because it has a black spot in its corolla which looks like a pupil; *Euphorbia,* having a milky juice, would be good for increasing the flow of milk; *Hypericum* having red juice ought therefore to be of use in hemorrhages, etc. It was noticed that some plants, either by their shape or color, brought to mind characteristics of the human body or a disease. It was surmised that this 'signature' defined the therapeutic action of the item in question. People thought it was a signature from God that this plant would heal diseases which affected that particular organ or system.

Despite the lack of scientific logic in this thinking, it often proves accurate. For instance, Dr. Hanschka thought about bamboo, experimented, and found it had qualities effective against degenerative processes in the spine, cartilage and connective tissue. *Bambousa arundinacea* is now used in cases of arthrosis, painful joints, cartilage fragility, and to strengthen the skin, hair, and arterial walls. See METAPHORICAL NATURALISM.

"God would not place a disease upon the Earth without providing a cure for it, and a clue to the cure's identity. He places a signature upon it by making remedies resemble the organs or maladies they can cure."— Paracelsus.

dolor (pl. dolores) pain, suffering, grief. 'Dolor faciei': facial pain.

domestic medicine medicine employed by lay people in the home. Though not a popular term now, it was very popular in the time preceding the rise of modern medicine in the early 20th century. Since there were few doctors and the training they received and the principles they practiced under were less than adequate, many doctors wrote 'domestic medical texts'. This allowed the lay person to try to take care of him or herself. The first such text was written by S. Bradwell (Phyfition), in 1635, *Helps for Suddain Accidents*. In 1765, Wm. Buchan wrote his *Domestic Medicine* which went through over 200 editions!

The People's Medical Adviser by R.V. Pierce, MD (1840-1914) was probably the most popular of all, selling more than 4.5 million copies over a seventy year period. At times this hardback was sold for 50 cents, at others, given away for free. It was primarily a sales vehicle for his Buffalo, NY based company, World's Dispensary Medical Association. Pierce was elected to the U.S. Congress in 1878. His son, V.M. Pierce, took over the company after his father died. By 1935, the Pierce empire was a shadow of its former self. Up until 1975 Pierce products continued to be manufactured, but they are no longer available.

Homeopathy was noted for its domestic medical side as well. F. Humphreys (1816-1900), prover of *Apis mel.* and *Plantago,* wrote *Humphrey's Mentor* (1858), which went through many editions and millions of copies. His book, too, was a vehicle to sell his products, called *Humphrey's Specifics.* It was quite a successful venture and the company is still in existence today. I.D. Johnson, M. Freligh, E. Guernsey, A. Lutz, C. Hempel, J. Ellis, B.L. Hill, J.H. Pulte, J. Laurie, and C. Hering were just a few of the homeopathic authors who penned domestic treatises. As another example, the rather lengthy title of Hill's book was *An Epitome of the Homeopathic Healing Art Containing the New Discoveries and Improvements of the Present Time. Designed for the Use of Families and Travellers; and as a Pocket Companion for the Physician* (1859). Hering's work was not intended for the household practitioner but for the practical situations which the doctor might encounter in his daily practice. It was entitled *The Homoeopathist, or Domestic Physician* (1835).

-doron a suffix which describes a group of anthroposophical medicines, e.g., *Digestodoron, Hepatodoron,* and *Menodoron*. It is from the Greek and means 'gift' or 'offering'. (It may be found in English names, too, such as

Theodore, 'gift of God'.) Thus *Cardiodoron* means 'gift for the heart'. These may also be termed 'type medicines' or 'typical medicines' in that the name matches a particular organic region. The dorons originated with R. Steiner (see ANTHROPOSOPHY) and his associates, Drs. Noll and Eisenberg. Dr. Noll, in particular, developed *Pertudoron* (pertussis), *Rheumadoron* (rheumatism), and *Infludoron* (flu). He is best known for *Infludo* which, like the other three, is a homeopathic combination product. *Infludo* contains six ingredients, *Phosphorus, Eupatorium, Bryonia, Eucalyptus, Aconite,* and *Sabadilla.*

dorsal referring to the back of an area, for example the dorsal portion of the hand (the 'back of the hand').

dorsum the back or upper surface.

dose the homeopathic dose is not one of weights and measures as is the case in allopathy, in which quantity is synonymous with dose. Dose in homeopathy refers to the force of impact of the remedy. The homeopathic dose means 'that particular preparation of the remedy employed', in particular the amount and/or form of that preparation. When asked, "What dose did you give?", the homeopath might reply, "I gave the 6th centesimal potency in dilution form, two drops dissolved in one tablespoonful of water and swished in the mouth three times a day for five days" or "I gave a single dose of 6 pellets of *Lachesis* 200C."

dosimetrics see ALKALOMETRY.

dossil a wad, as in a dossil of lint or cotton.

Douglas' abscess an abscess of the FOSSA DOUGLASII *(vide).*

Dover's powder a pain reliever and diaphoretic agent containing ipecacuanha, opium and lactose. After Thomas Dover, British physician (1660-1742).

Down's syndrome (mongoloidism, trisomy 21) a common birth defect usually associated with moderate mental retardation and various physical malformations. It is due to the presence of an extra chromosome.

dowsing a quest for information, often using devices such as pendulums or forked sticks. This information can be for personal benefit or on behalf of others, and it appears to come to the dowser through means other than the five senses. Though its method is unusual and perhaps mysterious, it is intelligence-based and informative. See RADIONICS.

Dr. Sehgal's rediscovery of homeopathy see SEGHAL'S HOMEOPATHIC METHOD.

drachm (dram) a unit of measure approximately equal to one teaspoonful in fluid measure or approximately 4 grams in solid measure.

drainage remedies remedies which promote the excretory functions of a particular organ or organ system, usually prescribed in low potency (3X, 6X) or in combination formulations. For example, frequent doses of low potencies of *Hepar sulp.* or *Chelidonium* would be useful to stimulate the functioning of the liver.

drastic a powerful and irritating laxative.

draughts drafts of air or wind.

dreams "The truly characteristic indications of a remedy are not only to be found among the physical and mental symptoms, but likewise among the dreams."—G.H.G. Jahr, *Therapeutic Guide.*

dregs the sediment of a liquid. The least desirable portion. A residue or small amount.

dromomania an insane desire to wander about from place to place, being unable to settle.

dropsical (edematous) affected by dropsy or the abnormal accumulation of fluid in tissues.

dropsy (edema) an abnormal accumulation of clear or yellowish fluids in tissues or a body cavity. The skin surface may become tense and hard and will indent when pressed.

drug picture the symptom picture which a homeopathic remedy presents; the essential characteristics of the actions of a remedy; the essence of the remedy. This 'picture' can be compiled from proving, toxicological findings and clinical experiences.

"[It was Kent who] developed 'pictures' of constitutional types of patients, i.e.: *Sulphur* as 'the ragged philosopher' etc. Later, his pupil, Margaret Tyler, developed this idea further in her book, *Homeopathic Drug Pictures,* and more recently Mr. George Vithoulkas, who studied with a student of Kent, has developed his own profoundly insightful 'essence pictures' along similar lines."—*The American Homeopath* 2:9, 1995.

druse the rupture of tissues with no surface lesion.

duce natura 'led by nature, with nature as guide,' 'the hints nature provides' (Latin).

Duchenne's disease (tabes dorsalis, childhood muscular dystrophy) a disease first described by Guillaume Duchenne (1806-1875), a French neurologist. (Duchenne also made important contributions in electrophysiology and is considered the founder of electrotherapy. He used faradism as early as 1830.) See TABES DORSALIS.

dum-dum fever see KALA-AZAR.

dumb ague (dumb chill) a subacute form of malaria with irregular attacks of fever without chills. A form of intermittent fever which has no well-defined 'chill'.

dumping syndrome (postgastrectomy syndrome) a syndrome characterized by flushed skin, sweating, dizziness, gastric discomfort, palpitations, cold sweats, weakness, headache, nonspecific pains, and an extreme fall in blood pressure, generally associated with persons who have had shunts of the stomach or a partial removal of the stomach. For example, a person who has had her stomach stapled (in order to lose weight) may experience this syndrome. Symptoms occur soon after eating when the contents of the stomach empty too rapidly into the duodenum (first part of the small intestine).

duodecimo (twelvemo, 12mo.) a sheet of paper folded into twelve pieces (leaves); a book printed on paper so folded, thus a small book (5" x 7.75").

duodenitis inflammation of the duodenum (first part of the small intestine).

Dupuytren's contraction/contracture a contracted state of the palm and fingers causing a permanent flexion of one or more fingers. Named after the renowned French surgeon Guillaume Dupuytren (1777-1835), who also was the first to classify the various degrees of burns and accurately describe the local effects of burns.

dusky somewhat dark; swarthy, or tawny.

dynamis force or energy; vital force. The life force of the individual, the level at which real causation of disease originates.

dynamization (potentization) the homeopathic process of serially diluting the remedy and succussing (shaking) it with each dilution. This in turn imparts an 'intangible' energy to the substance and /or releases innate healing power in the substance.

dysacousis/dysacusis 1) pain in the ear from exposure to sound. 2) The loss of the ability to discriminate words, syllables, or the understanding of words and/or the inability to process the details of sound even though the person can hear and is sensitive to sound.

dysaphia an impairment of the sense of touch.

dysbasia difficulty of any kind in walking.

dysbiosis a state of malfunctioning, especially in the intestinal region, meaning that food is not properly digested, the digestive apparatus is abnormal or inhibited in function, and the wrong bacterial flora are present in the bowels.

dyschezia a clinical sign characterized by difficult or painful expulsion of feces and usually associated with lesions in or near the anal region or even in the colon.

dyscrasis/dyscratic/dyscrasic 1) an abnormal, morbid or sick state of the body. 2) disease. 3) "That element of weakness transmitted from parent to child which of itself, produces certain definite results, and which renders [the individual] more susceptible to the ordinary diseases, and also changes the normal course of those diseases."—George Royal (1902). See CACHECTIC.

dysecoia difficulty of hearing or deafness.

dysentery a disease marked by frequent watery stools, often with blood and mucus and characterized by pain, tenesmus, fever, and dehydration. There are many variations (amebic d., bacillary d., viral d., bilharzial d.).

dysidrosis (dyshidrosis, pompholyx) a rare disease, with vesicular eruptions of the hands and feet.

dysmenorrhea (dysmenia) painful menstruation.

dysmnesia a naturally poor or an impaired memory.

dysontogenesis a defective development of the individual.

dysopia impaired sight.

dysorexia a diminished or perverted appetite.

dysosmia an impaired sense of smell.

dyspareunia painful or difficult sexual intercourse.

dyspepsia disturbed digestion. Indigestion.

dysphagia difficulty in swallowing.

dysphemia stuttering or stammering.

dysphoria restlessness or a sense of being ill at ease.

dysplasia (alloplasia) the replacing of normally dominant cell types in an organ or tissue by other cell types usually not found there or at that time in the tissue development.

dyspnea breathing which is labored or difficult. Shortness of breath.

dystocia a difficult childbirth.

dystonia a state of abnormal (either hypo- or hyper-) tonicity in any of the tissues.

dystrophia the progressive changes that may occur as a result of poor or defective nutrition. A wasting away.

dysuria difficult or painful urination.

E E E **E** E E E

e.g. (exemplia gratia) 'for example'.

EAP (electro-acupuncture) a general, almost non-specific term, as it may refer to an electrical current applied to acupuncture points or to the vast and ever broadening field of EAV (electro-acupuncture according to Voll). See EAV.

eau de Luce 'water of Luce'. An alcoholic mixture of oil of amber and ammonia.

EAV (electro-acupuncture according to Voll, EAP, EDS, GSR) a bioenergetic diagnostic and treatment method developed by Dr. Reinhold Voll (1909-

1989). Electrical resistance is measured at acupuncture points using a direct current (DC) test circuit. Extremely low or high resistances indicate dysfunction in the meridian being tested (e.g. lung or small intestine).

"EAV is the use of modern electronic instruments to *measure* acupuncture points, and from those measurements draw *diagnostic* conclusions about related organs, tissue systems and bodily functions. Points found to be abnormal (and thus reflecting bodily disturbances) can be brought back to 'norm' by treatment with micro-electronic currents generated by most such instruments. However, as you know from needle acupuncture, purely external stimulation very often is not sufficient to bring back lasting balance to the meridians. The reason for this is twofold, in that often the actual cause of the problem was not completely determined, or, the underlying pathology is so great that internal intervention is needed, such as the administration of well-indicated herbs or other remedies. The proper dispensing of medications also enables effective therapy to be continued between treatments.

"The key concept from the last paragraph is that of being able to *measure* acupuncture points. Taking all this a step further, it was found that specific points change their measurement readings when substances (such as vitamins, supplements, herbs, homeopathics, or even allopathics) are introduced into the measurement circuit. By placing samples of various substances a practitioner works with, one-by-one into a special holder (honeycomb) connected to the diagnostic instrument, the practitioner can evaluate which of the remedies will be most effective for the patient—*before* their administration, and *before* the patient leaves the office. Singularly or in combination, medications can be tested not only for effectiveness, but also for tolerance, to eliminate adverse side effects. This is termed medication testing. The ability to test the biocompatibility of remedies prior to taking them, plus its potential in food and allergy testing is, as one can well imagine, what has primarily stirred up so much interest in German Electro-Acupuncture techniques."—Walter D. Sturm, PhD., Occidental Institute Research Foundation.

There is now a vast array of instrumentation (VEGA, INTERRO, ACU-BASE OMEGA, etc.) which combines testing and medication screening with computer program diagnostics to diagnose and indicate forms of treatment. ETD (energetic terminal-point diagnosis), BFD (bioelectronic function diagnostics), SEG (segmental electrograms), bioresonance diagnosis and therapy (MORA, Nogier, Indumed, BICOM, TRICOM, MULTICOM and laser therapies) are all bioenergetic therapies. LISTEN, another EAV testing and diagnostic method, was recently developed by James Hoyt Clark of Utah, USA. It is a very comprehensive electronic testing method.

The VEGATEST, VRT (Vegetative Reflex Test), ART (Autonomic Resonance-Test) developed by Dr. H. Schimmel is one of the latest bioelectronic methods, as is SEG (segmental electrography). SEG does not operate on acupuncture-based information but "objectively shows regulative status of the biological system, tendencies toward chronic-degenerative disorders and malignancies (even before manifestation is in the final states), detect focal situations, etc." Another researcher, Dr. Franz Morell of Germany, did early EAV work. He developed a 'Minimal Test Preparation List' and a 'Punch Card' system.

EAV could be likened to a tree with Dr. Voll, Rife, Abrams, and Mathews being the trunk and other researchers and instrumentation constituting the various branches. One could perhaps refer to this vast field as resonance therapeutics or harmonic therapies.

Perhaps the earliest prelude to this vast field can be traced to A.P. Mathews, who said, in 1903, "Every excess of action, every change in the physical state of the protoplasm of any organ, or any area in the embryo or in the eggs, produces, it is believed, an electrical disturbance."—quoted in Barbara Brewitt, 'Quantitative Analysis of Electrical Skin Conductance in Diagnosis: Historical and Current Views of Bioelectric Medicine', *J. of Naturopathic Medicine,* 6:1, p. 66-75, 1996. Later, in the mid 1900s, Rosendal and, in particular, Harold S. Burr, et. al. at Yale University published many papers on bioelectric potential and its significance as an indicator of physiological states such as cancer, wound healing, central nervous system activity, drug use, sleep, etc. Burr found that "significant differences existed between the normal physiological electrical potential and that of pathological tumor formation and cancer."

The work of R.R. Rife needs to be mentioned as he also conducted brilliant seminal work in this as well as related areas. He discovered various oscillatory rates of microbes and used these rates to destroy pathogens.

This entry is not meant to be a definitive explanation; it is included to provide a succinct yet workable definition of this vast and ever-changing field. You may wish to consult the works of Julian N. Kenyon, specifically *Modern Techniques of Acupuncture, Vol 3.*

Also, it should not be confused with electroacupuncture (EA) which is the application of electrical current directly to acupuncture needles. This enhances the effects of acupuncture and by selectively choosing frequencies it is possible to release a variety of neuropeptides, e.g., 2 hertz stimulation releases beta-endorphin, a pain relieving substance. EA was first demonstrated by G. Hiraga of Japan in 1764. Consult *Beyond Yin and Yang* (1992, G. Ulett). See VOLL, RADIONICS, ACUPUNCTURE, BEV.

ebullition effervescence. A boiling or bubbling up, such as when blood rushes to the face or hot flashes.

eburnate ivory-like; hard, compact and white, as in an 'eburnate exostosis' or 'The bone has undergone eburnation.'

ecbolic a medicine which accelerates parturition (childbirth).

ecce medicus 'behold the doctor'.

ecchymosis bruise, black and blue spot. A purplish patch caused by extra-vasation (leakage) of blood into the skin. Ecchymoses differ from petechia only in size. Petechia are smaller. If the bruise has turned to a violet-black color, give *Ledum;* it finishes what *Arnica* started.

eccoprotic a laxative or a cathartic.

eccritic promoting the excretion of waste matter.

echolalia repetition of what others have said as if echoing them.

echte heilweg 'genuine healing' (German). *'Heilweg'* should be spelled *'Heilung'*.

eclampsia (puerperal convulsions) 1) sudden attack of convulsions especially occurring in the latter part of pregnancy or during labor. 2) a scintillation (flashing of light) which appears to the epileptic person before he has a seizure.

eclectic picking out from different sources what appears to be of highest value or most useful.

Eclecticism was actually a medical movement in the 1800s whose found-ing father was C.S. Rafinesque. Wooster Beach, John King, John Scudder, John Uri Lloyd, and Harvey Felter were major figures in Eclecticism. Thomsonianism and physio-medicalism are often lumped into or associ-ated with eclecticism but in reality the three are separate. To be sure, however, all used herbs and moved distinctly away from the drastic thera-peutics (bleeding and purging, etc.) of their more orthodox colleagues. Eclecticism (American Reformed School of Medicine) used high quality, refined herbal medications (in particular Lloyd's Specifics) whereas the other groups used more crude forms. The Eclectic Medical Institute of Cincinnati, founded in 1845, taught the eclectic approach *and* was one of the finest medical schools in the country at that time. For an interesting account of herbalism, read *Herb Doctors* (W. Boyle) available from Eclec-tic Medical Publications, 14385 Southeast Lusted Rd., Sandy, OR 97005. According to Cleveland's *Pocket Lexicon* (1855), eclectic physicians were those who professed to be liberal in their views, independent of party, and favored progress and reform in the profession. For the finest treatment of the eclectics please consult *Medical Protestants: The Eclectics in Ameri-can Medicine, 1825-1939* (J.S. Haller, Jr.) See THOMSONIANISM, PHYSIOMEDICALISM.

ecmnesia a loss of memory for recent events.

economy as it pertains to medicine, the efficiency to which an organism carries out its functioning. If a person digests his/her food in an 'economical' manner, s/he does so by expending the least amount of energy to carry out the process. If digestion is slow and labored the economy is said to be 'labored'.

ectal outer or external.

ectasia dilation of a blood vessel.

ecthyma an inflammatory skin disease attended by an eruption of large, flat pustules that ulcerate and become crusted. They vary in size from 0.5-2cm in diameter and are surrounded by a distinct inflammatory areola. The lesions are usually found on the legs and thighs, and occur in crops which persist for an indefinite period.

ectropion/ectropium the turning of a part inside out. See EVERSION.

eczema (tetter, salt rheum) an inflammation of the skin, of acute or chronic nature, presenting varied shaped lesions (dry or moist) and often accompanied with itching and burning.

eczema capitis (humid tetter, scall) eczema affecting the scalp.

eczema madidans a form of eczema characterized by large, raw, weeping surfaces studded with red points; associated with vesicular eczema.

eczema rubrum an inflammation of the skin with exudation of lymph marked by raw surfaces studded with red points.

eczematous pertaining to eczema.

edema pedum edema or fluid accumulation in the lower extremities or legs.

edematous (anasarca, ascites, dropsy, hydrops) relating to or marked by an abnormal accumulation of fluid in the tissues.

EDS electro-dermal screening, essentially the same as EAV. Points on the skin are 'checked' via an electric probe in order to diagnose illness. See EAV, VOLL.

effect to cause to be. That which comes directly from something which can properly be termed a cause. 'Apply the ointment to the affected area to effect a cure'!!?

effete exhausted of vitality or force. Ineffective, worn out. Characterized by unproductive self-indulgence or decadence.

efflorescence an unnatural redness of the skin.

effluxion a miscarriage prior to three months of pregnancy (also called 'abortion' in the old literature).

effluvia an exhalation, especially one of bad odor or injurious influence. Disagreeable odors, fumes or exhalations from decaying matter.

effusion the act of pouring out. Loss of body fluid by rupture of the containing vessel or sac.

egesta (dejecta) excreta, feces, excrement.

Ehretism a system for maintaining bodily health developed by Arnold Ehret (1866-1922). The main emphasis of his teachings is the elimination of mucus from the body. In order to accomplish this he advocated fasting, eating foods which formed little or no mucus in the body, vegetarianism and physical activity. "Mucus accumulates especially in the heating channel (stomach and bowels) of this tube-machine, and slowly clogs up the channel and filters (glands). The sum total of this defilement causes chronic defects, makes one grow old and is the main factor in the nature of all disease."— *Rational Fasting* (Ehret, 1926). He also wrote *Professor A. Ehret's Mucusless Diet.*

ejaculatio praecox premature ejaculation.

elective affinity the specific location or seat of action of a medicine. For example, *Belladonna* affects primarily the brain and nervous system, *Aconite* the heart, *Rhus* the skin, *Glonoin* the vascular system. Rademacher used this as a basis for his system of therapeutics.

electro-acupuncture (EAP) see EAV, VOLL.

electro-dermal screening (EDS) see EDS, EAV, VOLL.

electro-homeopathy see MATTEISM.

electuary a medicinal paste or lozenge which consists of the drug/herb mixed with honey and then placed in the mouth and swallowed.

eleemosynary pertaining to alms or the giving of alms.

elephantiasis (phlegmasia malabarica, elephantiasis arabum, elephantiasis indica, pachydermia) a chronic, often extreme enlargement and hardening of the cutaneous and subcutaneous tissue, especially of the legs and scrotum, resulting from lymphatic obstruction, and usually caused by a nematode worm, *Wuchereria bancrofti.*

elinguid tongue-tied, without the power of speech.

emaciation a wasted condition of the body. A loss of flesh, leanness.

emansio mensium amenorrhea; delayed menstruation.

embrocation the act of moistening/lubricating and then massaging/rubbing the diseased or affected part with oils, spirits, or liniments; also the actual substance used to rub the affected part.

emesis vomiting.

emetic an agent which causes vomiting.

emiction diuresis, urination.

emmenagogue an agent which stimulates the menstrual flow.

emmenia the menses.

emphysema a lung disease characterized by enlargement, overdistention, and destructive changes in the alveoli or air sacs. This overdistention causes great difficulty in breathing out (expiration) and thus the breathing is labored. An increased susceptibility to infection results. It also meant, at one time, a 'windy swelling' (a swelling caused by the diffusion of air into the tissues).

empiricism experience as a guide to practice or to the therapeutic use of any remedy rather than theories or scientific deduction or investigation. The view that experience, especially of the senses, is the only source of knowledge.

emprosthotonos (tetanus anticus) a tonic muscular spasm in which the body and head are forcibly flexed forward.

empyema the presence of pus in any cavity. If not specified then it usually occurs around the lungs (pyothorax).

empyocele a suppurating tumor of the scrotum; a collection of pus in the scrotum.

empyreumatic the disagreeable odor of decaying organic substances.

emunctory a cleansing agent. Discharging waste; excretory.

enanthesis the skin eruption of a disease, e.g., the skin eruption of scarlet fever or herpes zoster.

enantiopathic (palliative) the allopathic method of treating diseases. Of contrary properties. See ALLOPATHY.

encephalitis (brain fever, cephalitis) an acute inflammatory disease of the brain due to direct attack by a virus or to hypersensitivity initiated by a viral infection. Symptoms include apathy, double vision, extreme muscular weakness, headache, drowsiness or convulsions, and perhaps neck rigidity.

encephaloma a brain tumor.

encephalomacia softening of the brain.

enchondroma benign cartilaginous growth occurring in parts, such as the glands, lungs, bones, etc., where cartilage does not normally exist.

encomium a eulogy, tribute or lofty praise.

encopresis the involuntary passage of feces.

endamoebic (entamoeba) referring to a genus of amoebic parasites which cause dysentery when found in the digestive tract.

endarteritis obliterans inflammation of the inner coating of an artery to such a degree as to completely stop or severely inhibit the flow of blood.

endemic referring to an affection or disease particular to a certain group of persons or locality. Widely prevalent on an ongoing or chronic basis.

endocarditis inflammation of the membrane which lines the inside of the heart and its valves.

endocardium the membrane lining the interior of the heart.

endocervicitis inflammation of the membrane of the uterine cervix.

enervate to weaken.

enervation weakness, lack of energy.

English cholera see CHOLERINE.

ennui boredom; listlessness and dissatisfaction resulting from lack of interest. Loathing of life.

enomania a craving for alcohol, alcoholic drinks (Gr. *oenos,* 'wine').

enosimania extreme and irrational terror.

ensiform appendix the appendix 'in the shape of a sword'. The appendix can also be called 'vermiform' or 'wormlike'.

ENT 'ears, nose and throat'. EENT stands for 'eyes, ears, nose and throat'.

entelechy complete development; full realization of any action.

enteralgia cramps, colic. Severe neuralgic pains in the intestines.

enteric fever see TYPHOID FEVER.

enteritis inflammation of the intestines.

entero-colitis inflammation of the intestines and colon.

enteroparesis diminished or arrested intestinal peristalsis as a result of flaccid intestinal musculature.

enteroptosis prolapse of the intestine.

enterorrhagia intestinal bleeding.

enterorrhea old term for diarrhea.

enterostenosis a narrowing of the intestine.

entia non multiplicanda praeter necessitatem (lit., 'things should not be multiplied more than necessary') an abbreviated statement of Occam's Razor, a philosophical axiom known also to biologists as the Law of Parsimony: "The least complicated answer to any particular question is likely to be the correct one."

entrails the intestines.

entropium (entropion) inversion of the margins of the eyelids. Eyelashes turn inward.

enuresis involuntary urination; bed-wetting, usually occurring at night. Incontinence of the urine.

epilation loss of hair.

epilepsy (falling sickness, status convulvius, malum caducum) a disorder of the CNS (central nervous system) whereby nerve cells explosively discharge, causing transient episodes of unconsciousness and psychic dysfunction, with or without convulsions.

ephelis (pl. ephelides) lentigo; a freckle, usually from the sun.

ephemeral of brief duration. Lasting just a day.

ephialtes (incubus) nightmare.

epihidrosis moderate sweating.

epicondyle a projection from a long bone near the end of the bone.

epicondylitis inflammation of an epicondyle.

epidemic an acute disease which spreads rapidly from place to place, affecting large numbers of persons. A contagious disease which spreads rapidly.

epidemic catarrh see INFLUENZA.

epidemy an epidemic disease.

epididymis a small excretory duct of the testicle.

epididymitis inflammation of the small excretory duct of the testicle.

epigastrium (scrobiculus cordis) pit of the stomach; the upper central region of the abdomen.

epigastrum the upper and middle part of the abdomen.

epileptiform 'convulsion-like'. Similar to the convulsions seen in epilepsy.

epilose having no hair.

epiphora a persistent overflow of tears. Watery eye.

epiphysis usually the end of a bone which during the growth process solidifies separately from the shaft or diaphysis.

epiphysitis inflammation of an epiphysis.

episcleritis an inflammation of the subconjunctival tissues of the eye or of the sclera itself.

episioitis inflammation of the vulva.

epistaxis (hemorrhagia narium, rhinorrhagia) nosebleed.

epithelioma (epidermoid carcinoma) a benign tumor of the skin (epithelial cells). Skin cancer.

epochal a point in time or a great event from which succeeding time is measured.

eponym a name formed or derived from that of a person known or assumed to be the first, or one of the first, to discover or describe a disease, symptom complex, theory, etc. For example, Dupuytren's contraction, Eustachian tube, Fletcherizing, etc.

epulis a small tumor of or under the gum, or of the periosteum of the jaw.

erethism an abnormal increase in nervous irritability or state of excitement or irritation. An unusually quick response to stimulus.

ergo therefore, consequently, hence.

ergotism (St. Anthony's fire) poisoning by a toxic substance contained in the fungus *Claviceps purpurea* following the ingestion of the contaminated grain. Symptoms of poisoning fall into two categories: a spasmodic form with contractions and cramps of the muscles and a form characterized by gangrene which causes lameness and necrosis of the extremities due to peripheral vascular constriction.

erosio portionis an erosion or wasting away of parts, e.g., erosio portio vaginalis.

erotomania abnormal sexual desire; nymphomania or satyriasis.

errhine (sternutatory) an agent which provokes a mucus discharge from the nose.

eructation belching; the raising of gas or of a small quantity of acid fluid from the stomach.

erysipelas (rose, St. Anthony's Fire, erysipelas faciei, ignis sacer) superficial cellulitis (fever and local redness), a contagious disease caused by group A beta-hemolytic streptococci. The lesion is usually well delineated, shiny red, edematous and tender. Vesicles and bullae often develop. Erysipelas often attacks a wound; if not entirely cleared up it can become a source (nidus) of continued periodic infections, often recurring year after year. High fever, chills, and malaise are common. It frequently occurs without obvious injury. If unchecked the infection may spread to deeper tissue producing necrosis, gangrene, pneumonia, nephritis, and meningitis. E. genarum would refer to the cheek area.

    'St. Anthony's fire' was actually a popular term for ergotism or gangrenous erysipelas contracted from eating grain contaminated with the ergot fungus. See ERGOTISM. This connection was elucidated by Tuiller in 1630. It is called 'St. Anthony's fire' because persons so stricken were cared for by the Order of St. Anthony in their hospices. So these terms are a confused and jumbled lot. 'St. Anthony's fire' in homeopathic literature refers to erysipelas and sometimes to gangrene. Yet be aware that 'St. Anthony's fire' may also refer to ergotism.

erysipelatous inflammation of the skin with accompanying fever, marked by erythema/redness of the skin.

erythema a morbid or unhealthy redness of the skin due to congestion of the capillaries.

erythema fugax a transient and diffuse reddening of the skin which occurs in excitable persons, usually as a result of emotional stimulus.

erythema multiforme a symmetrical red eruption of papules or vesicles, usually confined to the back and the dorsal surfaces of the forearms and legs. The lesions are closely aggregated but vary in size and arrangement. There are many variations of e. multiforme, including Fiessinger-Leroy's syndrome, dermatostomatitis, Steven-Johnson syndrome, ocular mucous membrane syndrome, etc.

erythema nodosum (dermatitis contusiformis) a redness of the skin marked by the formation of painful nodes, especially on the shins, lasting a few days to a few weeks.

erythema solare sunburn.

erythematodes (lupus erythematodes) see LUPUS ERYTHEMATOSUS.

erythematous marked by or related to redness. Redness of the skin caused by excessive quantities of blood in the skin, generally occurring with skin injuries, inflammations and infection.

erythematous tonsillitis (red angina) a generic description of a red sore throat and inflammation of the tonsils.

erythism see ERETHISM.

erythrasma an eruption of reddish-brown patches especially in the armpits and groin, usually associated with the fungus *Microsporon*.

erythrism redness of the hair with a ruddy, freckled complexion.

erythrocyanosis irregular reddish blue markings on the skin, usually reticular (like a fine network) in arrangement, due to a circulatory disturbance of the skin.

erythromelalgia (Mitchell's disease, Gerhardt's disease, red neuralgia, rodonalgia) a cutaneous vasodilation of the feet (rarely of the hands) characterized by redness, mottling, changes in skin temperature, and neuralgic pains.

erythropsia a visual disorder in which everything appears red.

eschar a dry scab or slough formed on the skin as a result of a burn or the action of a caustic substance.

escharotic a substance capable of producing a scab or sloughing off tissue.

esculent edible. Fit to be eaten.

esophagectasia (oesophagectasia) a dilation of the esophagus of unknown origin.

esophagismus spasm of the esophagus.

esophagus (oesophagus) the membranous, muscular tube which connects the pharynx (back of the mouth) to the stomach allowing food, etc. to enter the body.

esophoria the tendency of one eye to deviate inward; a convergent squint.

essence the true characteristic or substance. See DRUG PICTURE. For example, the essence of *Vanadium* is "the idea that they have to be successful, but they are not allowed or they are incapable. They feel obliged to live up to many tasks, but they are confused as to what tasks and why."—*Vanadium metallicum* (*Homoeopathic Links*, 2/94, p. 11).

Essiac an herbal formula of Native American origin (Ojibwa). It was brought to public attention as a cure for cancer by Renee Caisse (1888-1978), an Ontario nurse, in 1922. In 1924 she used it on her aunt, who was thought to be in the final stages of inoperable stomach cancer. She drank the tea for 2 months, recovered and lived for twenty more years. Essiac ('Caisse' spelled backwards) consists of four ingredients: sheep sorrel *(Rumex acetosella),* burdock *(Arctium lappa),* slippery elm inner bark *(Ulmus fulva),* and turkey rhubarb *(Rheum palmatum).* Renee's life is documented in *Calling of An Angel* (G. Glum). *The Essence of Essiac* (S. Snow) presents a lot of information on the recipe and herbs in general.

Charles A. Brusch, M.D., personal physician to Pres. John F. Kennedy, worked with Renee from 1959-1962. It is postulated Caisse communicated with or knew of Hoxsey, a physician who advocated alternative treatments for cancer. See GERSON THERAPY.

estivate to be dormant.

eston aluminum acetate (an insoluble powder, used as a dusting powder).

estruation sexual excitement or passion.

et seq. 'and the following' or 'and so forth'.

ethmoid a bone of the skull forming the upper bony nose. One of the sinus cavities.

etiology the science of the cause of diseases. The etiology of a disease is the same as the cause.

eucrasia health or a state of well-being. See HEALTH.

euonymin a glucoside from a tree, *Euonymus atropurpureus* (wahoo bark), used as a cathartic.

eustachian tube (auditory canal) the canal, lined with mucous membrane, connecting the pharynx with the ear drum.

First described by the Italian anatomist Bartolomeo Eustachio (1524-1574). Eustachio's genius was never truly recognized for two reasons: 1) he was a contemporary and critic of Vesalius, and 2) his opus on anatomy was completed in 1552 but wasn't published until 1714, because he showed his work to the Pope who, disapproving of dissections, locked it away in the Papal Library. Pope Clement XI discovered Eustachio's opus and gave it to his personal physician, Giovanni Lancisi, who then had it published. Eustachio' work is more anatomically correct and less artisticly flamboyant than Vesalius'. Eustachio discovered the thoracic duct, the adrenals, and the abducens nerve, and he gave the first accurate description of the uterus.

euthanasia an easy or painless death, or the method of effecting it.

eutocia an easy childbirth.

evanescent transitory, vanishing or likely to vanish.

evectics the art of acquiring bodily health and vigor.

eventration a protrusion of the intestines through an opening in the abdominal wall.

eversion (ectropion) a turning outward as of the eyelid. The lid is folded upon itself, exposing the conjunctival surface or sulcus. This may be done manually in order to inspect the conjunctiva of the eye.

exacerbation an aggravation of the condition, symptoms, or disease. An increase in the severity of a disease or amount of symptoms.

exanthemata the characteristic skin eruption of an eruptive fever such as measles or scarlet fever.

exanthemic fever fever with accompanying eruptions. May refer to scarlatina.

excogitate to discover or work out by thinking.

excoriated abraded, raw, chafed, or worn off. Superficial abrasions of the skin caused by scratching or scraping, e.g., scratched atopic eczema, scratched insect bites and scabies.

excrement waste material expelled from the body after digestion; feces.

excrescence any outgrowth, wart, nodule or eruption from the surface.

exedens (lupus exedens) a tubercular skin disease which is characterized by brown colored skin eruptions or bumps.

exfoliated epithelium a condition in which the top layers of skin scale or fall off.

exfoliating dermatitis (Wilson's disease, pityriasis rubra) an acute or chronic inflammation of the skin, in which the epidermis is shed more or less freely in large or small scales.

exfoliation the falling off or the peeling back in layers or scales.

exocervicitis an inflammation of the outer part of the cervix.

exophthalmic goiter (Grave's/Basedow's/Flajani's/Marsh's/Parson's/Parry's disease) a condition marked by prominence of the eyeballs, enlargement of the thyroid gland, tremor, rapid heart action, muscular tremor, and nervous irritability.

exophthalmus protrusion of the eyeballs in hyperthyroidism

exordium a prelude or introduction. The beginning or introductory part intended to prepare the way for what follows.

exostosis a bony tumor, node or growth, springing from the surface of a bone, most commonly in the form of ossification of muscular attachments. As Kent described it, exostosis is a disruption in the body's ability to distribute the minerals which build bone. Those minerals, primarily calcium and phosphorus, are not distributed evenly throughout the body, thus bone substance may be absent in one part of the body while overgrowths might occur in another. Softening of the bone and defective bone formation will be found. For example, the keynote 'late learning to walk' actually means the child knows how to walk but can't because the leg bones are weak. 'Tardy development of bone tissues.'

extend to continue to another, perhaps remote, location, as in 'the pain in my wrist extends into my fingers'. Here the focus of the pain is in the wrist but travels to the fingers. This sort of symptom may need to be differentiated from the radiating one. See RADIATE.

extirpation the complete removal of an organ or a part. To root out, eradicate. To destroy wholly.

extravasation leakage out of a blood vessel into surrounding tissues.

extremis relating to the end; perhaps to the end of life.

exudation the oozing of fluid from blood vessels into tissues or cavities.

exudative pleurisy inflammation of the lining of the lung with subsequent fluid leakage.

exutory see ISSUE.

exutorium something which detoxifies and/or causes drainage or fluid movement.

eye-memory memory chiefly of what is seen.

eyegum the moist or semi-dry mucus in the eyes, corners of the eyes, or on the lashes.

F F F F F F F

face ague (facial neuralgia) see FACEACHE.

faceache (tic douloureux, face ague, prosopalgia, trigeminal neuralgia) spasmodic facial neuralgia. A form of trigeminal neuralgia due to degenerative changes in the nerve. Facial pain along the nerve trunk. Severe, paroxysmal bursts of pain in one or more branches of the trigeminal nerve, often induced by touching trigger areas in or about the mouth.

facetious playfully jocular; humorous and flippant.

facial paralysis/palsy see BELL'S PALSY.

facies cadaverica see HIPPOCRATICA.

facies hippocratica see HIPPOCRATICA.

factitious artificially made rather than a product of nature. Not natural.

fag enervation, fatigue, exhaustion, weariness.

faradic (faradism) relating to induced and rapidly alternating electrical currents of medium voltage and amperage used to cause contraction of weakened muscles or to treat paralysis. One electrode is placed near the muscle's origin and the other electrode near the point of insertion. Enough current can be generated by 2 or 3 dry-cell batteries.

Electricity was used therapeutically in the late 19th and early 20th centuries. After Michael Faraday (1791-1867), an English scientist who declined knighthood and the presidency of the Royal Society. He discovered electromagnetic induction in 1831. Faraday was a giant in science, especially in the field of physics. The British Prime Minister came to visit Faraday and asked him what use would come of his discoveries. Faraday replied, "I don't know, but I wager that your government will tax it some day!" Compare GALVANIC.

farinaceous food starchy food. Food made from flour or grains ('farina': a fine meal prepared from cereal grains and used as a cooked cereal or in puddings). Having a mealy or powdery texture.

farrago medley, jumble, or hodgepodge. A mixture composed of various materials.

fascicle small bundle or cluster.

fatuity stupidity.

fauces the throat or pharynx area. The passage from the mouth into the throat. A cavity behind the tongue, palatine arch, uvula and tonsils from which the pharynx and larynx proceed.

favus (tinea capitis) a fungal skin disease characterized by the presence of round, sulfur-yellow, cup-shaped crusts having an odor. Usually affects the scalp.

favus convertus pustular ringworm, or ringworm of the scalp.

febricula simple, continued fever.

febrifuge an agent which decreases or lessens fever.

febrile feverish

febris (pl. 'febres') fever.

febris flava yellow fever.

febris helodes a fever characterized by profuse sweating.

febris nervosa nervous fever. See TYPHOID FEVER.

feculent foul or fecal. Full of foul matter or sediment.

felon (panaritium, whitlow, panaris, paronychia) an abscess or inflammation of the finger tip, especially around the nail. Phlegmonous inflammation of a finger or toe.

ferruginous relating to or containing iron; chalybeate.

ferrum salitum iron salts.

festina lente accelerate slowly, make haste slowly.

festination an acceleration of gait seen in paralysis agitans or other nervous conditions.

fetid/foetid foul, offensive, disagreeable, stinking (odor).

fetor strong odor; strong stench.

fetor oris bad breath.

fever 1) a contagious and usually short-lived enthusiasm/eagerness. 2) an abnormally high body temperature. When periodic, fevers are described as quotidian (every day, or every 24 hours), tertian (every other day, or every 48 hours), quartan (every third day, or every 72 hours), or quintan (every fourth day, or every 96 hours).

fever blister see COLD SORE.

fibrinous stringy.

fibroid a tumor of muscular fibers. Resembling or composed of fibers or fibrous tissue.

fibroma a fibrous tumor.

fibrositis inflammation of fibrous tissue (a term used to denote aching, soreness, or stiffness in the absence of objective abnormalities).

ficus fig. May denote a fig wart or reddish, fleshy excrescence.

fidgets a state of restlessness.

Fiessinger-Leroy's syndrome (dermatostomatitis, Steven-Johnson Syndrome) see ERYTHEMA MULTIFORME.

fifty-millesimal potency (Q-potency, LMs) see POTENCY.

fig wart (condyloma) a wart which looks like a fig, or sprig of cauliflower and usually serves to indicate the presence of the sycotic miasm.

filament a delicate thread. 'Filamentous' would mean thin or stringy.

filariasis a disease caused by the presence of filaria (a genus of the Nematoda worm) living parasitically in the subcutaneous connective tissue and serous cavities of the host; it occurs in tropical and subtropical regions. Elephantiasis is an example of a disease caused by filaria.

filch to steal or pilfer.

filz lause pediculus pubis. Lice. 'Crabs'.

Fincke potency see POTENCY.

finesse delicacy of discrimination.

fissures deep cracks or splits in the skin due to bending or stretching dry, inelastic skin, as in athlete's foot and late atopic eczema.

fistula an abnormal passage or connection between two body cavities or to the surface, e.g., anal fistula, hepatic fistula. A sinuous ulcer.

fistula in ano anal fistula.

fistula Steno's duct (ductus parotideus, ductus incisivus) a fistula affecting Stensen's duct (the parotid duct, leading from the parotid gland, located near the ear, to the roof of the mouth).

flaccid lacking firmness; soft and limp, flabby.

flank the section of flesh between the last rib and the hip; the side.

flash phenomenon see NEURAL THERAPY.

flat repertorisation a term of recent appearance which simply refers to finding the simillimum through repertory consultation, namely repertorisation.

flatulence abdominal gas or flatus. The presence of an excessive amount of gas in the stomach and intestines. The first 'modern' book on flatulence was written in 1582 by the Flemish researcher and physician Jean de Feyens (*De Flatibvs Humanum corpus molestantibus*). Before this, Hippocrates and others theorized that flatus was caused by the inhabitation of the human body by animal or nature spirits. Feyens correlated it to nature by comparing it to the atmospheric movement of clouds and mists. He rightly recommended carminatives and offered nearly forty recipes in his book.

flatus gas in the stomach or intestine; expelled gas from the anus.

fleck typhus see TYPHUS.

Fletcherizing the practice of completely chewing the food to the point where all taste of the food is lost. Advocated by American author Horace Fletcher (1849-1919), who also recommended that one abstain from eating food until driven to eating by hunger.

In 1895, Fletcher's health was so broken that he was unable to get health insurance. He began a study of nutrition, finding that if he chewed his food very thoroughly his health improved. He lived on food that cost him eleven cents a day and consisted of milk, maple sugar and prepared cereals eaten under his rules, namely: chew all the taste out of solid food until it has become liquified, eat only when hungry, sip and taste all liquids which have taste, and never eat when angry or worried. The public nick-named him 'The Great Masticator'. He combined his thoughts on masti-cation and positive thinking into a book entitled *Physiolic Optimism* (1908) and also wrote *How I Became Young at 60*, as well as several other books. As you may well imagine, he regained his health and on his fiftieth birthday took a 200 mile ride on his bicycle. 'Fletcherism' and 'fletcherize' are associated terms.

flexion the act of bending; the condition of being bent.

flexor carpi ulnaris one of two muscles which flexes the wrist joint.

flexor surfaces the surfaces exposed when the palm is turned upward; also the back of the legs (the calf and hamstring muscles).

floaters see MUSCAE VOLITANTES.

floccillation (floccitatio) see CARPHOLOGIA.

flocculation test see HENSHAW FLOCCULATION TEST.

flocculent having a fluffy or woolly appearance. Made up of or containing woolly masses. Flaky.

flocculi flaky masses resembling tufts of cotton or wool.

florid of a bright red color, noting certain cutaneous lesions.

flower essence a general term for a liquid prepared by immersing a flower in water and then exposing it to sunlight or heat. The healing properties from that particular flower become infused into the liquid. The liquid is then bottled for later use. See BACH FLOWER REMEDIES.

fluor albus (leucorrhea, whites) a white or yellowish purulent discharge from the vagina, "resembling water in which meat has been washed."

flux the menstrual flow. To flow or cause to purge, evacuate or cleanse. A morbid discharge of fluid matter. 'Blood flux' refers to dysentery.

fluxion potency see POTENCY.

fly-blisters (cantharides, 'Spanish flies', *Cantharis/Lytta vesicatoria*) a bleeding method in vogue in the 1800s along with cupping, leeching, scari-fication and venesection. A paste was made of the powdered flies (also used was the potato fly/bug/beetle, *Leptinotersa decemlineata)* and ap-plied as a plaster. It supposedly operated as a general stimulant by provok-ing the physical loss of fluids via the blisters created. It was said to relieve torpor by diverting blood away from the area of inflammation to the blis-tering area. It could alter the circulation in feverish patients and perhaps act as a counter-irritant.

Oftentimes once the skin was blistered with the plaster, a cantharide ointment was applied to keep the blisters 'running' for as much as five days. Turpentine as well as the actual powdered beetles may also have been added at various points.

Tincture of cantharides was used internally as a diuretic, yet often produced uncomfortable symptoms such as abdominal pain, bloody urine, dysuria, and cardiac arrhythmias (due to the cantharidin), leading to death. As it was a powerful lower urinary tract irritant (topically or internally), it could induce prolonged and profound erections and hence its reputation as an aphrodisiac. Also the source of the remedy *Cantharis*.

foetida foul smelling; having a rank or foul odor.

foetor ex ore (halitosis) offensive breath; bad breath.

follicle a simple tubular gland. An old term for a lymphatic nodule. A crypt or minute cul-de-sac or lacuna, such as the depression in the skin from which the hair emerges.

follicular pharyngitis (granular pharyngitis, clergyman's sore throat) a form of chronic pharyngitis (inflammation of the pharynx) in which the mucous membrane has a granular appearance.

follicular tonsillitis inflammation of the tonsil whereby the tonsillar canals are inflamed and project as whitish points from the surface of the tonsil.

folliculitis inflammation of follicles (simple tubular glands). Sebaceous follicles are probably the commonest follicles to be affected; they are small sebaceous glands of the skin which open into the hair follicles.

fomentation the application of heat and moisture to a part to relieve pain, reduce inflammation or induce perspiration.

fomites (plural of fomes) a substance such as clothing which is capable of absorbing and transmitting disease contagium. Clothes which have been in contact with an ill person.

fontanelle a membranous space between the cranial bones in fetal life and infancy. There are six fontanelles in the human fetus, so called because they move in a rhythmical fashion, much like a fountain. Even in adults the cranial bones move to a rhythm and can be manipulated. At one time 'fontanelle' may also have meant an issue (see ISSUE) or an artificial ulcer created for the discharge of blood (humors) from the body. The word comes from the French *fontaine,* meaning 'fountain'.

foot and mouth disease (hoof and mouth disease, aphthae epizooticae, epidemic stomatitis, aphthous fever) an infectious disease of cattle characterized by a vesicular eruption in the mouth and pharynx, chill, fever, and marked prostration; the disease is communicable to man.

foot rot a contagious disease, in sheep and cattle, characterized by chronic inflammation of the foot, ulceration, softening of the hoof, discharge of a fetid odor, and lameness.

foramen a perforation or opening, especially in a bone.

foreboding a dark sense of impending evil; a premonition or apprehension.

formication a sensation as if ants were running over the skin.

fortnight a period of 14 days.

fossa Douglasii (Douglas' cul-de-sac, excavatio rectouterina) a pocket formed by the deflection of the peritoneum from the rectum to the uterus.

fossa navicularis the terminal dilated portion of the urethra in the glans penis. The area of the expanded urethra. The cavity behind the vaginal opening.

fossa a pit, cavity or shallow groove as in an organ of the body. A depression usually more or less longitudinal in shape.

Fothergill's pain (facial neuralgia, tic douloureux, Fothergill's disease) see FACEACHE. After the Quaker John Fothergill (1712-1780), a British physician who called attention to the effect weather has on certain diseases. He also gave the first clear description of migraine in 1777.

Fowler's solution (ague-drop, potassium arsenite solution, liquor potassii arsenitis, arsenical solution) a solution used in malarial affections and chorea, as a convenient way of administering arsenic. Introduced by T. Fowler, an English physician (1736-1801).

foudroyant dazzling, stunning, or overwhelming.

Fourierism a social structure espoused by French author and socialist reformer F.M. Charles Fourier (1772-1837), according to which society would be organized into associations large enough for industrial and social needs.

foxglove *(Digitalis purpurea)* 'foxglove' is derived from the Anglo-Saxon word *foxesglew* or fox music, in reference to the ancient musical instrument it resembled. The dried leaf of this plant was introduced into medicine by British physician Withering, in 1785. Its activity is due to the principle glycoside, digitoxin. It is a strong heart stimulant which increases the contractility of the heart tissue. It also lengthens the refractory period of the heart. As a result of these two actions the heart may diminish in size.

fraenum/frenum a fold of tissue or mucous membrane that limits the movement of any organ.

framboesia (yaws, pian) an infectious, nonvenereal disease of the tropics caused by *Treponema pertenue*; characterized by an initial cutaneous lesion (mother yaw) on the hand or foot followed by one or more crops of multiple, crusted raspberry-like lesions. As the disease progresses it may affect bone, usually about the nose and mouth. This is the tertiary stage or gangosa. It does not produce central nervous system or cardiovascular involvement. Serologic (serum) tests for syphilis are positive.

Frederick's disease locomotor ataxia in children. See LOCOMOTOR ATAXIA.

fremitus a palpable vibration. A vibratory sensation conveyed to the hand resting on the chest or other part of the body.

frog tongue a salivary tumor under the tongue. See RANULA.

frontal eminence the frontal bone on either side of the forehead.

frowsy untidy.

fulgurating lightning-like; used to describe sudden excruciating pain.

fulguration (electrocoagulation) the destruction of tissue, usually by means of electricity. Here a special electrode is used which consists of a needle and probe. Sparks are discharged from the needle point directly into tissues. All sorts of skin growths can be removed in this way. 1 or 2 treatments are necessary to destroy small growths such as warts.

fulminant (fulgurant, foudroyant) occurring with great rapidity; lightning-like swiftness.

functional disease a disease which affects the healthy functioning of an organ or area without any change in structure or anatomy. See ORGANIC DISEASE, FUNCTIONAL MEDICINE.

functional medicine according to H.W. Schimmel, the leader/founder of this field, "functional medicine [FM] is a branch of the healing arts that deals with the bio-energetic events which precede and accompany the morphological and biochemical alterations of a disease. FM employs energy-oriented diagnostic methods for the evaluation and measurement of the function, bioenergetic status and of the regulatory capability of individual organs as well as of the connective tissues.FM methods aim to reveal the energetic events leading to an advanced diagnosis. It can be utilized then for the prevention of morphologic and biochemical disturbances of a disease or, in the face of a fully developed disease, it can provide the proper therapeutic guidance."—*Townsend Letter for Doctors* (Jan. 1995, p. 85)

Dr. Schimmel is the founder of the VEGATEST, an EAV test method, as well as the co-author of *Functional Medicine, Vol. I: The Origin and Treatment of Chronic Diseases* (Schimmel/Penzer, 1996, Haug.) See KERN MERIDIAN COMPLEXES.

FM is officially recognized in Germany and listed in health insurance manuals. FM recognizes the energetic *and* morphological aspects of disease as a holism. Physicians who practice this type of medicine almost always use electronic instrumentation (i.e., Voll, VEGA, SEG, etc) to diagnose and treat illness. This form of medicine falls under the broad category of Resonance homeopathy. Dr. Schimmel discovered, isolated, and analyzed resonance relationships between the homeopathic single remedies and complexes, organ structures, and microorganisms. He developed specific homeopathic remedy combinations to treat these as well as viral and fungal infections. The researcher Dr. M. Buthke conducted experiments in this area, culturing the pathogenic microorganisms of patients on agar diffusion plates and then exposing them to Resonance Remedies, which had a fungicidal effect.

Royal R. Rife (1888-1977) conducted seminal work in the mid-1900s on the energy frequencies of microbes. By increasing the intensity of a frequency which resonated with microbes, Rife would increase their natural oscillations, causing them to distort and disintegrate. Rife termed this frequency the mortal oscillatory rate (MOR), which did no harm to surrounding tissues.

Dr. Jeffrey Bland is active in this field. Consult his CD 'Essentials of Functional Medicine'.

functional medicine complexes complex homeopathic remedies based on Dr. med. Helmut Schimmel's theories and researches into resonance homeopathy (EAV, etc.)

fundus the part farthest removed from the opening of the organ. The posterior portion of the interior of the eyeball. A 'red fundus' means that when the physician looks into the eyeball he sees that the back portion of the eyeball's interior is red and inflamed.

fundus oculi the posterior portion of the inner surface of the eyeball.

fungoid fungus-like.

fungus hematode a spongoid or soft cancer. One source says a medullary sarcoma. A soft, bleeding malignant tumor which may appear as if it were a fungus.

funicular neuralgia nerve pain originating from a bundle of nerves. It is hard to be more specific as funicular (funiculus) is such a broad term.

funnel-breast/chest a state in which the chest narrows sharply toward the abdomen.

furfuraceous branny, scaly, scurfy; composed of small scales, like dandruff.

furor uterinus (L., 'uterine madness/frenzy/passion') see NYMPHOMANIA.

furuncle a boil or cutaneous abscess usually as a result of an infection to a hair follicle or a cutaneous gland.

furuncular otitis inflammation of the inner ear caused by a furuncle/boil.

furunculosis a condition marked by the presence of furuncles (small boils, 2mm or less in diameter), or a condition in which new crops of furuncles follow repeatedly after the healing of preceding crops.

furunculus malignans see CARBUNCLE.

G G G G G G G

gait the manner of walking, running, stepping or pacing, e.g., a rambling/rapid/ spastic gait.

galactogogue an agent promoting the secretion or production of milk.

galactophorous ducts the excretory ducts of the glands of the female breast, which terminate in the papilla or nipple.

galactopyretus see MILK FEVER.

galactorrhea an excessive flow of milk. A continued discharge of milk from the breast in the intervals of nursing or after the child has been weaned.

gald (galde, gawld, gauld) a painful swelling, pustule or blister. A sore or wound produced by rubbing or chafing. May also refer to a state of mental irritation or exasperation.

galloping consumption (phthisis florida) a rapidly spreading form of pulmonary tuberculosis.

galvanic (Voltaic) pertaining to galvanism, which is direct current electricity produced by a chemical reaction rather than electricity produced by heat, friction or induction. 'Galvanization' is the transmission of a direct current of low force through any part of the body for the purpose of diagnosing or treating disease. Here low voltage (40-80v) and low to medium amperage are used.

Luigi Galvani (1736-1798), an Italian physiologist, conducted experiments with frogs showing that electricity can be produced from chemical action/reactions. Unrelated but interesting is the fact that electrical currents can be set up in the mouth when different metals are used in dental restorative work. Here electrical potential differences of 500 millivolts can occur. See HIGH FREQUENCY CURRENT, FARADIC.

Another variety of healing with electrical current is the use of high-frequency current. Here a low amperage, high voltage, high frequency current is passed through a specific part of the body, which increases the volume of blood and lymph flowing to those parts of the body. This results in increased oxygenation and nutritive stimulation of tissues. It also aids in the removal of waste products. There are two forms of this type of current, that of Tesla and of D'Arsonval. The Tesla Coil releases a high voltage, low amperage current, the D'Arsonval uses the opposite.

Nikola Tesla (1856-1943) is a very interesting figure in the history of electricity and physics. He held many patents for motors, transmission of electric power, lighting, high frequency apparatus and circuit controllers, radio, telemechanics, turbines, etc.

ganglion a group of nerve cells, such as one located outside the brain or spinal cord.

ganglium tendinosum a ganglionic cyst attached to the sheath of a tendon.

gangrene death of a part due to a lack of blood supply in that area. It is usually due to disease or injury. The decomposition of organic matter under the influence of microbes accompanied by the development of disagreeable odors (putrefaction). The products of putrefaction are gases (ammonia, methane), acids (acetic, lactic, butyric), and other toxic substances such as indoles, phenol, and ptomaines (cadaverine, putrescine, etc.).

gaol fever see TYPHUS.

garrulous loquacious, talkative, wordy.

gastralgia stomach pain or discomfort.

gastric fever (febris gastrica) a fever in which the inflammation of the stomach is the primary characteristic.

gastricism (dyspepsia) upset stomach.

gastritis inflammation of the stomach.

gastroataxia (sordes gastricae) a derangement of the stomach.

gastrodynia stomach pain or ache.

gastroenteritis (enterogastritis) inflammation of the stomach and intestine. Symptoms include fever, abdominal cramps, nausea/vomiting, diarrhea, and headache.

gastromalacia a softening of the walls of the stomach.

gastroptosis prolapse or a downward displacement of the stomach.

gathered breast inflammation and suppuration of the breast which is particularly apt to occur during nursing. *Bryonia* is almost a specific in this case.

gavage the administration of liquid nourishment through the stomach tube.

gemmotherapy a method of drainage (see DRAINAGE) in which glycerine macerates are prepared in the 2X potencies from fresh buds of certain trees or vegetable tissues in the process of growing and dividing. This form of therapy is thought to stimulate similar processes in the various organs of the body.

general symptoms those symptoms which pertain to the patient as a whole, e.g., "I feel better in the summer, or with warmth." See entry under SYMPTOMS.

"Among the generals, the symptoms of the first grade are, *if well marked,* the *mental symptoms.* These take the highest rank, and a strongly-marked mental symptom will always rule out any number of poorly-marked symptoms of lesser grade. Second in grade, after the mental symptoms, and his reaction to mental environment, come, *if well marked,* such general symptoms of the patient as his reactions, *as a whole,* to bodily environment: *to times and seasons, to heat and cold, to damp and dry, to storm and tempest, to position, pressure, motion, jar, touch, etc.*

"The third-grade general symptoms are the *cravings* and *aversions.* But to be elevated to such rank they must not be mere likes and dislikes, but longings and loathings.

"Then next in importance comes, in women, the *menstrual state,* i.e., general aggravation of symptoms *before, during and after* the menses. Of lower rank comes the question of menses *early, late* and *excessive.*"—

M. Tyler & Sir John Weir, *Repertorising.*

genodermatosis congenital anomalies/disorders of the skin.

genu the knee.

genupectoral The knee-to-chest position.

genu valgum (tibia valga, genu introrsum, genu inversum, knock-knee) an inward curve of the femur and stretching of the internal lateral ligament of the knee-joint, occurring as a result of an unnatural growth of the inner condyle. Thus the knees come close together and the feet are widely separated.

genu varum (bandy-leg, tibia vara, genu arcuatum, genu eversum, genu excurvatum, genu extrorsum, bow-legs) a wide separation of the knees, with the legs bowed outward. The tibia and femur are bowed in proportion to the severity of the condition.

genus epidemicus the combined symptoms of a large group of people afflicted with a disease or epidemic. This combined symptom list is then used to find the remedy best suited to treating those persons so afflicted without having to devote the time necessary to repertorize each and every person. It is sort of an 'epidemic simillimum'.

The 'remedy epidemicus' is a remedy found to be curative in a majority of people suffering from the same disease (as in epidemics). Thus it is possible to administer the remedy to a vast number of people without taking each person's case history.

Hahnemann used genus epidemicus in 1799 with an outbreak of scarlet fever. "Usually the physician does not immediately perceive the complete picture of the epidemic in the first case that he treats, since each collective disease reveals itself in the totality of its signs and symptoms only after several cases have been closely observed. Nevertheless, an observant physician can often come so close after seeing only one or two patients that he becomes aware of the characteristic picture of the epidemic and can already find its appropriate homeopathic remedy."—*Organon*, Aphorism 101.

Max Stoll (1742-1787) of Swabia and Thomas Sydenham (1624-1689), the Father of English Medicine, did seminal work on this subject and could have influenced the thinking of Hahnemann. Sydenham, one of the main founders of epidemiology, espoused his theory of 'epidemic constitutions', maintaining that "contagious diseases are influenced by cosmic or atmospheric influences which may change their type—that they may spring from miasms, from the bowels of the earth, that they may have long periods of evolution and seasonal variations, and that some diseases may be mere variants or subvarieties of others."—*History of Medicine*, 4th (Garrison, p. 270)

German measles see RUBELLA.

Gerson therapy a method of cancer treatment developed by German born physician Max Gerson (1881-1959). In advance of conventional medicine, Gerson advocated a healthy diet and the elimination of toxins. He prohibited smoking, alcohol, animal fat, smoked and pickled foods. His suggested diet included an abundance of fruits, carrot juice, vegetables (13 glasses of freshly squeezed vegetable and fruit juices, one glass consumed every hour) and foods containing Vitamin C, fiber and beta-carotene. He also advocated coffee enemas. His method of treatment evolved out of his successful results with treating skin tuberculosis through low-salt dietary management. *A Cancer Therapy* (M. Gerson, 1958)

Gerson first used his diet for cancer in 1928. Another important aspect of his approach concerned the balance of potassium and sodium in the body. He sought to eliminate dietary sodium and replace it with potassium, thereby altering the internal environment which supported the tumor.

Other cancer therapies flourished, two of the more popular being those of Contreras and Hoxsey. Ernesto Contreras used laetrile, a modified vegan diet, proteolytic enzymes and antioxidant supplements. The latter primarily relied on botanical agents—the Hoxsey Formula—to combat cancer. See Harry Hoxsey's *You Don't Have to Die* (1956). The Hoxsey formula has been in use for nearly 100 years and consists of potassium iodide, licorice root, red clover flowers, burdock root, stillingia root, berberis root, poke root, cascara amarga or sagrada, prickly ash bark, and buckthorn bark.

Another doctor, albeit lesser known, William D. Kelley, DDS, publicly offered his method ('Kelley ecology') after he used it to recover from his own metastatic pancreatic cancer. In principle, it is basically like the Gerson treatment except with a greater reliance on pancreatic enzymes. Actor Steve McQueen tried Kelley's method when he developed cancer, but he ultimately succumbed. Kelley wrote *One Answer to Cancer: An Ecological Approach to the Successful Treatment of Malignancy* (1969). A New York physician, Nicholas Gonzalez, championed Kelley's work and blended it with his own theories about typology, namely sympathetic types and parasympathetic types (*One Man Alone: An Investigation of Nutrition, Cancer, and William Donald Kelley*, 1987).

L. Burton, G. Naessens, E. Revici, S. L. K. Csatary, G.H. Earp-Thomas, R. Burzynski, and Wm. B. Coley (1862-1936) are other personalities of significance within the anti-cancer movement. Iscador, an injectable preparation from the mistletoe plant, is a popular anti-cancer agent in Europe. See COLEY'S TOXINS, ESSIAC.

See James P. Carter's interesting *Racketeering in Medicine: The Suppression of Alternatives* (1992).

gerontoxon see ARCUS SENILIS.

GHP see GOOD HOMEOPATHIC PRACTICE/SCORE.

giddy characterized by instability or hilarity; fickle, wild, thoughtless, heedless. Also having lost the power of preserving balance of the body and thus wavering and inclined to fall.

gill a unit of measure, approximately 1/4 of a pint.

gin drinker's liver (hob-nailed liver) see NUTMEG LIVER.

gingival referring to the gums.

glabella the hairless space between the eyebrows. The smooth prominence, most marked in the male, on the frontal bone above the root of the nose between the eyebrows.

gladiolus (corpus sterni) body of the sternum (breastbone). The middle and largest part of the sternum.

glairy resembling the white of an egg, as in 'glairy mucus'.

glanders (farcy, equinia) a highly contagious acute or chronic disease of horses and mules communicable to dogs, goats, sheep, and man but not to cows. It is caused by *Malleomyces mallei*. Symptoms produced are fever, inflammation of mucous membranes (particularly of the nose), enlargement and hardening of the regional lymph nodes, and the formation of nodules which have a tendency to coalesce and then degenerate to form deep ulcers. In man the disease usually runs an acute febrile course and terminates fatally.

glandular fever (infectious mononucleosis) an infectious disease of childhood, characterized chiefly by fever, swelling of the cervical lymph nodes, and enlargement of the liver and spleen; it lasts usually two or three weeks and has a favorable prognosis.

glans the apex (head) of the penis. The very vascular body that forms the apex of the penis. A conical acorn-shaped structure.

Glauber's salt (vitriolated soda) hydrated sodium sulfate. In material doses, it was used as a cathartic in the 1800s. Listed in the homeopathic materia medica as *Natrum sulfuricum*. It was first introduced about 1650 by the German chemist J.R. Glauber, M.D. (1603-1668).

glaucoma a disease of the eye characterized by high fluid pressures within the eyeball, damaged retina, hardening of the eyeball, and partial or complete loss of vision.

gleet (blennorrhagia, blennorrhea) a slight mucopurulent discharge (usually the chronic stage of urethritis) from the urethra; or the disease which produces this discharge, also called chronic urethritis.

globule (pellet) the small round ball of sugar upon which the appropriate homeopathic dilution is impregnated. Before the medication is sprayed onto the globule/pellet it is often called 'placebo'. Once impregnated it becomes the medication and may be dissolved directly in the mouth or dissolved in water and then taken in teaspoon or tablespoon doses or sipped. The size of globules varies from a poppyseed to a pea and in homeopathic pharmaceutical terms are referred to as 10, 20, 30, 35, 40, 50, 60 (smallest to largest). Of course any size may be manufactured but these are the standard sizes in use. "I gave just one pellet of the No. X" means the practitioner gave one pellet, size 10 (poppyseed size).

globus hystericus (apopnixis) a sensation as if a ball was caught in the throat or as if the throat were compressed. Often a symptom of hysteria.

glomerulonephritis inflammation of the kidney. Here the primary disturbance is in the functional unit of the kidney, the glomerulus. Hypertension, convulsions, edema, nitrogen retention and acidosis may result.

glossitis inflammation of the tongue.

glossoplegia (glossolysis) paralysis of the tongue.

glottis 1) that area in which the vocal structures of the larynx may be found. 2) the small oblong aperture or opening between the vocal cords.

glucoside (glycoside) any member of a series of compounds which when hydrolyzed (broken down when allowed to react with water) yield a sugar and another compound.

gluteal referring to the buttocks.

glutei (gluteal, gluteus) pertaining to the buttocks.

glutinous adhesive, sticky, pasty.

glycosuria sugar in the urine.

goitre (goiter, bronchocele, struma) a chronic enlargement of the thyroid gland, not due to a neoplasm, occurring endemically in certain regions where iodine is deficient in the diet (especially mountainous regions) and sporadically elsewhere.

gonagra gout in the knee.

gonarthritis inflammation of the knee-joint.

gonarthrocace tuberculosis or inflammation of the knee-joint.

gonitis inflammation of the knee.

gonorrhea a specific infectious inflammation of the mucous membrane of the urethra and adjacent cavities, due to *Neisseria gonorrhoeae*. It is characterized by pain, burning urination, a profuse mucopurulent discharge, and may be accompanied by complications such as prostatitis, periurethral abscess, epididymitis, cystitis, purulent conjunctivitis. It may also cause arthritis, endocarditis, and salpingitis.

gonorrheal orchitis inflammation of the testes caused by gonorrhea.

Good Homeopathic Practice/Score a method or criteria for evaluating homeopathic cases, presentations and papers. This method has been suggested by Peter Konig, an Austrian homeopath. He offers a somewhat complex system of case scoring based on his 'Criteria of Quality and Comparison of Homoeopathic Prescriptions and Cases of Chronic Diseases'. For example, a case might be scored *GHP 5/10 (1,3)*. Briefly this would mean that the case has garnered 5 out of 10 points based on Konig's elaborate suggestions. The 1 refers to 'remarkably deep changes in the life of the patient are observed, maybe a complete and new orientation in life', while the 3 refers to 'a distinct homoeopathic initial reaction (initial aggravation) is observed.' It is too complicated to discuss here but is nevertheless interesting from many standpoints. One could glance at the 'case score' to get an idea of what the case was like. Consult 'A Proposal for a Good Homeopathic Score', P. Konig, *Homeopathic Links,* 9:4, p. 193-195, 1996.

gooseskin (cutis anserina, horripilation) gooseflesh, goosebumps.

gossypium genus of the plant from which cotton comes.

gracile slight or slender. Gracefully slender.

grafting the method, discovered by Korsakoff, of making medicated pellets from unmedicated pellets by placing a medicated pellet in contact with the unmedicated ones. It was found that all the pellets became medicated. This is not a preferred method of preparation as there is no quality assurance. Since this method has not been scientifically validated, the final product cannot be accurately evaluated. It is best to purchase remedies from homeopathic pharmacies; they are inexpensive and their quality is assured.

Grahamism the nutritional and wellness teachings espoused by the 19th century temperance leader, Sylvester Graham (1794-1851). Part of his life was devoted to traveling and lecturing on diet and lifestyle. He advocated whole grain breads and flours, plenty of vegetables and fruits, pure water, fresh air, daily exercise, as well as hard mattresses. Whole wheat flour or 'graham flour' became popular and 'graham crackers' are still well-known today.

His ideas were formulated into a 'Science of Human Life' which said that all illness could be prevented by proper personal hygiene. He stressed specific rules concerning diet, dress, sex, cleanliness, etc.

Wm. Alcott had similar ideas and was a contemporary of Graham. Alcott postulated that "meat 'atoms' were less stable than vegetable atoms because meat decomposes more quickly than vegetables in the body, thus linking a longer lifespan with a vegetarian diet."—*The Great American Medicine Show* (p. 63, 1991)

grain 1) the seed or seedlike fruit of the cereal grasses. 2) a minute portion or particle. 3) a unit of weight (abbreviated as gr.) approx. 65 milligrams, originally based on the weight of a 'grain of paradise'. Grains of paradise are the seeds of a reedlike herb from West Africa used as a flavor and carminative. They are pungent and contain paradol, which is related to ginerol.

grain itch see PRAIRIE ITCH.

Gram's solution/stain a mixture of iodine, potassium iodide in water and used to stain bacteria as an aid to identification, either Gram - or Gram +.

grand mal seizure (generalized epilepsy, major epilepsy, idiopathic epilepsy, epilepsia gravis) a form of epilepsy or seizure characterized by a loss of consciousness and tonic spasms of the muscles. Repetitive generalized clonic jerking follows, after which the individual is confused and then falls into a deep sleep.

granular pharyngitis (angina granulosa) see CLERGYMAN'S SORE THROAT.

granulated liver see CIRRHOSIS.

granulating forming small, fleshy, bead-like grains on the surface of a wound while healing, as in g. ulcers.

granulation formation into grains or granules. The formation of minute, rounded, fleshy projections on the surface of a wound in the process of healing.

granulocytopenia see AGRANULOCYTOSIS.

graphospasm see WRITER'S CRAMP.

gratis freely, free of charge.

gravedo frontal sinusitis.

gravel sandlike, granular calculi or stones in the gall bladder, kidney, or bladder. An unconsolidated mixture of uric acid and calcium oxalates/phosphates which forms the substance of urinary stones and often passes with the urine.

Graves' disease (exophthalmic goiter, thyrotoxicosis, Parry's disease, Basedow's disease, hyperthyroidism) a disease caused by excessive production of thyroid hormone and characterized by an enlarged thyroid gland, protrusion of the eyeballs (exophthalmos), tachycardia, nervous excitability, loss of weight, muscular weakness and a tendency to intense, acute flareups called thyroid crises or storms. There is excessive excretion of nitrogen and calcium leading to osteoporosis and disturbances in calcium metabolism.

Dr. R. J. Graves (1796-1853) observed and described this syndrome in 1835. He asked that his epitaph read, 'He fed fevers'.

gravid pregnant.

green vitriol ferrous sulfate. Often used to treat anemias.

green sickness see CHLOROSIS.

gressus gallinaceus the walk or gait of a domestic fowl or chicken.

gressus vaccinus the walk or gait of a cow.

gripe a sharp pain in the bowels, colic, tormina (severe colic or griping intestinal pain). Bellyache.

grippe (influenza, Russian influenza) the flu.

groats grains which have been dried, hulled and broken-up. With wheat groats the fragments are bigger than grits.

grocer's itch an obstinate psoriasis or eczema usually of the hands.

grosso modo 'in great form or manner'.

grub see COMEDO.

gruel a thin, watery porridge. For example, an oatmeal gruel is made in the following way: 1 oz. of finely ground oatmeal is boiled with 3-4 pints of water, strained and cooled. Pour off the clear liquid from the sediment and drink. To improve its flavor add sugar, lemon juice or wine.

grumous like a clot of blood; thick and viscid.

gulae the throat (or more precisely, the front part of the throat).

gullet pharynx and esophagus. The throat.

gumboil (parulis) an alveolar abscess. A small boil or abscess on the gum. The recurrent infection of the gums with boil formation.

gumma (pl. gummae) a tumor, usually of syphilitic origin, so called from the gummy nature of its contents. It is a well-defined mass a centimeter or more in diameter, with a tendency to encapsulation and surrounding fibrosis. It has a consistency of firm rubber or gum.

gutta a drop, roughly a minim of water, but varying greatly according to the nature of the liquid and the form of the vessel from which it falls.

gutta rosacea (carbuncled face) see ACNE ROSACEA. "His face is all bubukles and whelks, and knobs, and flames of fire."—Shakespeare.

gutta serena see AMAUROSIS.

guttatim drop by drop.

guttur the throat. 'Guttural' refers to sounds made in the throat.

gynatresia closure of the vagina by a thick membrane.

gynecomastia the presence in the male of large breasts.

gyrosa (sham-movement vertigo) dizziness accompanied by an impression as if the body was rotating or if objects were revolving around the body.

gyrospasm spasmodic rotatory movements of the head.

H H H H H H H

habromania (amenomania) delusional insanity in which the delusions are of a cheerful or joyous character.

haemalopia the effusion of blood into the eye. Blood-shot eye. *Nux vomica* is almost a specific for this condition.

haematidrosis 'bloody sweating'. The escape of blood into the sweat glands from the capillaries.

haematocele a blood tumor. Accumulation of blood in the scrotal tissues.

haematoma, hematoma a focalized leakage of blood which soon clots to form a solid mass and becomes encapsulated by connective tissue.

haematoporphyrinuria the presence of hematoporphyrin in the urine. An old term for a metabolic disorder of the porphyrins.

haemoderm the blood. The blood as a tissue.

haemoptoe bloody cough. See HEMOPTYSIS.

haemostatic stopping the flow of blood.

haggard appearing worn and exhausted. Emaciated, gaunt. Wild and unruly; uncontrolled.

Hahnemann, Samuel Christian Friedrich (1755-1843) the German (Saxon) born physician and pharmacist who founded homeopathy and is considered its father. He received his medical degree from Erlangen University in 1779 and developed his theories, publishing them in 1796 in Hufeland's *Journal* and then in his opus *Organon of Rational Medical Doctrine* (*Organon der Rationellen Heilkunde*; later editions were titled *Organon of Medical Art*), 1810, Dresden. Thereafter he gained many followers and detractors as the many moves he made in his lifetime testify to. He lived in Leipzig and while in Cothen was court physician to the Duke of Anhalt-Cothen. In 1835, he settled in Paris, living out the rest of his life teaching and practising his beloved homeopathy. His other important works are: *Materia Medica Pura* (6 vol., 1811-1821, Dresden), his four volume treatise on chronic disease, *Die Chronishen Krankheiten* (1828-1830, Dresden) and his *Lesser Writings* edited by J.E. Stapf (1829-1834, Dresden/Leipzig). See HUFELAND'S JOURNAL.

Hahnemannian one who practices homeopathy according to Hahnemann's dictates, viz. using the law of similars, the minimum dose, and the single dose. Also termed classical homeopathy. In repertorization Hahnemann attached primary importance to generals and modalities, strong evaluation based on the concomitants, the use of physical generals, and mentals to differentiate.

Hahnemann cocktail a liquid given to drunks who were brought into the Hahnemann College Hospital. It consisted of *Nux vomica* and *Capsicum,* 10 drops of each in a tablespoonful of spirits of ammonia.

Hahnemann schema (regional plan, 'symptomatology of a drug') the arrangement of rubrics in a repertory following a natural anatomical arrangement, namely mind, vertigo, head, eyes, vision ... back, extremities, sleep, chill, fever, perspiration, skin, generalities.

halitosis (foetor ex ore) bad breath.

Hallion's law the basis of organotherapy: the concept that extracts of a healthy organ, when administered to an ill person with a diseased organ, exert on that same organ a stimulating influence. For example, if it is found that the liver functioning of an alcoholic is severely compromised, liver extracts from healthy animal tissue may be given to 'remind' the diseased liver how to function or to support that functioning. See ORGANOTHERAPY.

halo the aura of majesty or glory surrounding a person, thing, or event. A circular band of colored light around a light source, as around the sun or moon. A red circle or boundary around skin eruptions. Though unrelated, *halo-* indicates salt or the sea, as in 'halobiont' (a plant or organism growing in a salty environment).

halloos shouts or calls of 'halloo', or simply to shout out to. Used to urge on hounds in a hunt.

halophagia salt eating. Craving for salt.

hankering longing for, craving, yearning.

hard palate the front portion of the roof of the mouth. It feels hard as compared to the rear portion of the roof of the mouth (soft palate).

hare-lip (labia leporina) a congenital fissure in the upper lip, often found in combination with a cleft palate.

hartshorn (aqua ammoniae, ammonium hydrate) ammonia water. Any volatile ammonium salt, such as the carbonate. *Cornu cervi*, the horn of a stag (hart), was the original source of ammonia or hartshorn spirit; now it is made synthetically. It is a mixture of ammonium bicarbonate and ammonium carbamate in water, which produces 30-34% ammonia and 45% carbon dioxide. It was used as a stimulant expectorant and reflex stimulant in doses of 200-600 mgs.

haruspicy divination through the study of the organs of a slaughtered animal.

Hashimoto's disease (struma, thyroiditis) a disease of the thyroid gland described by H. Hashimoto (1881-1934), a Japanese physician. It is the infiltration of the thyroid gland with lymphocytes, resulting in progressive destruction of thyroid tissue and thus hypothyroidism.

hauteur loftiness of manner or bearing; haughtiness of demeanor.

hawking an explosive expiration made to clear the throat of mucus.

healing crisis the point at which disease symptoms are at their worst and then the course of the disease can proceed in two directions: death or irreversible damage or recovery. A simple example of a healing crisis can be seen in the flu. A person slowly develops symptoms, which worsen to reach an apex. Then the sweat or flu breaks and the person goes on to recovery.

healing by first/second intention see UNION BY FIRST/SECOND INTENTION.

health (eucrasia) according to the World Health Organization (WHO), health is defined as 'a state of complete physical, psychic, and social well-being and not merely the absence of illnesses and infirmities'. See HOLISM.

"Health is a matter of perfect equilibrium, perfect balance; trifling circumstances may sway it, and even as seemingly trifling circumstances may sway it, so may it be balanced by the least possible in medication, which may, in conditions of perfect health, cause the same loss of balance, or a corresponding loss of equilibrium."—H.A. Roberts, *Principles and Art of Cure by Homoeopathy.*

heartburn (water brash, pyrosis) burning eructation. See WATER BRASH.

hebdomadal referring to a group of seven. A period of seven days, or a week.

hebephrenia a type of emotional syndrome which occurs in young persons around the age of puberty consisting of a regression of behavior to an infantile or primitive state. Silliness, unexplained laughter and smiling, masturbation, untidiness and seclusiveness are the primary manifestations. First described by Ewold Hecker (1843-1909).

Heberden's disease see ANGINA PECTORIS.

hebetude dullness, lethargy.

hectic habitual. A term often used to describe the constant fever of tuberculosis: an afternoon rise of temperature, accompanied by a flush on the cheeks, occurring in active tuberculosis. Of, relating to, or having an undulating fever, as in diseases such as tuberculosis or septicemia.

helcology the study of the cause, prevention, and treatment of ulcers.

helminthiasis the condition of having intestinal worms.

heloma (clavus, corn) a callosity on the hand or foot.

helleborism the treatment of disease by purging with hellebore, a drastic purge (both cathartic and emetic).

hematemesis vomiting of blood.

hematocele a tumor formed by the leakage and collection of blood in a part, especially in the scrotum or in the pelvis.

hematochyluria the presence of both blood and chyle in the urine.

hematoma auris (othematoma, insane ear) a blood-cyst or tumor of the ear. A purplish, rounded, hard swelling of the auricle, due to an effusion of blood between the cartilage and perichondrium; it may be the result of trauma or occur spontaneously in the insane.

hematoporphyrinuria the excretion of hematoporphyrin into the urine, occurring as a result of the decompostion of hemoglobin.

hematuria the presence of blood in the urine.

hemaxis blood-letting. See BLEEDING.

hemeralopia (day-sight, night-blindness) an inability to see at night. Vision which is better during the day. Compare NYCTALOPIA.

hemicrania migraine. Pain on one side of the head.

hemi-cranial referring to half of the head.

hemianopsia/s blindness in one half of the visual field. May be bilateral or unilateral.

hemiopia a defect of sight in which the person sees only one-half of an object.

hemiparesis a slight paralysis of one side of the body.

hemiplegia paralysis of one side of the body and of the opposite side of the face. Or simply paralysis of one side of the body.

hemming clearing the throat. Often used with 'hawing' (the sound made by a speaker during a pause to collect his thoughts). 'Hemming and hawing' thus means hesitating or stalling for time.

hemopathy (hematopathy) a blood disease. Any abnormal condition or disease of the blood or blood-forming tissues.

hemophilia (bleeder's disease) a potentially fatal sex-linked, hereditary disease occurring only in men but carried by women, characterized by prolonged coagulation time and thus abnormal bleeding.

hemoptysis bloody expectoration from the larynx, trachea, bronchi, or lungs.

hemoralopia (hemeralopia) a defect of vision in which the person sees perfectly well all day, but in evening or morning perceives little or nothing at all. Compare NYCTALOPIA.

hemorrhage bleeding. The escape of blood from blood vessels. Most commonly capillary hemorrhage, as in nose bleeds or in the lungs.

hemorrhagic diathesis a constitutional tendency towards bleeding.

hemorrhagic fever (Manchurian hemorrhagic fever, Korean hemorrhagic fever) a condition characterized by an acute onset of headache, chills and high fever, sweating, thirst, photophobia, coryza, cough, myalgia, arthralgia, and abdominal pain with nausea and vomiting. This phase is then followed by capillary hemorrhages, edema, oliguria and shock.

hemorrhagica (hemorrhage) bleeding; the escape of blood from a torn or injured blood vessel.

hemorrhoids anal-rectal varicose veins.

hemosialemesis the spitting up of blood and saliva.

Hensel's tonicum an iron preparation consisting of equal parts of the ferric and ferrous oxide salts. Hensel created a number of physiological preparations: Haematin Iron 1-5, Precipitated Sulphur 1-5, Phosphate of Calcium Magnesium 1-5, Physiological Salts, Amorphous Silicic acid 1-5, Physiological Earths 1-5, and Nerve Salt.

Hensel's Physiological Theory for Treatment was at first thought to be the same as Schuessler's, but it is the opposite. Whereas Schuessler says cell health needs to be built up, Hensel argued that cells are part of a continued consumption and mutation of substances. Health rests on transmutation of the individual: "Unless substances are used up, there can be no renewed growth and the peculiarity and law of animal life lies just in this as indeed Schuessler, contradicting himself, concedes when he says: 'By the side of the origin of new cells the destruction of the old ones by the infuence of oxygen takes place.' Nevertheless he rests on the declaration of Virchow: 'The essence of disease is the changed cell.' " Hensel was not a homeopath. His major work was *Macrobiotic: Our Diseases and Our Remedies; for Practical Physicians and People of Culture* (c. 1883).

Henshaw flocculation test (serum flocculation test) a test, developed by George Russell Henshaw, M.D. (1896-1985) in the middle of the 20th century, to aid in the selection of the remedy. A visible flocculation zone (looks like fluffy cotton) develops in the serum when in contact with the correct homeopathic remedy. In Dr. Henshaw's researches he used this test to confirm or differentiate between well-chosen remedies. It was also used to determine the ideal potency. Later he changed the name of the test to Serum Remedy Sensitivity Test. He published a seven page preliminary report, 'A New Method of Determining the Indicated Remedy by a Flocculation Test of the Serum', in the *JAIH*, Sept. 1932. Garth W. Boericke also conducted research in the area: 'A Lipoid Flocculation Test for the Selection of the Homeopathic Remedy' (*The Hahnemannian*, Journal of the Homeopathic Medical Society of the State of Pennsylvania, Oct/Dec., 1956, p. 120.)

hepar adiposum fatty liver. See CIRRHOSIS.

hepatalgia liver pain; pain in that region.

hepatic referring to the liver.

hepatitis inflammation of the liver caused by infectious or toxic agents, characterized by jaundice, hepatomegaly, fever, and other systemic manifestations.

hepatization the conversion of tissue into a firm, jelly-like substance resembling the liver; usually used to refer to the lungs during pneumonia.

herbaceous referring to a plant with a non-woody stem which dies down at the end of a growing season; or referring to an herb (a plant with medicinal qualities); or green and leaflike in appearance or texture.

Hering's Law the concept that during homeopathic treatment of a disease, symptoms disappear in an orderly manner. That is, symptoms improve from above downwards, from vital to less vital organs, from the most recent to earliest symptoms and the symptoms disappear in reverse order to their appearance. It was first described by Constantine Hering (1800-1880) in his preface to Hahnemann's *Chronic Diseases* (1845). In this preface, Hering describes his observations on how diseases progress to a cure.

J.T. Kent coined the term Hering's Law (of Cure), when he described the progress of cure in his lectures. Actually as more and more clinical data is analyzed one finds that, "With the simillimum most symptoms begin to improve simultaneously and disappear in the reverse order of their appearance, and not necessarily from above downwards and from inside outwards."—Andre Saine, *Simillimum* (1991, 4:4, p.35).

hermeneutics a philosophical method that deals with the interpretation of the historical, social, psychological, etc. aspects of our world.

herpes 'a spreading skin eruption'. An eruption of groups of deep-seated vesicles on red, inflamed bases.

herpes circinatus/bullosis (dermatitis herpetiformis, dermatitis multiformis, Duhring's disease) a chronic disease of the skin marked by a severe, extensive, itching eruption of vesicles and papules which occur in groups; spontaneous healing rarely occurs except in children. Relapses are common.

herpes labialis (herpes facialis, cold sore, fever blister) herpes of the lips. A form of herpes simplex, an affection marked by the occurrence of one or more deep vesicles on the border of the lips, external nares, or on the glans penis or vulva.

herpes preputialis herpes of the prepuce (the free fold of skin that covers the head/glans of the penis).

herpes progenitalis herpes simplex of the genitals.

herpes simplex an infection by the herpes simplex virus *(Herpesvirus hominis)* marked by the eruption of one or more groups of vesicles on the border of the lips, at the external nares, or on the glans, prepuce, or vulva. Such infection commonly reappears during other febrile illnesses or even physiologic states such as menstruation. Also called, according to site, a cold sore on the lips, h. facialis, h. genitalis, h. preputialis, etc.

herpes zoster (zona, shingles, cruels, ignis sacer) an acute painful inflammatory disease of the skin, consisting of grouped vesicles corresponding in distribution to the course of the cutaneous nerves.

herpes tonsurans (porrigo furfurans, tinea tonsurans, tinea capitis) ringworm of the scalp; a fungus infection caused by species of *Microsporum* or *Trichophyton*.

herpetic vulvitis a herpes-like eruption of the vulva.

herpetic herpes-like. Having the characteristics of the herpes syndrome.

Hertoghe's syndrome the loss of hair at the sides of the eyebrows.

hetaera (pl. hetaerae) a concubine or courtesan. An educated slave.

heteroisopathics a therapeutic method consisting of giving the ill person remedies prepared from substances in his environment which appear to play a role in his illness.

heteropathic (allopathic) the treatment of disease by administering medications or therapies which produce different symptoms in healthy subjects from those of the disease being treated. See ALLOPATHY.

heu prisca fides 'oh, old fashioned trust' (Latin).

hidebound (diffuse symmetrical scleroderma) with rigid, hard, thickened skin.

hidrose (hyperhidrosis, sudoresis) excessive sweating.

hidrosis pedum excessive sweating of the feet.

'high flyers' ('transcendentalists') a term used in the late 1800s by proponents of low-potency homeopathy when they referred to high potency believers.

hilar glands glands at the hilum of the lungs, that area where blood vessels and bronchial tubes enter the lungs, at the level of the 4th or 5th thoracic vertebrae. The hilar glands are not glands per se, but lymph nodes. The term 'hilar glands' was coined in the late 19th century and is actually a misnomer. (This, no doubt, has happened quite a bit in the past, e.g., Peyer's glands.)

hilarity noisy merriment, joyousness, glee, gaiety.

hilum (hilus) a depression at the edge or on the part of an organ where the nerves and vessels enter and leave.

hippocratic (facies hippocratica, facies cadaverica) an appearance of the face, first described by Hippocrates, indicative of the rapid approach of death. The nose is pinched, temples hollow, eyes sunken, ears leaden and cold, lips relaxed and the skin pale.

Hippocrates of Cos (c.460-c.357 BCE) was a Greek physician who traveled widely in the eastern Mediterranean and is considered the father of medicine. Little is actually known of this important teacher yet his influence was immediate and long-lasting. He left a vast amount of writings ('Hippocratic Corpus'), much of which was probably written by others. The best known of his works, *Aphorisms*, is probably genuinely Hippocratic. The 'Hippocratic Oath', still the oath taken by physicians in this country, is the most widely known of his writings and consists of two parts: the first is a covenant concerning the relationship of the apprentice to the teacher and the obligations the pupil has to his teacher; the second constitutes the ethical code of the physician.

Hirschberg's test a test designed to determine the amount of strabismus in a patient. It is estimated from the position of the corneal reflection of a candle flame or flashlight held one foot from the patient's eye. The clinician places his own eye near the light source and looks just over it. From the German ophthalmologist J. Hirschberg (1843-1925). See STRABISMUS.

Hirschsprung's disease a habitual constipation of young children due to enormous congenital hypertrophy and dilatation of the lower portion of the colon. The disease is named after the Danish physician Harold Hirschsprung (1830-1916), who described it in 1887. However, Dr. F. Ruysch (1638-1731), a Dutch physician, mentioned it (case #92) in his treatise some 170 years before Hirschsprung!

hirsute covered or coated with hair; hairy.

hirsutism a condition characterized by growth of hair in unusual places and in unusual amounts.

hob-nail liver see CIRRHOSIS.

Hodgkin's disease (pseudo-leukemia) cancer of the lymph nodes and system. A chronic, progressive, usually fatal, inflammatory disease characterized by enlargement of the lymph nodes, spleen, and often the liver and kidneys. Occurs twice as often in men as in women.

Hodgson's disease an abnormal dilation of the aortic arch associated with aortic valve insufficiency. Joseph Hodgson (1798-1869), a British physician, first described this heart disease in 1815.

Hoffman's anodyne (compound ether spirit NF IX) a mixture of ethyl oxide, alcohol, and ethereal oil (a volatile liquid consisting of equal volumes of heavy oil of wine and ether), used as a carminative to expel flatulence in teaspoonful-sized doses.

holism (organicism, wholism) a belief system based on the doctrine that the individual (or situation) must be studied or viewed as a whole (physically, emotionally, mentally, and spiritually). Thus, treating the ill person must be based on this premise. Holistic medicine is based on the awareness of Oneness. To quote Dr. R. Ornstein, a pioneer of the holistic model: "We are psycho-physiological beings animated by spirit. . . We are a unity of spirit, mind and body, where rhythm, melody, and harmony permeates a multidimensional universe. The Universe is a hologram, a mental construct, a creation of consciousness itself." Along this line R. Twentyman, a British philosopher and homeopath, made this comment about the homeopathic remedy: "The mirror image changes consciousness." A very early examination of holistic health was Dr. Abraham ben Isaac Wallich's *Sepher Refu'ot (Harmonia Wallichis Medica)*, published in 1700. In this book he endeavored to show that diseases of the spirit correspond to those of the body and require similar treatment.

homaccord see POTENCY CHORD.

homar short for *Homarus*, the digestive fluid of the lobster.

homeopathic surgery an archaic term used by homeopathic surgeons who performed surgical operations and used homeopathic remedies to "control erysipelas, fever, and other sequences in surgery, lessening the mortality and making recovery possible in otherwise fatal cases."

Famous homeopathic surgeons of yesteryear include W.T. Helmuth, C.E. Fisher, C. Adams, C.M. Beebe, W.H. Bishop, H.R. Chislett, N.W. Emerson, W.E. Green, J.E. James, J.M. Lee, T.L. Macdonald, W.B. Morgan, G.H. Palmer, S.B. Parsons, E.H. Pratt, G.W. Roberts, J.K. Sanders, G.F. Shears, W.B. Van Lennep, C.E. Walton, D.G. Wilcox, S.F. Wilcox, H. Wilson, and M. Macfarlan.

homeopathy (homoeopathy, *homoopathie*) a holistic therapeutic medical science based upon the teachings of Hahnemann. The primary precept, the law of similars, is used to treat ill persons (animals, also) using minute doses of potentized substances. Other concepts central to homeopathy include Hering's Law, symptom classification, hierarchy of symptoms, potencies, repertory use, case taking, materia medica, and various models which attempt to explain disease, constitutions, typology, etc.

Succinctly, homeopathy is a therapeutic medical science which holistically treats illness and inherent constitutional problems by applying the 'like cures like' principle and using minute quantities of specially prepared substances; these substances can be from the plant, animal, or mineral kingdoms. *Simplex, simile, minimum* (single remedy, law of similars, minimum dose) are the three principles on which homeopathy is based.

It has been suggested that Moses was the most ancient healer to use homeopathic principles. From the Bible: "The Hebrew came to Mara, where the water was bitter. Some complained: 'What shall we drink?' Moses prayed and after the prayer he threw a bitter branch into the bitter water; and the water turned sweet!—For God is not like the humans, who can soothe the bitter only with sweet: with the bitter he makes the bitter sweet."—*Illustrierte Geschichte der Medizin* (1990, p. 2237, as communicated in *Homoeopathic Links*, 1/91, p. 22).

See also the introductory essay on homeopathy.

homeoprophylaxis the administration of homeopathic remedies to induce in the patient an immunity against a particular disease.

homeops a term popular in the 1800s which allopaths used to refer to homeopaths.

homeostasis a state of physiological equilibrium produced by a balance of functions and of chemical composition within an organism.

homeovitic a term coined by Eliz. Bellhouse to describe how her flower remedies, Vita Florum, worked. A 'like vitality' principle.

hominy a coarse corn meal.

homologous having the same form or function.

homotoxicology an integration of the information provided by the basic medical sciences with the principles of homeopathy in order to create l) a greater understanding of health and disease, and 2) remedies of a more curative activity. Homotoxicology is, according to adherents, a bridge between allopathic and homeopathic medicine. There is no easy definition of homotoxicology but in general, complex remedies are used rather than single and they may include any of the following: potentized enzymatic catalysts, suis-organ preparations, extensive nosode preparations, potentized allopathic drugs, homeopathic remedies in potency chords and complex formulations.

Homotoxicology attempts to explain disease not just in the traditional manner but by understanding the phases of disease (humoral and cellular) in combination with various embryonic germ layers. This association can be seen in the often cited chart, the Table of Homotoxicosis, which systematically charts the course of a disease through six phases (excretion, reaction, deposition, impregnation, degeneration, neoplasmic). Thus it is an aid in prognosis as well as choosing the treatment based upon which phase the person is in. For instance, a person who starts smoking starts in the excretion phase. As the individual continues to smoke, acute inflammation is the reaction, which then becomes chronic. Bronchial asthma occurs next and is emblematic of the impregnation phase. The lung begins to degenerate as pulmonary emphysema sets in and, if the abuse continues, pulmonary cancer (neoplasmic phase) can result. Homotoxicologists would say this whole evolution is one disease and not separate entities.

For a more detailed explanation read Dr. Hans-Heinrich Reckeweg's opus *Homotoxicology* (1948) and his *Homotoxicology: Illness and Healing Through Anti-Homotoxic Therapy* (1980), Dr. David Bianchi's *An Introduction to Homotoxicology* (1992), and Ivo Bianchi's *Principles of Homotoxicology* (1989). See MOLECULAR PATHOLOGY.

homotoxone (homotone) a term commonly used in homotoxicology (see HOMOTOXICOLOGY). It is postulated that when toxins ('homotoxins' is the term coined by Dr. Reckeweg) are formed, enzymatic systems couple them to form a homotoxone (a neutralized substance) which is then eliminated.

hookworm disease see ANKYLOSTOMIASIS.

hooping cough see WHOOPING COUGH.

hordeolum (pl. hordeola) a stye; an inflammation of a sebaceous gland of the eyelid usually the size of a barley-corn (approximately 1/8 inch in diameter).

hormesis (hormoligosis) a term coined by researchers C.M. Southam and J. Ehrlich in the early 1940s to describe the stimulatory effects induced by very low levels of toxic substances. For example, the natural anti-cancer defenses can be stimulated by minute amounts of cancer-causing chemicals. In other words, minute quantities of toxic substances stimulate growth in living organisms. See ARNDT-SCHULZ LAW.

hormoligosis a term coined by T.D. Luckey to characterize substances which were stimulatory at low doses, neutral or slightly inhibitory at modest dosages and toxic at high doses.

horny corneous, of the nature or structure of horn, a substance composed chiefly of keratin.

horripilation (gooseskin, cutis anserina) gooseflesh, goosebumps. The bristling of body hair.

hospital fever see TYPHUS.

hourglass contraction the central constriction of a hollow organ (stomach, uterus, etc.).

housemaid's knee (synovitis, prepatellar bursitis) an inflammation and swelling of the bursa (a small sac interposed between parts that move upon one another) just behind the knee-cap. It is due to traumatism in persons who spend a lot of time on their knees.

Hufeland's journal the journal edited by Christoph Wilhelm von Hufeland (1762-1836), a magnanimous and kindly physician who was a friend and doctor to Goethe, Herder, and Schiller. Through 'his' journal *(Journal der praktischen Arzneikunde),* which he edited for some forty years, he corrected misconceptions about phrenology, Mesmerism and other subjects of a controversial nature. He did so with homeopathy when, in 1796, he published Hahnemann's paper, 'Experiment On a New Principle of Discovering the Curative Powers of the Drug Substances'. In this first published work, the term 'homeopathy' is coined and the concept of similars is outlined. Homeopaths owe a debt of gratitude to this enlightened pioneer of medical journalism.

Hufeland wrote a very popular book on personal hygiene, *Hufeland's Art of Prolonging Life* (1797). It was translated into most of the European languages.

Hufeland was "one of the most successful and respected physicians of his time, graduated in medicine from Gottingen in 1783. He initially succeeded his father and grandfather as court physician at Weimar where he came to know as patients and friends Goethe, Schiller, and their brilliant circle. In 1793 he was called to Jena as professor and went to Berlin in 1800 as royal physician, director of the medical college, and chief physician at the Charite. Hufeland was a leading figure in 19th century medical journalism, editing four journals, and was also a prolific author. ... His outspoken support for vaccination played a major role in its eventual adoption in Germany."—*Heirs of Hippocrates,* # 1183.

humid asthma (pituitous asthma) asthma with profuse mucus and expectoration.

humid tetter see ECZEMA CAPITIS.

humors one of four fluids which comprise the body and determine the health and temperament, according to the ancients. They were blood, phlegm, yellow bile (choler), and black bile (melancholer). Disease occurred when one or more of these humors was diseased or out of balance. According to humoral pathology, the cause of all disease is rooted in an imbalance of the bodily humors. Hippocrates (c.460–c.357 BCE) and Galen (131–201 ACE) were great advocates of this theory (see CELLULAR PATHOLOGY and MOLECULAR PATHOLOGY).

Some more modern scholars place importance on this theory by saying that there are four temperaments (sanguine, phlegmatic, choleric, and melancholic, respectively). An interesting theory, not just for idle thought, but for deep reflection. The founder of anthroposophy, Rudolf Steiner, discusses the temperaments in great detail in his works. Consult Francis X. King's *Rudolf Steiner and Holistic Medicine* for a lucid, and interesting introduction into anthroposophy. See ANTHROPOSOPHY.

Huneke's flash phenomenon see NEURAL THERAPY.

hunger weakness, pain, and discomfort which is caused by the need for food. This is different from 'appetite' which simply means the desire for food.

Hunterian chancre a syphilitic chancre.

"When pressed between the finger and thumb, [it] feels like a piece of cartilage... Its edges are seldom raised above the surface, but commence abruptly and pass in a shelving, sloping, direction to the bottom of the ulcer, which dips down deeply into the subjacent textures, and thus acquires its well-known, contracted cup shape. The surface of the ulcer, instead of looking moist, and discharging freely, like the soft chancre, is generally dry, or covered with a kind of scab."—S. Yeldham, *Homeopathy in Venereal Diseases*, p. 73.

"[It is] dense and hard ... the shape of half a pea... Every indurated, genuine Hunterian chancre is at first soft, the induration generally only showing itself five or six days afterwards, although it may ... appear in the first twenty-four hours."—Jahr, *The Venereal Diseases*, p. 75.

A Scottish surgeon, John Hunter (1728-1793), in an unsuccessful attempt to differentiate gonorrhea from syphilis, inoculated himself with what he thought was gonorrhea and acquired a syphilitic chancre.

hyacinth a plant, perhaps a lily, gladiolus, or iris, that, according to Greek mythology, sprang from the blood of the slain Hyacinthus.

hyaline glassy appearance.

hydatid a watery vesicle or cyst usually seen under the eyelids, but which can appear in other parts of the body, especially the liver. A hydatid cyst of the liver is composed of the larval stage of a worm, *Echinococcus granulosus*. The larvae may remain dormant for quite some time, even decades, before rupturing, allowing its contents to spread into the system. It is only then that the patient becomes symptomatic, developing jaundice, lung complications, anaphylactoid reactions, etc.

hydrargyrism see HYDRARGYROSIS.

hydrargyrosis (hydrargyrism, mercurialism) the morbid effects of mercury poisoning.

hydrargyrum mercury. Hg is the chemical abbreviation for mercury.

hydrargyrum metallicum *Mercurius sol.*, quicksilver. See MERCURY.

hydrargyrus see CALOMEL.

hydrarthrus see HYDARTHROSIS.

hydarthrosis (hydarthrus) a white swelling of a joint. A uniform swelling round the joint, of the color of the skin, and extremely painful. Mostly affects the knee joint. A serous effusion into a joint.

hydraemia a condition of the blood in which the fluid content is increased but the total amount of the blood does not increase proportionately.

hydragogue a purgative that causes copious liquid discharges; causing the discharge of watery fluid.

hydroa any skin disease characterized by vesicles or bullae.

hydrocele a collection of clear fluid in a cavity; specifically, such a collection in the scrotum.

hydrocephaloid an increase in the volume of cerebrospinal fluid within the skull, with "symptoms similar to hydrocephalus. The child grows restless, utters plaintive cries, rolls its head, commences to squint and falls into a stupor—a state of things which Marshall Hall has designated by the name of 'hydrocephaloid', in contradistinction to hydrocephalus acutus, which is of an inflammatory nature."—Raue, *Special Pathology,* p. 469.

hydrocephalus an abnormal accumulation of fluid in the cerebral ventricles, causing enlargement of the skull and compression of the brain.

hydrogenoid one of the three constitutions put forth by Edward von Grauvogl (1811-1877). It is characterized by an excess of water in the tissues and blood and a heightened sensitivity of the patient to cold and dampness; it corresponds to the sycotic miasm of Hahnemann (1755-1843). The two other Grauvogl constitutions are CARBO-NITROGENOID (psoric) and OXYGENOID (syphilitic).

hydrogogue a substance which causes the loss of fluids.

hydrolipoplexic tending to accumulate an excess of fluids and lipids (fats) in the body, especially in the abdomen and thigh regions.

hydronephrosis (dropsy of the kidney) a collection of urine in the pelvis of the kidney as a result of obstructed outflow. The pressure of the fluid will, in time, cause atrophy of the kidney structure, eventually destroying the kidney.

hydropathy a misnomer. See HYDROTHERAPY.

hydrophobia (canine madness, lyssa) 1) rabies in man. 2) an abnormal fear of water.

hydropic edematous; relating to the accumulation of fluid.

hydrops (edema, dropsy, hydropsy) accumulation of watery fluids.

hydrops genu water on the knee. See HYGROMA PATELLA (housemaid's knee).

hydrorrhachis edema of the spinal cord, an increase in the cerebrospinal fluid between the membranes and the cord or in the central canal or cavities formed in the cord substance. May sometimes refer to spina bifida.

hydrosalpingitis (hydrosalpinx) an accumulation of watery fluids in the Fallopian tube with an accompanying inflammation.

hydrotherapy (hydiatry, hydropathy) the use of water as a form of therapy to cure illness.

It is a very powerful therapy and of some use in virtually all diseases. Ablutions, compresses, water packs/dressings, sheet packs, medicinal baths, steam treatments, douche baths, jet baths, salt glows, percussion douche, enemas, and fomentations are just a few of the many water therapy techniques. This subject is too vast to begin to cover, so you may wish to consult Drs. Boyle and Saine's excellent book, *Naturopathic Hydrotherapy* (Eclectic Medical Publishing, 14385 Southeast Lusted Rd., Sandy, OR 97005).

hydrothorax a collection of watery exudate in the lungs.

hydrotis dropsy of the ear. An effusion in the internal ear.

hydruria (polyuria) the excretion of a greatly increased amount of watery urine without a proportional increase in the solid portion.

hyganthropharmacology homeopathic provings. See PROVING.

hygroma (cystic lymphangioma) a serous cyst, usually found on the side of the neck, but rarely in the axilla or groin. A dilated or varicose condition or tumor of the lymphatics.

hygroma patella a tumor on the knee composed of lymph fluid and blood.

hygrostomia salivation.

hyperaesthesia an abnormal sensitivity to stimuli, particularly pain. Excessive sensibility.

hyperazoturia the excretion of an excessive amount of urea.

hyperchlorhydria (hyperhydrochloria) the presence of or an excessive secretion of an abnormal amount of hydrochloric acid (HCl) in the stomach.

hyperemesis excessive vomiting.

hyperemesis gravidarum the uncontrollable vomiting of pregnancy.

hyperemia an increased content of blood in a part. Congestion.

hyperidrosis (hyperhidrosis, polyidrosis) excessive or profuse sweating.

hyperlaxity a greater than normal degree of freedom of movement in extension of the joints.

hypermetropia (hyperopia) farsightedness (the ability to see distant objects more clearly than closer ones). An abnormal refraction of the eye causing the rays of light to focus behind the retina.

hyperosmia an exaggerated sense of smell.

hyperostosis hypertrophy (abnormally excessive growth) of a bone.

hyperphagia over-eating.

hyperphoria tendency of one eye to deviate upward from its normal position.

hyperplasia excessive formation of tissue. An increase in the size of tissue or organ due to an increase in the number of cells.

hyperpyrexia an extremely high fever.

hypersalivation excessive production of saliva. 'Waterbrash' and 'hypersalivation' may have been used synonymously by some early authors.

hyperthermy an above-normal body temperature.

hyperthyroidism an abnormal condition brought about by excessive functional activity of the thyroid gland. See GRAVES' DISEASE.

hypertrichosis the excessive growth of hair; abnormal hairiness.

hypertrophy excessive growth, growth to an abnormally large size.

hyphema blood in the anterior chamber of the eye.

hypnosis a state similar to sleep but induced by a practitioner, resulting in the susceptibility of the subject to suggestions, including curative ones. "Putting him to sleep so he thinks he sleeps when he's really awake."—an Arikari-Hidatsu medicine woman.

hypochondria 1) that section of the abdomen lying below the ribs. 2) low spirits, melancholia, fear, anxiety, and feelings of gloom. A feeling that something awful is about to happen. See HYPOCHONDRIACAL.

hypochondriacal a morbid concern about the health and exaggerated attention to any unusual bodily or mental sensations; an unfounded belief that one is suffering from some disease. Comes from the Greek 'hypochondrion', because the imaginary disease is often referred to the stomach region. The hypochondriac's symptoms are usually referred to as being 'all in the mind', and in our society not worthy of much attention. However, this can be looked at in another way, namely, that the person is announcing his life suffering in the language of bodily symptoms. In its own words, so to speak, the body is expressing concerns about its life circumstances.

"All of life's experiences speak to us, whether the language be that of dreams, emotions, or bodily responses. . . . A patient produces symptoms until someone hears him and listens to what he is speaking about, or until he figures out his body's messages for himelf."—G. Epstein, *Healing Into Immortality* (1994).

hypochondrium the region of the abdomen at each side of the lower ribs.

hypodynia a slight pain.

hypogastrium the lowest of the three median regions of the abdomen, above the pubic bone and below the navel.

hypoglobular anemia (hypocytosis, cytopenia, oligocythemia) the lack of cellular elements in the blood.

hypoglycemia low blood sugar. An abnormally small concentration of glucose (sugar) in the circulating blood.

hypomania a moderate degree of maniacal exaltation and exaggerated overactivity followed often by a period of depression. Moderate behavioral changes may also occur.

hypopion (hypopyon) effusion or accumulation of purulent matter (pus) in the anterior chamber of the eye.

hyposphyxia abnormally low blood pressure with sluggishness of the circulation.

hypostatic pleuritis inflammation of the lining of the lungs, which causes congestion and stagnation of the blood in the capillaries or larger vessels due to gravitation; often seen in the lungs of a person long in bed with an exhausting disease, and in the leg veins of those who stand a lot.

hyposthenia weakness.

hypotension low pressure, as in low blood pressure.

hypothenar the fleshy eminence on the palm of the hand just below the thumb.

hypothermy (hypothermia) subnormal temperature of the body.

hypothymia despondency; depression of spirits, a diminution of the intensity of emotions.

hypoxia low levels of oxygen in the tissues and blood.

hypsarrhythmia an abnormal, chaotic heart rhythm usually found in patients with infantile spasms.

hysometra (hydrometra) dropsy or edema of the womb/uterus.

hysteralgia (hysterodynia, metralgia, metrodynia) pain in the uterus.

hysteria a nervous disorder accompanied by extreme emotional excitability and lack of control, especially in fits which alternate between laughing and crying. This disorder was formerly believed to be confined to just young women but is now known to affect either sex, and thus is no longer called 'hysteria', but 'histrionic personality disorder'.

From the Greek *hustera*, 'womb'. In ancient Greece it was believed that hysteria was common in women, originating in the womb.

hysteria clavus a state of excitation where lancinating pains are felt from the top of the head backwards.

hysteria globus a state of excitation where it feels as if a ball is caught in the throat. 'I was so excited it felt like my heart was in my throat.'

hysteroptosis (hysteroptosia, metroptosia) prolapse of the uterus, falling of the womb; a downward displacement of the uterus.

hystricism (hystriciasis, ichthyosis hystrix) an extreme form of ichthyosis, usually occurring in elevated patches. See ICHTHYOSIS.

ib. (ibid., ibidem) 'in the same place'. Used in footnotes and bibliographies to refer the reader to the entry just previously cited.

i.e. (id est) 'that is'.

iatrogenic relating to an abnormal state or condition produced by a doctor by his administration of poor treatment (either procedures or drugs).

ichor/ous (sanies) a burning, thin, acrid, pus-like discharge from an ulcer, wound or sore.

ichthyol (ichthyolum, ammonium ichthyol, ichthammol) a brownish oil obtained by the distillation of bituminous coal. From the Greek *ichthys*, 'fish'; fossils of fish are often found in the coal or shale, thus the name. Used in ointment form as an antiseptic and drawing salve.

ichthyosis (fish-skin disease, xeroderma) dry, hard scaliness of the skin, like fish scales, usually worse in the winter. Generally sweat is diminished as are oily (sebaceous) secretions.

icteric pertaining to jaundice, especially the yellow-colored skin.

icterus (morbus arcuatus, jaundice) yellowness of the skin. See JAUNDICE.

ictus a stroke, a beat or a blow, as in 'ictus cordis' (heart beat) or 'ictus paralyticus' (a stroke of paralysis). 'Solis ictus' is sunstroke.

idem the same.

idiopathic of unknown or spontaneous origin, as in 'idiopathic disease' (a disease in which no causative factor is recognized).

idiosyncracy an unusual characteristic of an individual (structural, physiological, temperamental, or behavioral, etc.). Also an unusual reactivity which an individual has to a substance or even remedy.

"If there were no idiosyncrasy there would be no homoeopathy. Every individual is susceptible to certain things; is susceptible to sickness, and equally susceptible to cure. Cure rests in the degree of susceptibleness."—*New Remedies* (J.T. Kent).

idiot according to the Binet-Simon intellect tests, a person congenitally without understanding or ordinary mental capacity. One who does not advance beyond the Binet age of 3 years. An idiot is unable to guard against common dangers and incapable of learning connected speech. The term 'idiot' is archaic and no longer used in the field of psychology. See BINET TEST.

ignis sacer (L. 'sacred flame') zona. See HERPES ZOSTER. This term may also refer to erysipelas.

ileac/iliac passion a disease with abdominal pain, vomiting of feces and spasms of the abdominal muscles. Similar to ileus.

ileocaecal pertaining to the ileum and cecum of the large intestine or that area/region of the abdomen.

ileum the third and last portion of the small intestine, about 12 feet in length, extending from the junction of the jejunum to the ileocecal valve.

ileus (passio iliaca) an obstruction of the bowel accompanied with colic pains.

ileus miserere a form of colic, a twisting pain in the region of the navel.

ilio-scrotal relating to the ilium and the scrotum or that area.

ilium the flank or loin area. The upper part of the innominate bone. The upper broad portion of the hipbone.

illuminist in homeopathic theory, one who believes that an acute disease is a curative response of the organism to its chronic problem. However, it has not been demonstrated that treating the acute disease suppresses the chronic disease.

imbecile an archaic term for one who is congenitally weak-minded, capable of some education, but not advancing beyond the Binet age of 7. See BINET TEST.

imperforate closed, without an opening.

imperious domineering; overbearing. Regal or imperial. Urgent or pressing.

impetigo (scrum-pox) a contagious infection causing pustular eruptions which ripen, rupture or become crusted. It occurs chiefly on the face around the mouth and nostrils. It may be further classified as i. simplex, i. contagiosa, i. vulgaris, or, according to the shape of the patches, as i. circinata, i. gyrata, or i. figurata.

impetigo contagiosa a form of impetigo with eruptions of flattish vesicles which develop into pustules.

imponderabilia remedies made from sources which have no mass, which exist only as vibrational energy—*X-rays, Magnet, Sun, Electricity,* etc.

"I have used the potentized *X-Ray* since 1897 when I laid a flint glass bottle containing absolute alcohol under a tube, which I personally used, and which was activated by my Meyervitz coil. This was given to my old friend, Doctor Samuel Cleveland, and he told me he gave it to Doctor Bernhardt Fincke of Brooklyn to potentize." - Wm. B.Griggs (*The Layman Speaks,* 14:1, p. 30 (1961)

impotent 'lacking virile power' (incapable of sexual intercourse, usually refers to males). Powerless; ineffectual. Lacking physical strength or vigor; weak.

impotentia virilis male impotence.

in der Rothen (Roten) Ruhr 1) red diarrhea. 'Ruhr' was an infectious diarrhea of two varieties—the amoebic or 'white diarrhea', and the bacterial or 'red diarrhea'. 2) in the socialistic Ruhr region of Germany.

in situ in the natural or normal place.

in toto in total.

inanition emptiness, exhaustion from starvation, a lack of food or a defect in assimilation.

inappetence lack of appetite.

incarnation the process by which abscesses or ulcers are healed: little grain-like fleshy bodies form on the surface of ulcers or wounds and serve the double purpose of filling up the cavities and bringing closely together and uniting the sides.

incipient beginning to be or to appear; becoming apparent. Just beginning.

incipient dementia dementia in the beginning stages. The start of the deterioration or loss of the intellectual faculties, the reasoning power, the memory, and the will; characterized by confusion, disorientation, apathy, and stupor of varying degrees.

incommode inconvenient; also, to inconvenience or disturb.

incontinence inability to retain, to control the excretory functions (usually refers to the bladder, e.g., 'an incontinent bladder').

incrassation a thickening or swelling.

incubus 1) nightmare. 2) an evil spirit which was believed to lie on women in their sleep and force sexual intercourse on them.

imperforate closed, without an opening.

incunabulum an artifact from an early period, usually before 1500. A book which was printed before movable type was invented, usually taken to mean before 1500. Also the infancy or early stage of something.

indefatigable untiring, incapable of being fatigued.

Indian continued fever a fever in which there are no intermissions in the temperature curve. The temperature is very constant, not varying more than $1-2^0$ F during 24 hours.

indican of or containing potassium salts. A general term for substances found in the sweat and in variable amounts in the urine, which when found in abnormal amounts can indicate protein putrefaction in the intestine.

indicanuria the presence of indicans in the urine.

indolent inactive, sluggish; painless or nearly so, as in 'indolent ulcer'.

inductive logic the principle of reaching a general conclusion by examining a small set of data. Reaching a conclusion by examining the particular and applying it to the general. For example, observing two trees with green leaves and concluding that all trees in the forest must have green leaves.

induration a hard spot or place. The hardening of a tissue or part.

inebriants intoxicants.

inebriety drunkenness, alcohol intoxication. 'Inebriate', a habitual drunkard.

inertia sluggishness; lack of movement, inactivity. An absence of contractility.

infantile paralysis see POLIOMYELITIS.

infarct an area of dead tissue resulting from failure of the local blood supply; also an obstruction.

inferior in anatomy, lower. Applied to structures nearer the feet, as contrasted to superior, nearer the head.

influenza (epidemic catarrh, epidemic catarrhal fever, grippe, *epidemisches schnupfenfieber*) an epidemic, often pandemic, disease characterized by inflammation of the mucous membranes of the respiratory tract, runny nose, mucopurulent discharge, fever, pain in the muscles and prostration. "A specific epidemic and endemic catarrh of the respiratory mucous membranes, marked by great prostration, an evenly high temperature, a tendency to complicative diseases, and a rapid development of pre-existing or co-existing pathological conditions."—*Medical Counselor,* 8/1/1885.

infra under, below.

inframammary below the mammary gland (breast).

infratoxic below the toxic level.

infusion something steeped or soaked in water without boiling in order to concentrate or extract the active ingredients.

ingesta the partially digested food in the stomach.

ingluvin (may be misspelled as influvin) a digestive substance similar to pepsin and obtained from the stomach of chickens. Therapeutically it relieves vomiting and aids digestion.

inguinal pertaining to the groin.

inimical antagonistic, harmful, or not conducive.

1) refers to a lack of harmony between two or more remedies. For example, *Nux vomica* and *Zincum* are inimicals; they should not be given at the same time as their actions oppose or antagonize each other. Another way in which inimical may be used is 2) "The inimical forces, partly psychical, partly physical, to which our terrestrial existence is exposed, which are termed morbific noxious agents, do not possess the power of morbidity deranging the health of man unconditionally; but we are made ill by them only when our organism is sufficiently disposed and susceptible to the attack of the morbific cause that may be present and to be altered in its health, deranged and made to undergo abnormal sensations and function, hence they do not produce disease in everyone, nor at all times."—S.C.F. Hahnemann.

innocuous (innoxious) harmless.

innutrition a lack of nutrition.

inoma a fibroid tumor, fibroma.

insensibility lack of awareness or consciousness. Without a sense of feeling.

insipid lacking flavor or zest; unpalatable. Lacking excitement or interest;

unstimulating, vapid.

insolatio sunstroke; excessive exposure to the sun.

insolent insulting in manner, speech, or behavior. Arrogant, impudent, impertinent.

insomnia sleeplessness or disturbed sleep; a prolonged condition or inability to sleep.

inspissated thickened by evaporation or absorption of fluid; as in scybalum, a hard round mass of 'inspissated' feces.

insufflation the act of blowing into, as blowing a gas, powder, or vapor into a body cavity.

integument an external covering or skin; the membrane covering the body and continuous, at the various orifices, with the mucous membrane of the alimentary, respiratory, and urogenital tracts.

intercalate to interpose or insert.

intercostal between the ribs.

intercranial within the head.

intercurrent in homeopathy, a remedy given to provide movement in a stalled case. For example, if *Sulphur* is given and provides some benefit, then when given again it doesn't seem to work. Then another remedy is indicated, given and does some work, then another remedy is given and does some work. Yet no remedy, despite being well chosen, seems to be clearing the case, the homeopath may choose an intercurrent to move the case on to a cure. Usually, but not always, the intercurrent is a nosode.

This subject may also be approached from another angle. More often than not, a single remedy will not cure a case (Boenninghausen and Hahnemann knew this *and* mentioned the use of intercurrent remedies), thus another remedy needs to be inserted between the primary one. This remedy is termed the interim or intercurrent remedy. For example, if *Rhus tox.* and *Bryonia* are indicated yet *Rhus* seems to be a bit more so, it will be given first, followed by *Bry.,* (if necessary) then *Rhus* again.

interdigital between the fingers or toes.

intermit to cease for a time.

intermittent (intermittent fever, ague, malaria) referring to a type of fever in which the temperature falls to normal at regular intervals, and then goes back up, e.g., ague.

intermittent fluxion potency see POTENCY.

interosseus between the bones. Lying between or connecting the bones.

interstitial nephritis an inflammation of the kidneys in which the interstitial connective tissue is chiefly affected. The interstitial connective tissue refers to the tissue responsible for maintaining the form and structure of an organ, in this case the kidney. By contrast, parenchymatous tissue is the tissue of the organ responsible for carrying out the purpose of that organ.

See PARENCHYMA.

intertrigo a red, edematous eruption or excoriation of the skin produced by friction or chafing of adjacent parts.

intraocular within the eye.

intromission insertion, the act of putting in, as of the penis into the vagina.

intumescence enlargement, swelling, puffiness.

intussusception the recurring of one part within another; especially of the passage of one part of the intestine into another. A telescoping of the intestine.

inunction the act of rubbing an oily or fatty substance into the skin; also the substance used.

inure to train, habituate, instruct in the proper use of.

invalidism a state of chronic ill-health.

inveterate chronic, long-seated, firmly established.

involution the return of an enlarged organ to its normal size.

ionthus see WHELK.

ipse dixit 'he himself said it' (an assertion without proof).

irascibility prone to outbursts of temper, easily angered.

iridescent producing a display of lustrous rainbow-like colors.

iridocyclitis inflammation of both the iris and ciliary body.

iridodiagnosis see IRIDOLOGY.

iridology (iridodiagnosis) a system of diagnosis which reveals pathological and functional disturbances in the body. It is based upon the noting of abnormal markings, structures, pigmentation, and color variations of the iris. For further information contact the NIRA (National Iridological Research Association), PO Box 31013, Seattle, WA 98103. Rayid, another iridological method founded by Denny Johnson, uses patterning of the iris to determine personality and genetic predispositions.

iridodonesis (hippus) a trembling of the iris.

Irish button syphilis.

irisin a resinoid from blue flag *(Iris versicolor)*, used as a cathartic and to stimulate the flow of bile.

iritis inflammation of the iris.

irregulars an archaic term often used by allopaths in the 1800s to refer to homeopaths.

irresolute hesitating, faltering, wavering, unresolved.

irritant contact dermatitis a nonallergic skin reaction resulting from contact with a primary irritant, such as an acid or alkali, which causes skin damage in all those directly exposed to it.

ischaemia/ischemia a local anemia caused by mechanical obstruction of the blood supply. If prolonged, death of tissue can occur.

ischialgia (ischias, ischioneuralgia, coxalgia, sciatica) pain in the hip-joint.

ischias see ISCHIALGIA.

ischias antica the anterior or front of the hip.

ischidrosis (anhidrosis) suppression of the perspiration.

ischuria retention or suppression of urine.

iso-organotherapy (sarcodes, opathery, organotherapy) the use of homeo-pathically prepared healthy organ substances to treat and therapeutically support that specific organ, such as using a 6X preparation of healthy liver tissue administered to a person with a cirrhotic liver. This homeopathic preparation acts to stimulate healthy liver processes and to support the liver in general. C. Hering advised using this method early in his career (1830s). See ORGANOTHERAPY, SARCODE, OPOTHERAPY.

isode an isopathic agent.

isopathic homeopathically prepared pathological materials, secretions, or ex-cretions which originate from the patient himself, such as making a ho-meopathic potency from the patient's urine and then administering it to the patient; or making a homeopathic remedy from the patient's boil and then administering that to the patient in order to treat the boil. A blood remedy could also be made and this has its own special term, AUTO–HEMOTHERAPY.

isopathy (*aequalia aequalibus curentur,* law of sameness) the employment of homeopathically prepared substances responsible for the disease itself. It is not based on the principle of *similarity* but on *sameness*, on the sub-stance being identical to the etiological agent, e.g., the use of pollens in allergic asthma, the use of *Arsenicum* to treat arsenic poisoning, or the use of potentized drugs to treat toxic side effects of those drugs (also called tautopathy). It is similar to desensitization but is better as desensiti-zation may result in an increased reactional capacity of the patient to aller-gens. Isopathy may help eliminate toxins which have accumulated in the patient.

Though the principles of isopathy were being put to therapeutic use by many others and much earlier in medical history, the term 'isopathy' is credited to Joseph Wilhelm Lux, a German veterinarian, somewhere around 1831-3. His first isode was a 30C dilution of a blood specimen from an animal with anthrax. Thus *Anthracinum* was created. More specifically *Anthracinum* is a nosode. In 1833 Lux wrote *Isopathik der Contagionen*.

Alexis Eustaphieve wrote a very early treatise on isopathy when he published, in 1846, *Homoeopathia Revealed. A Brief Exposition of the Whole System Adapted to General Comprehension. 2nd Ed. with a Sketch of Isopathia.*

Father Denys Collet (1824–1909) was another early advocate of isopathy. He wrote *Isopathie, Methode Pasteur par Voie Interne.* He suggested another category of preparation, serotherapeutic isopathy or serotherapy. This consists of homeopathic remedies of immune serum, e.g. Marmorek (homeopathic remedy prepared from the antituberculous serum from a patient with tuberculosis). O.A. Julian did much work in this area and wrote *Dynamized Micro-Immunotherapy* (1977).

Kruger, Nebel, Roy, Munoz, Fortier-Bernoville, Brotteaux, Schmidt, Schimmel, Parrot, Speight, Vannier, Voll, Reckeweg, H.C. Allen (*The Materia Medica of the Nosodes*, 1910), O.A. Julian (*Materia Medica der Nosoden*, 1960), and others did important work in this area.

The definitions in this area can become confusing. For instance, a nosode can also be an isode (isopathic remedy) or it can be used to treat totally unrelated symptoms which are not isopathic. This is because the definition of nosode is "a homeopathic preparation which consists of extracts of pathological materials, pathogenic cultures, human or animal metabolic products, or pathologically abnormal organs or tissues suitably dispensed in sterile, dilute, and potentized form according to homeopathic methodologies. By way of examples, *Tuberculinum* is a nosode prepared from the lesion induced by the Koch mycobacterium, *Variolinum* the nosode prepared from matter obtained from a smallpox pustule, and *Carcinosin* the nosode from a carcinoma, and so on."—*Homeopathy: A Frontier in Medical Science* (Bellavite, 1995).

Strict adherence to the definition of isopathy makes it fundamentally different from homeopathy. Since isodes were never proven on healthy human subjects, one does not know the full range of symptoms it can produce and no case individualization was performed. The isode was just given based on the identical nature of disease and isode.

isotherapy see ISOPATHY.

issue a 'wick' made of an absorbent material (horse hair, linen thread, silk) which, when placed in a wound or cut, allows that area to be drained of fluids. 'Seton' and 'issue' are actually one in the same and were used frequently by allopaths in the 18th and 19th centuries. They thought that the outlet created would allow the disease to come or drain out of the body.

iterative repeating or being repeated.

J J J J J J J

jactitation (jactation) 1) bragging, boasting, public declaration. 2) an extreme restlessness or tossing of the body.

jail-fever see TYPHUS.

jaundice (icterus, morbus regius) yellowness of the skin, mucous membranes, and secretions, due to bile pigments in the blood. Jaundice may be due to any number of causes, the most familiar to us being hepatocellular: the destruction of liver cells by toxic agents (alcohol particularly), thus the liver cannot perform its role of detoxification, allowing toxins to pour into the system, contributing to the yellowness of the skin as a symptom of liver dysfunction.

Jenichen/'Jenichen potencies' after J.C. Jenichen (1787-1849), who was entrusted by many practitioners in Germany with the preparation of remedies in high potency. He prepared them, in what seems to us today, odd potencies (12M, 400C, 800C, 7M, 40M, etc.) Jenichen suggested that the remedies gain their curative power from the succussion and not the dilution. Jenichen's potencies were used by Hering, among others, and at one time sold by Boericke & Tafel. Their effectiveness was unquestioned.

In 1846 Jenichen wrote to Stapf, a fellow homeopath:

"The words of our friend Gross, 'but where does this lead? where is the limit?' spurred in me—since we have no *a priori* knowledge and can obtain insight only through experimentation— . . . the decision to increase the potency of arsenic from 2500 to 8000, and my faithful arm and muscle power carried me through 165,000 vigorous succussions. . . . It will now doubtlessly be very interesting to you to determine if Ars. 8000. is still effective, or if the limit has been surpassed at this point or even before."— quoted by G. v. Keller in *Classical Homeopathic Quarterly,* 3:4, 1990, p. 125.

jugular the prominent vein on either side of the neck which can be seen and easily palpated or touched.

K Korsakovian potency, after Korsakoff. See POTENCY. May also be used to indicate Kent's *Repertory,* e.g. 'K. 368' means page 368 of Kent's *Repertory.*

kala-azar (dum-dum fever, oriental sore, espundia, visceral leishmaniasis, tropical splenomegaly) a chronic and usually fatal disease characterized by irregular fever, enlarged spleen, hemorrhages, dropsy, and emaciation. It is caused by *Leishmania donovani,* a protozoan, and mainly effects the populations of tropical Asia. 'Oriental sore' refers to the cutaneous variety, while the muscosal-cutaneous form is called 'espundia'.

keloid (cheloid) a fibrous, excessive formation of tissue, usually at the growth site of a scar, elevated, rounded, white, occasionally pink, firm and with ill-defined borders.

kenophobia (cenophobia, agoraphobia) a fear of being in open spaces.

Kentian after J.T. Kent (1849-1916) who said, "There are no diseases, only sick people." 'Kentian' refers to practicing homeopathy using the law of similars, the minimum dose, the single dose, repertorizing to find the remedy and giving added importance to mental and psychic aspects, too. In Kent's method of repertorization he placed primary importance on mentals, generalized less, and considered physical generals as secondary. He would consider particular symptoms in order to differentiate remedies.

"The symptoms of supreme importance to the case, that expressed the very deepest level of the patient's disturbance, were often the mental symptoms, which required the higher attenuations."—*The American Homeopath* (2: p. 9, 1995)

'Kentian' also means using the higher centesimal potencies (200c, 1M, 10M, etc.) a single time, giving the remedy dry in the mouth, then waiting for several weeks to several months; as opposed to 6th edition prescribing in which a remedy in a Q (LM) potency is given in water daily. See POTENCY.

keratectasis (keratoconus, staphyloma) protrusion of the cornea.

keratin an insoluble fibrous protein which forms fingernails, horn, feathers and hair, and which gives fibers their elasticity.

keratitis inflammation of the cornea.

keratomycosis disease of the cornea due to the presence of a fungal growth.

keratosis (callus) any disease of the skin characterized by an overgrowth of the skin.

Kern meridian complexes complex homeopathic formulae developed by Dr. Helmut Schimmel (founder of the VEGATEST method) and Kern Pharma, Inc. According to literature these 'meridian complexes' "influence energy flow through the organs as associated with the corresponding acupuncture meridians, vessels and chakras ... to release and regulate blocked energy circulation in the patient." See EAV, RADIONICS, BEV.

ketonuria see ACETONURIA.

keynote a symptom which is so apparent, or striking that it strongly suggests or points to a single remedy. For example, pain in the right shoulder blade points to *Chelidonium*.

"The predominating symptom which readily directs attention to the totality."—H.N. Guernsey. See keynote symptoms under SYMPTOMS.

kinetosis (cinesia) see CINESIA.

king pin rubric see SEHGAL'S HOMEOPATHIC METHOD.

king's evil see SCROFULA.

kleptomania (cleptomania) an uncontrollable impulse to steal without needing the item taken. The objects stolen are usually of symbolic value only, being petty and useless.

knock knee see GENU VALGUM.

Koetschau's hypothesis/law (type effect hypothesis) a more precise version of the Arndt-Schulz law: small doses stimulate; moderate doses stimulate, then depress, with a return to normalcy; large doses produce a very brief stimulant effect followed by severe depression and death.

This hypothesis was formulated by German physician Karl Koetschau in the 1920s. See ARNDT-SCHULZ LAW, WILDER'S LAW.

Koplik's spots (Filatov's spots) small red spots on the mucous membrane of the mouth with a bluish-white speck in the center, occurring early in measles before the skin eruption and considered a confirming sign of the disease.

Korsakoff potency see POTENCY.

Korsakoff's psychosis see DELIRIUM TREMENS.

koumiss fermented milk, yogurt. See KUMYSS.

KR acronym for Kent's *Repertory*, e.g., 'KR-157' means Kent's *Repertory*, p. 157.

kraurosis shriveling and drying of a part.

Kretschmer typology a classification of four physiological constitutions developed by Dr. Kretschmer: 1) leptosomatic or asthenic (thin and tall person with narrow shoulders, a long, narrow and flat thorax and a narrow long head), 2) athletic (broad, protruding shoulders, solid high head, large thorax, taut belly, the shape of the trunk tapers off downward, prominent musculature and coarse build), 3) pyknic (medium-sized and thick-set figure, a soft, broad face, with short neck, obesity with a rounded belly, and a low, vaulted chest), and 4) dysplastic (different or unsymmetrical bodily shapes and endocrine imbalances).

kryptorchism (cryptorchism) a developmental defect whereby the testicles fail to descend into the scrotum and remain in the abdomen or inguinal canal.

kumyss (koumiss, koumyss, milk wine) a fermented milk product, perhaps a thin, watery yogurt. "A sparkling beverage prepared from pure, sweet milk, containing all the nutritive elements in a readily digestible and highly assimilable condition."—Boericke & Schreck product catalogue (1870). B & S put it up in champagne bottles. "It may appear curdled, shake and with use of champagne tap it comes out as a creamy foam."

Kupffer's cells reticuloendothelia cells which line the liver sinuses and phagocytize (eat) foreign proteins/particles (bacteria, viruses, etc.) and also form immune bodies. The blood from the gastrointestinal tract, laden with nutrients as well as foreign bodies and other impurities goes directly to the liver, which then purifies it before allowing it to go out into the general circulation. Kupffer cells aid this filtering process. After Karl Kupffer (1829-1902), a prominent German anatomist.

kwashiorkor a malnutrition syndrome most commonly seen in children between the ages of 6 months and 4 years and most prevalent in Third World or the developing nations.

"Distinguishing features: Apathy and peevishness, retardation of growth, changes in the pigmentation of the skin and in the pigmentation and texture of the hair, muscular wasting, oedema and fatty, necrotic or fibrotic changes in the liver. Nutritional dermatoses are commonly but not invariably present. Etiology: Kwashiorkor is generally considered to be the result of severe protein deficiency arising from the intake of a diet low in protein and relatively high in calories, usually supplied as carbohydrates. Secondary deficiencies of individual vitamins may develop. The diagnosis of kwashiorkor is usually made at the oedematous stage. Kwashiorkor must be distinguished from marasmus. The relation between the two seems to depend largely on the adequate calorie intake and the excess carbohydrate in the diet of the former. In both cases there is an acute deficiency of protein. Prognosis: The mortality in untreated cases is very high. But response to treatment is fairly good."—Kichlu & Bose, *A Text-Book of Descriptive Medicine (with Clinical Methods and Homeo-Therapeutics)*, p.955-7.

kyllosis clubfoot. See TALIPES.

kyphosis (cyphosis, humpback, hunchback) angular curvature of the spine, the convexity of the spinal curve being posterior, usually situated in the thoracic region, and involving few or many vertebrae. It may be a result of such diseases as tuberculosis, osteoarthritis, or rheumatoid arthritis of the spine, or an improper posture habit.

kysthitis (colpitis) inflammation of the vagina.

labia plural of labium, 'lip'. May refer to the rounded folds of tissue forming the boundaries of the vulva.

labia leporina see HARE-LIP.

labio-glosso-pharyngeal hemiplegia a partial or one-sided paralysis of the lips, tongue and pharynx.

labyrinthine see MENIERE'S DISEASE.

labyrinthitis an acute infection or irritation of the inner ear, with severe nausea, vomiting, exhaustion, and dizziness.

lachrymose producing tears, tearful.

lachrymal fistula a fistula opening into a tear duct or the lachrymal sac. A fistula is an abnormal duct or passage from an abscess, cavity, or hollow organ to the body surface or to another hollow organ.

lachrymal pertaining to the tears or to the organs secreting and conveying the tears. Relating to weeping.

lachrymation tearing. Secretion of tears to excess.

lactatio (lactation) the time of suckling; when the infant suckles at the breast.

lacteals see CHYLE.

lactiferous tubes (galactophorous ducts) the tubes which carry or convey milk.

lactis pertaining to milk.

lacto-pepsin a digestive aid prepared from pepsin (10 parts pure pepsin, 7.6 parts pancreatin, 50 parts lactose, 5 parts malt extract, 2.6 parts lactic acid, 10 parts 25% hydrochloric acid, and 20 parts glycerin. To this enough powdered tragacanth is added to make a pill-mass).

lactorrhoea (galactorrhea) excessive flow of milk. See GALACTORRHEA.

lactose (milk sugar) a somewhat sweet sugar extracted from milk and used, in various proportions, to make homeopathic pellets.

laesio capitis an injury of the head (Latin *laesio,* 'wound, blow, lesion').

lagophthalmus (oculus leporinus) a condition in which the eyes cannot be entirely closed.

lancet a surgical instrument of a variety of shapes, usually very sharp, sharp-pointed and double-edged, used in venesection, opening abscesses and cutting in general.

lancinating stabbing, piercing, sharply cutting; as in 'lancinating pains'.

land scurvy see PURPURA HEMORRHAGICA.

Landry's paralysis acute ascending paralysis. A flaccid paralysis beginning in the muscles of the legs and spreading upward to involve the arms and other muscles of the body. Named after the French physician B.O. Landry (1826-1865), who first described it.

languid weary, drooping from exhaustion. Weak, feeble, faint or sickly.

languor sluggishness, heaviness.

lanugo the down-like hair covering the fetus. Also the fine hair covering most of the body in adults (except the hair on the head).

laparotomy (celiotomy) incision into the abdomen or loin or through any part of the abdominal wall.

lapis infernalis (lapis imperialis) silver nitrate.

lardaceous resembling lard (the white solid or semisolid rendered fat of a hog), as in 'lardaceous kidney'.

laryngismus stridulus (asthma thymica, crowing convulsions, Kopp's asthma, Millar's asthma, Weichmann's asthma, spasmodic croup) a spasmodic affection of the larynx seen most commonly in young children characterized by a sudden crowing inspiration followed by an arrest of respiration of several seconds duration, with increasing cyanosis, and ending with long, loud, whistling inspirations. See MILLAR'S ASTHMA.

It was described by J.H. Kopp (1777-1858), a German doctor, and John Clarke, a leading London obstetrician and pediatrician. Clarke's book, *Commentaries on Some of the Most Important Diseases of Child: Part the First* (1815) contains the "first exact description of laryngismus stridulus."— Garrison & Morton.

laryngitis inflammation or infection of the larynx. Hoarseness, irritation and loss of voice may occur.

lascivious of or characterized by lust. Exciting sexual desires.

lassitude weariness, heaviness, exhaustion, lethargy. A state of exhaustion or weakness; debility.

lateral in anatomy, side. At, belonging to, or pertaining to the side. Away from the midline of the body or limb, as opposed to 'medial'.

lateritious/latericeous resembling brick dust.

laudable healthy; formerly said of a copious pus thought to indicate an improved condition of the wound. A creamy yellow, non-odorous pus secreted by a healthy granulating surface indicating that the healing process is proceeding along a favorable course.

laudanum tincture of opium, primarily used in the 19th century to allay pain, decrease restlessness, and induce sleep. The 1820 USP (United States Pharmacopoeia) formula contained 6% opium. Today's modern formula contains 10% opium or 1% morphine, but it is seldom used.

lave to wash or bathe. To wash or lap against.

lavement washing or bathing.

law of initial value See WILDER'S LAW.

laxity a relaxed state.

lazaretto a leper hospital. A place of detention for persons afflicted with contagious diseases or quarantined. A lazar is a person infected with a filthy or pestilential disease.

lead colic (painter's colic, colica saturnina) chronic intestinal pains and constipation caused by lead poisoning.

lecanomancy the act of divination by the inspection of water in a basin.

lecherous given to promiscuous sexual indulgence, lewd, sensual.

lectophobia fear of speaking or lecturing.

left-sided remedies remedies whose chief activity is centered upon the left side of the body, e.g., *Arg. nit., Brom., Cina, Clematis, Graph., Lachesis, Phos., Sepia, Sulphur,* and *Thuja.* However, as with right-sided remedies, this fact does not preclude prescribing a left-sided remedy for a right-sided complaint. Matching the overall picture of the remedy, especially the mental and emotional elements, can supersede the importance of left- or right-sidedness.

legasthenia (congenital alexia) the inability to understand something read. Intelligence and neurological findings may be within normal limits yet the person is unable to understand what s/he reads.

lege artis the legal art or legitimate art.

leishmaniasis see KALA-AZAR.

lema (sebum palpebrale) the sebaceous secretion of the Meibomian glands of the eyelids, which lubricates the lids.

lentescent of a slow nature.

lenticular pertaining to or resembling a lens or lentil (i.e. double-convex). Having a lens-like or crystalline appearance (referring to the skin).

lentigo (p. lentigines) a freckle; a circumscribed patch of pigment, small in size, occurring mainly on the face and hands.

lepra an old term for leprosy.

leprominium the leprosy nosode.

leprosy (Hansen's disease, lepra) a disease dating back to biblical times, the nature of which is uncertain, but which might have been psoriasis or a leucoderma. A chronic, infectious disease occurring almost exclusively in tropical and subtropical climates, caused by *Mycobacterium leprae,* and characterized by mutilating lesions of the skin and subcutaneous tissues (tubercular l.) or of the nerves (anesthetic l.). A Norwegian physician, G.A. Hansen (1841-1912), isolated the bacteria in 1871.

leptospirosis see WEIL'S DISEASE.

lesion injury or impairment from a disease, usually well-circumscribed and well-defined.

lethargy sluggishness, apathy, indifference.

leucemia see LEUKEMIA

leucocythemia see LEUKEMIA.

leucocythemia splenica leukemia with marked enlargement of the spleen.

leuco-phlegmatic a term applied by the older medical writers to a dropsical habit of the body (the tendency of the body to retain fluids). Sluggish. Refers to a temperament characterized by want of tension of fiber and general inertness of the physical and mental powers. Dropsical diathesis.

leucocytosis an increase in the white blood cell count which is normal during pregnancy, pathologic in many infections and toxemias.

leucoderma (milk-skin, vitiligo) absence of skin pigmentation in patches or bands.

leucoma (albugo) a white opacity of the cornea, usually dense and opaque.

leuconychia (leucopathia unguium, canities unguium) white spots on the nails.

leucoplakia (smokers' tongue, buccal or lingual psoriasis, ichthyosis linguae) the occurrence of irregular white patches on the tongue (l. lingualis) or cheek (l. buccalis). Thickening of the tongue may also occur.

leucorrhea (whites, fluor albus) a whitish or yellowish purulent discharge from the vagina.

leukemia (leucemia, leucocythemia) a disease of the blood marked by a persistent increase in the amount of white blood cells (leucocytes) and associated with changes in the spleen and bone-marrow or in the lymphatic glands. Leucocytes (neutrophils, eosinophils, basophils, lymphocytes, monocytes, etc.) are 'the mobile units of the body's protective system'. Each has varying functions, e.g., the granulocytes and monocytes protect the body against invading organisms by ingesting them.

levantine 1) a closely woven sturdy silk fabric. 2) referring to an area of the Eastern Mediterranean. 'Levanter', a strong easterly wind in the Mediterranean area.

levitate to rise into the air and float in an apparent defiance of gravity. In the repertory under 'Generalities, vertigo, floating'.

lex talionis punishing a crime with a like act ('an eye for an eye').

libertinism promiscuity, acting without moral restraint; can imply either 'freethinking' or 'profligate, dissolute' (more often applied to a man, whereas promiscuity is more often applied to a woman). One who acts without moral restraint is a libertine.

libidinous having sexual desire.

libido innate sexual drive or energy.

lichen planus an eruption of flattened papules of a reddish color and shining surface, occurring singly or grouped in patches of varying size and shape; the eruption occurs chiefly on the flexor surfaces of the extremities, but may involve the trunk or the mucous membranes. Itching may be slight or severe. The disease may be acute and widespread or chronic and localized.

lichen propicus (prickly heat) see MILIARIA.

lichen ruber (pityriasis rubra pilaris) a chronic, mildly inflammatory skin disease in which firm, sharp papules form at the mouths of the hair follicles with horny plugs in these follicles. Scaly patches are then formed.

lichen scrofulosorum an eruption of reddish papules, single or aggregated in patches of varying size, occurring in scrofulous subjects.

lichen simplex (papular eczema) an inflammation of the skin, of acute or chronic nature, presenting papular lesions, moist or dry, and often accompanied with itching, burning, and various paresthesias.

lichenification diffuse hyperplasia of the layers of the skin that is produced by repeated rubbing, which accentuates the normal skin furrows and rhomboid lines.

Lieberkuhn's glands (crypts of Lieberkuhn, Galeati's glands, intestinal glands) tubular glands found in the intestinal mucous membranes of the small and large intestine, first described by the German anatomist J.N. Lieberkuhn (1711-1756).

Liebig's law of the minimum see AVOGADRO'S NUMBER.

lienitis inflammation of the spleen.

lienteric diarrhea-like. 'Lienterica', a diarrhea with undigested food present. Stools having the appearance of being undigested.

limbus a border or margin. To be 'in limbo' is to be in an inbetween state, neither here nor there.

lime water (liquor calcii hydroxidi) an aqueous solution of calcium hydroxide used as an antacid.

limpid clear; characterized by transparent clearness, pellucid. Calm and untroubled, serene.

linea a line.

linea nasalis the line extending from the edge of the nose, creating a semicircle around the mouth.

lingua the tongue.

lingual pertaining to the tongue, or tongue-shaped.

lipoma (adipoma) a fatty tumor. A sebaceous cyst.

lipothymia fainting.

lippitude (lippitudo) soreness of the eyes; being bleary-eyed. Blepharitis with a gummy secretion causing the margins of the eyes to adhere.

liquor potassae (potassium hydroxide) a slightly diuretic solution primarily used to relieve the pains of gastric acidity.

lithaemia (uricemia) the presence of excessive amounts of uric acid in the blood.

litheosis a condition marked by having stones, usually urinary or bile stones.

lithiasis the formation of stones of any kind, especially bile or urinary/kidney stones.

lithic pertaining to calculi or stones; pertaining to lithium.

lithontriptic (lithotriptic) an agent which dissolves a calculus or stone in the bladder or urethra.

lithotherapy a form of homeopathic therapy in which various semi-precious and precious gemstones/minerals are potentized and used to treat various diseases.

The French homeopath Max Tetau was the great popularizer of this therapy. Low potencies (3x - 9x) of gems and minerals are administered because of their ability to remove or cause the elimination of the associated metal, which—proponents of this therapy maintain—is in chelated form in the body. Dr. Tetau maintains:

"There is a crystalline structural analogy between the mineral and the chelate from the metal ion to be liberated. As an example: It is because the chelating complexes entrapping calcium and phosphorus have a crystallographic structure belonging to the quadratic system, and not to the hexagonal system, that in the treatment of osteoarthrosis of the vertebral column and in senile osteoporosis, dynamized quadratic feldspar, and not triclinic feldspar, is used, in addition to potentized Apatite, which is phosphate of calcium, containing ions of carbonate, fluoride, chloride, and/or hydroxyl, the major constituents of bones and of teeth."—H. Gaier, *Thorson's Encyclopedic Dictionary of Homeopathy,* 1991, p. 330-31.

This therapy attempts to normalize that best results are obtained with the use of the 8x potency. These lithotherapeutic agents have not undergone homeopathic provings but are prescribed exclusively on their pathological associations, e.g., Rhodonite for insomnia or Versailles chalk for senile osteoporosis and decalcification.

lithotomy an operation to remove a kidney stone.

litmus a blue coloring matter obtained from *Roccella tinctoria*, a species of lichen, the principal component of which is azolitmin. It is used as an acid-base indicator, pH 4.5 red, 8.3 blue. Currently produced by H.F. Kimel of Precision Labs in Cincinnati, who purchases the lichens from a Dutch company and boils them in a 55 gallon garbage can. The product is then applied to paper and packaged in vials.

liver spots see CHLOASMA.

livid pale, ashen; also black-and-blue, cyanotic.

livor a black and blue mark.

lixiviate to wash or percolate the soluble matter from.

LM potency (Q, quinquagintamillesimal) the 50 millesimal potencies of the 6th Edition of the *Organon*. LM in actuality means 50M (50,000C), yet somehow has come to mean the Q potencies of Hahnemann. See PO-

TENCY.

local symptom see entry under SYMPTOMS.

localized sensation see 'local symptom' under SYMPTOMS.

lochia the discharge from the vagina of mucus, blood, and tissue debris, following childbirth.

lockjaw (clenched jaw) a firm closing of the jaw due to tonic spasm of the muscles of mastication (chewing) from the disease of the motor branch of the trigeminal nerve. An early sign of tetanus.

locomotor ataxia (tabes dorsalis) see TABES DORSALIS.

logwood (hematoxylon) the heart-wood of *Haematoxylon campechianum*, a tree of Central America. It is astringent and tonic, used therapeutically in diarrheas (at doses of 0.6 to 2.0g.). However, it is chiefly used as a dye in bacteriology.

loin(s) the lower part of the back. The flank, the part of the side and back between the ribs and the pelvis.

loquacious very talkative.

lordosis an abnormal forward curvature of the spine, usually in the lumbar region.

Loschmidt's number the number of molecules in 1 ml of gas at 0^0 C and 1 atmosphere of pressure; Avogadro's number divided by 22,400. From J. Loschmidt (1821-1895), a Czech chemist and physicist. Some incorrectly equate Loschmidt's number with Avogadro's number. See AVOGADRO'S NUMBER.

loth a unit of weight formerly used in Germany, Switzerland, Holland, and Austria, roughly equivalent to half an ounce.

low fever see TYPHUS.

low form of disease a serious disease which is in remission or not too serious at the moment.

lubricous (lubricious) 1) elusive or slippery. 2) lewd.

ludicrous laughable or hilarious through obvious absurdity, incongruity or unreasonableness.

lues (Latin for 'pestilence') syphilis.

lumbago a painful, inflammatory rheumatism of the tendons and muscles of the lumbar region.

lumbodynia see LUMBAGO.

lumbricoides resembling an earthworm, vermiform. A round worm parasitic in the human intestine, *Ascaris lumbricoides*.

lumpy jaw see ACTINOMYCOSIS.

lunar caustic (silver nitrate, argentum nitratum, silver caustic) a caustic used principally as for warts, disinfecting wounds, as an anthelminthic and in the eyes of newborns to prevent gonococcal ophthalmia (erythromycin ointment is now used in newborns instead).

lunatic an insane person, a madman (from the Latin *luna*, 'moon'.)

lung fever pneumonia

lunula the opaque whitish semi-lunar area near the root of the nail (Latin, 'little moon').

lupia 1) an encysted tumor. 2) a genus of diseases which 'molest' (destroy) the affected part.

lupoid referring to a lupus-type eruption.

lupus 1) generally refers to lupus vulgaris (tuberculous lupus). Tuberculosis of the skin, occurring in the form of reddish brown tubercles, aggregated in the form of nodules or patches. (From the Latin *lupus*, 'wolf' referring to the appearance after being disfigured by the disease, especially around the nose and ears). 2) a malignant ulceration often destroying the nose, face, etc.

lupus erythematosus (lupus sebaceous, lupus erythematodes, erythematodes, lupus superficialis, seborrhea congestiva, ulerythema centrifugum) an eruption of flat red papules, usually with a small white scale in the center of each, occurring in patches on the face, scalp and often on each cheek with a bridge extending over the nose ('butterfly eruption'); scarring follows healing of the eruption. This can actually be quite a serious immunological disease and may become systemic (disseminated). Then it becomes an inflammatory disease of the connective tissue. Fever, malaise, fatigability, joint pains or arthritis, red, inflamed skin, lesions on the face, neck and upper extremities, anemia, pleurisy, and lymphatic problems occur.

lupus hypertrophicus that variety of lupus in which new connective tissue formation predominates over the destructive process, and markedly raised, thick patches result.

lupus non-exedens tuberculosis of the skin, occurring in the form of reddish brown tubercles, but without the formation of exudates.

lupus vorax 1) eating hungrily, ravenously, or voraciously like a wolf. 2) a malignant sore. See NOLI ME TANGERE.

Luschka's tonsil the pharyngeal tonsil, from the German anatomist Herbert Luschka (1820-1875).

luxation a dislocation, as in the luxation of a joint. See SUBLUXATION.

luxus excess of any sort.

lycorexia 1) emaciation accompanied by a good appetite. 2) a feeling of satiation after eating very little.

lymphadenitis inflammation of a lymph node.

lymphadenopathy a general term for any disease process which affects lymph nodes and the lymphatic system.

lymphangioma a tumor of lymph nodes and/or lymphatic vessels.

lymphatic pertaining to a lymphatic vessel or to the lymph.

lymphatic drainage draining or purging the lymphatic system of built-up toxins. This can be accomplished by the use of specific homeopathic remedies noted for their organ-stimulating and drainage activity. Massage techniques and exercise also promote the clearing of lymph fluids and lymphatic cleansing. See MANUAL LYMPHATIC DRAINAGE.

lymphatism 1) a condition of the body characterized by sluggishness in the vital processes and functions. Having the lymphatic temperament (sluggish and phlegmatic). 2) a condition of excess lymphoid or tonsillar structures.

lyophilization 'freeze drying'. A process of dehydration, as water is removed from frozen material by sublimation (in this case the frozen water is sucked away by the use of a vacuum), leaving the raw material. This material, if stored in airtight opaque containers free of air and water vapor, can be kept almost indefinitely.

lypemania melancholy; a depressive insanity.

lypothymia melancholia.

lysis 1) the gradual subsiding of disease symptoms. 2) destruction of red blood cells, bacteria, etc.

-lysis a suffix indicating destruction or dissolution

lyssophobia 1) fear of going mad. 2) fear of rabies.

lyterian indicating the end of a disease.

M M M M M M M

macabre gruesome; grim and horrible; ghastly.

macula (pl. maculae) a small discolored patch or spot on the skin, not elevated above the general surface, 1cm or less in diameter.

madarosis a loss of the eyebrows or of the eyelashes.

made-stone (bezoars) a stone used to extract ill or evil influences from wounds or a possessed individual.

magna est veritas et praevale bit 'truth is great and goes powerfully'.

magnetized massaged, rubbed or stroked. Mesmerized.

mal-de-mer sea sickness (French).

malacia 1) a softening of tissues. 2) a depraved appetite.

malady disease or disorder (Latin *mal*, 'bad').

malaise a general feeling of illness, often accompanied by discomfort and restlessness.

malar of the cheekbone or upper jaw.

malar bone the frontal cheek bone.

malaria (intermittent fever, paludism, swamp fever) an infectious disease characterized by cycles of chills, fever, and sweating, transmitted by the bite of the infected female anopheles mosquito.

malariotherapy a type of therapy used for some sixty years, 1918-75, to treat neurosyphilis (syphilis of the brain). In this case and in some cases of Lyme's disease the spirochetes invade the brain tissues, resulting in an extremely difficult infection to cure. Enter malariotherapy: here a curable form of malaria is induced in the patient by injecting a small amount of malaria-infected blood. After three weeks, drugs are given to cure the malaria. It was found that this induced malaria stimulates the production of immune substances (interleukins and interferons) which in turn could cross the blood-brain barrier to destroy the spirochetes.

malarial cachexia see CACHEXIA MALARIA.

malaxis ventriculi (gastromalaxia) a softening of the stomach.

malignant depending on the context, this word does not necessarily mean cancerous. It can be used in a descriptive manner to denote severity. For example, some authors have used 'malignant furuncle' synonymously with 'carbuncle'.

malinger to fake/feign sickness.

malingerer a person who fakes having a disease or illness.

malis any parasitic disease.

malleation a sort of hammering movement of the hands against the thighs which might be considered a tic.

malleolus (pl. malleoli) the ankle. The rounded protuberance on either side of the ankle joint.

Malphigian bodies/corpuscles (renal corpuscles) the beginning of the urinary tubules of the kidneys. They are a mass of arterial capillaries encased in a capsule and attached to a tubule in the kidney. From the Italian anatomist Marcello Malpighi (1628-1694), who is also considered the father of histology. Depending upon the context, this term may also refer to lymph nodules surrounding the capillaries in the spleen.

Malta fever see MEDITERRANEAN FEVER.

malum disease.

malum caducum epilepsy.

mammae breasts.

mammillitis (thelitis) 'Paget's disease of the nipple'. Inflammation of the nipple.

mandamus a mandate (Latin, 'we decree').

mania a mental disorder characterized by great psychomotor activity, excitement, a rapid passing of ideas, exaltation, and an inability to focus attention.

mania-a-potu (delirium tremens, DT's) an alcoholic psychosis marked by unusual symptoms such as epileptiform seizures, confusion, illusions, anxiety, rage, violent criminal tendencies, and sometimes hallucinations; it is usually followed by amnesia of the episode. In sensitive individuals this may occur only after a small amount of alcohol is consumed. (From the Latin, 'mania from drinking').

manual lymphatic drainage a gentle whole-body massage designed to stimulate the lymphatic system to carry away excessive fluid and thus poisons/waste products which accumulate in the loose connective tissue. This technique was developed by Dr. Vodder and his wife in 1932 and is quite popular in Europe, especially Walchsee, Austria. *Textbook of Dr. Vodder's Manual Lymphatic Drainage* is the first of three extensive volumes written on the subject (Vol. I is by E. and G. Wittlinger and Vol. 2 and 3 by I. Kurz).

manubrium sterni (episternum) the first or upper piece of the sternum (breastbone). 'Manubrium' means 'handle, hilt, that which is grasped in the hand'. The sternum is perceived as being sword-shaped, with the manubrium or hilt on top.

Map of Hierarchy a term central to the homeotherapeutic philosophy of American homeopath Paul Herscu. Dr. Herscu has applied this 'map' in his treatment of children. It "...relates to the states, [phases], or remedies children go through as they progressively get worse or vice versa, as they move towards health and cure. As the child's pathology worsens, they carry over some of the symptomatology of the previous remedy state, resulting in a picutre which may be a combination of two. His map provides a model from which you can see this, and thus may help in the selection of the most appropriate remedy." - *Homeopathy Today* (1997, 17:4, p. 16)

It is an aspect of his overall method of analysis "...based on the idea that every remedy, every illness, every patient has a cycle or pattern within it. If we can identify or understand that cycle or pattern, then we can see how all the symptoms fit together. Each of these cycles in composed of segments, these being major themes which run through the symptoms." - *Homeopathy Today* (1997, 17:4, p. 15) For further elaboration consult Herscu's latest book *Stramonium* (1997).

M.A.P. an acronym for a combination homeopathic remedy containing three molds, *Mucor, Aspergillus,* and *Penicillium.* It is quite useful for hayfever treatment.

mapped tongue (geographic tongue) a patched-looking tongue, with smooth patches surrounded by raised grayish edges.

marasmus a gradual wasting away of the body from insufficient, imperfect foods or from poor absorption of foods. Extreme emaciation or general atrophy, occurring especially in young children, which may not be due to any specific or obvious cause.

"Marasmus arises from subsistence on a diet which is deficient overall, and in which there is no excess of carbohydrate. The marasmic child is much underweight. The muscles are grossly wasted. The skin is thin to the pinch, since the sub-cutaneous fat is lost, and is tightly stretched over the bony prominences and the protuberant belly. Oedema may occur in the extremities, but is not pronounced. Changes do not occur in the hair and skin texture, unless there are concurrent specific deficiencies. The liver and pancreas are usually normal. Marasmic children usually retain their appetites and are consequently easy to feed."—Kichlu & Bose, *A Text-Book of Descriptive Medicine, with Clinical Methods and Homeopathic Therapeutics*, p. 957. 'Marasmus senilus', wasting away of old age. Cf. KWASHIORKOR.

Marmorek the anti-toxic serum derived from a patient suffering from tuberculosis (as in 'serum of Marmorek'). Some references say it is the same or very similar to Tuberculin Koch.

marsh ague an intermittent fever of persons residing in marshy areas and attended with alternating cold and hot fits or spells.

marsh gas (methane, fire damp) a gas occurring as a natural product of decomposition in stagnant pools or marshes.

maschalopanus an indurated swelling of the axillary glands.

masseter the muscle which raises and lowers the jaw. The jaw muscle, the muscle used in chewing.

mastitis (mazoitis) inflammation of the breast.

mastodynia pain in the breasts.

mastoid process the pointed bone directly behind the ear lobe. That region behind the ear.

mastoiditis inflammation of any part of the mastoid process.

materia medica (pl. materia medicae or materia medicas) 'medical matter'. The branch of medical science which studies the origin and preparation of drugs, their doses, and their mode of administration; also, the drugs themselves. In homeopathy, a reference work listing remedies and their therapeutic actions. 'Materia Medica Pura' means that the information comes solely from provings and not from clinical or toxological symptomatology. See PROVING.

There are many homeopathic materia medicas, the most well known being Boericke's, which came out in 1901 (2nd edition, 1903; 3rd, with repertory, 1906: 5th, 1912; 6th, 1916; 8th, 1922; 4th and 7th editions, dates unknown). There are others: *Dictionary of Practical Materia Medica*

(J.H. Clarke), *Guiding Symptoms of Our Materia Medica* (C. Hering), *Encyclopedia of Pure Materia Medica* (T. Allen), *Clinical Materia Medica* (E.A. Farrington), *Synoptic Key* (C.M. Boger), *Manual of Pharmacodynamics* (R. Hughes), *Essentials of Homeopathic Materia Medica* (J. Jouanny), *Textbook of Materia Medica* (A. Lippe), *Homeopathic Materia Medica for Nurses* (B. Woodbury), *Phatak's Materia Medica* (S. Phatak), *Study of Remedies by Comparison* (H.A. Roberts), etc.

There are two kinds of materia medicas, ones like Hering's and Allen's which are compilations of raw proving data and those like Boericke's, Kent's, Nash's, etc. which are good digests. In its most basic form, a materia medica consists of quotes from the persons who 'proved' the substance. When homeopathy was in its infancy the number of drugs or remedies in the materia medica was very small. It was relatively easy to go remedy by remedy and look up symptoms in order to find the curative remedy. However, as the science expanded it was necessary to find a better way to retrieve all these 'quotes' or symptoms, therefore an index was needed. And thus the repertory was born. See REPERTORY.

"The approach to the study of the case and the approach to the study of the materia medica are essentially the same—the materia medica is the facsimile of the sickness."—H.A. Roberts, *Principles and Art of Cure by Homoeopathy.*

"There is no road to the practice of homoeopathy—whether it is the clinical road or the symptomatic road—which does not entail close and constant study of the Materia Medica."—J.H. Clarke, *The Prescriber.*

"All the diseases known to man have their likeness in the Materia Medica, and the physician must become so conversant with this art that he may perceive this likeness."—J.T. Kent, *Lectures on Homoeopathic Philosophy.*

materia peccans morbid or poisonous material which was believed to contaminate the body if it accumulated (Latin, 'offensive matter', lit. 'sinful matter').

material doses (appreciable doses, physiological doses, large doses) doses which are not homeopathic. Doses which contain active medicinal material and rely upon that to bring about therapeutic activity. For example, the typical aspirin tablet contains 325 mg of aspirin, a material level of active ingredient, whereas homeopathic *Aspirin* would not contain any measurable amount of aspirin.

materialism the philosophical opinion that physical matter is the only reality and that everything in the universe, including emotions, thoughts, the mind and even the will, can be explained using physical laws. According to this philosophy, physical wellbeing and worldly possessions are the greatest good and value in life.

matrix (extracellular matrix, ground substance) the colloidal substance or bodily 'sea' in which the entire human organism resides. Accordingly, once this 'sea' is understood, regulated and brought into balance, health can be realized. This theory is proposed principally by Alfred Pischinger, M.D., a professor at the University of Vienna, and elaborated in his book *Matrix and Matrix Regulation: Basis for a Holistic Theory in Medicine* (1991).

"Every cell in the body is embedded in a thin layer of semiliquid gel. This is the extracellular matrix, the playground of Holistic Medicine. All cells are cared for and regulated by this nurturing gel. It gets its consistency from a microscopic three-dimensional collagenous mesh. The liquid milieu inside this mesh is a meeting place for the systems that control all the major functions of the body. It is the matrix that enables us to adapt to a changing environment. Cells are not adaptable; each one is a closed system, with fixed behaviors that are set by their genes. The matrix, on the other hand, is an *open dissipative system*, able to juggle many interacting influences so that they function together, defying the forces of chaos.

"The mesh is the first structure to react to any change of environment, and that reaction affects everything else that goes on in the matrix. It has a remarkable ability to develop rhythmic patterns of contraction, that promote the best possible adaptation to adverse conditions. Those patterns can spread throughout the entire matrix, and they can be self-perpetuating. The effect of a pinprick can be traced as it spreads—it takes about four hours to go from head to toe. A very small but constant irritation, such as a badly healed scar, can set the stage for chronic disease."—*Townsend Letter for Doctors and Patients,* May 1997.

Matteism a system of medical therapeutics developed by an Italian researcher, Count Caesar Mattei, in the 1800s. He called it electrohomoeopathy but the only semblance it has with homeopathy resides in the fact that most of 'his' remedies are potentized.

Matteism is a pathological theory of his own and no remedy provings were done whatsoever. Basically, Mattei felt that disease came out of derangements of either the blood or lymph, and that cancer was a combination of both. Thus he developed remedies (he never said how they were produced or where they came from) to be taken internally often in very frequent doses, and, as the occasion arose, to be applied to various points on the body. In order to facilitate the practitioner's practice of electro-homeopathy, he provided charts and tables in his books to indicate where the remedy should touch the body. His remedies included *Anti-scrofolous, anti-canceroso, anti-angioitics, lord,* and *marina.*

Early books on the subject include *Electro-homeopathic Medicine: A New Medical System, being a popular and domestic guide founded on experiences by Count Caesar Mattei* (translated by R.M. Theobald) and *The Principles of Electro-homeopathy. A New Science Discovered by Count C. Mattei of Bologna* (American edition, 1883).

Matteism was not looked upon favorably by the homeopathic community: "This monstrous imposture, which its inventor has not been ashamed to baptise, with the greatest effrontery, electro-homoeopathy, in giving to his mysterious preparations the form of our globules; this audacious counterfeit, I say, which took birth at Bologna from the diseased brain of an eager dreamer, has extended itself like a hideous plague all over Italy, and from thence overflowing into the rest of Europe, has enveloped Switzerland (where one can already count two forms of Matteism), France, and above all Russia, where this ridiculous system of therapeutics, primitive to a degree alike in theory and in practice, seems to have found the territory most favourable to its diffusion, probably owing to the little scientific culture of the well-to-do classes of that country."—Bernard Arnulphy, M.D. (*Transactions of the International Homoeopathic Convention*, London, July, 1881, p. 80–81).

maw worm *(Ascaris vermicularis)* the thread-worm.

maxilla (pl. maxillae) the upper jaw bone.

Mayr method/cure a method developed by F.X. Mayr (1875-1965) for diagnosis and treatment of the unhealthy abdomen. Central to his theory of illness is the functioning of the intestinal organs. Thus he established diagnostic criteria for the healthy and unhealthy abdomen, such as shape and firmness, sensitivity to pressure, intestinal position, and gas content. He also established connections between digestive disturbances, posture and the condition of the skin. His method of treatment involves fasting, special diets, exercise, hydrotherapy, abdominal massage and intestinal cleansing.

mazoitis (mastitis) inflammation of the breast.

McBurney's point the point of tenderness in appendicitis, five or six centimeters above the right anterior superior iliac spine, on a line drawn from this point to the navel.

mealy granular, mottled, flecked with spots.

measles (morbilli, rubeola) a disease which (after exposure and an incubation period of two weeks) begins with coryza, cough, conjunctivitis, and spots in the mouth (Koplik's spots). A few days later chills, fever, and a red maculopapular eruption appears first on the face or behind the ears. Three days later the eruption fades and is followed by a branny desquamation. It is caused by a virus, and one attack confers immunity.

meatus an opening, passage or canal, as in the external and internal meatus of the ear.

meconium the first intestinal discharges of the newborn infant, greenish in color and consisting of epithelial cells, mucus, and bile.

meddlesome inclined to interfere or intrude in people's affairs or business.

medial in anatomy, toward the midline of the body, as opposed to lateral (on the side or away from the midline). Relating to the middle or center. For example, the clavicles (collarbones) are lateral to the sternum (breastbone), which is medial.

Mediterranean fever (brucellosis, Malta fever, Rio Grande fever, undulant fever) a remittent febrile disease caused by infection with bacteria of the genus *Brucella*. In humans it causes weakness, loss of weight, and anemia. It rarely spreads from person to person, but spreads readily from animal to animal and from animal to man. See UNDULANT FEVER.

medorrhoea a discharge from the reproductive organs, usually meaning gonorrhea. 'M. urethralis' means gonorrhea, 'm. virilis' means gonorrhea of the male urethra.

medullary pertaining to the bone marrow; pertaining to a central cavity.

megrim migraine or dull headache affecting one side of the head, in the region of the temple. Not to be confused with 'megrims' (vertigo in horses).

Meibomian gland (tarsal gland) one of the sebaceous glands on the margins of the eyelids which secretes a lubricatory fluid.

mel honey.

melancholia a mental disorder characterized by extreme depression, apathy, gloom, fear, brooding and painful delusions. Activities are usually inhibited, although the patient may show psychomotor overactivity or may have many depressive ideas that shift rapidly.

"A form of insanity whose essential and characteristic feature is a depressed, i.e., subjectively arising painful emotional state, which may be associated with a depression of other nervous functions."—Lilienthal, *Medical Counselor,* 6/15/1885, p. 233.

Melanchthon one who is a leader in the reforming of ideas. An eponym after Philipp Melanchthon (Philipp Schwarzerd, 1497-1560), a German humanist. He was a contemporary of Martin Luther and an important figure in the Lutheran Reformation.

melanomania an unusual passion for music; the habit of singing incessantly.

melanosis the abnormal deposit of melanins (brown-black pigments) in the various parts of the body.

melena/melaena (melenemesis, morbus niger) black vomit. May also mean the passage of dark-colored tarry stools, due to the presence of blood altered by the intestinal juices.

melitis inflammation of the cheek.

melicera a cyst or tumor which contains matter of a honey-like consistency.

melituria see DIABETES MELLITUS.

meloncus a particularly violent ulcerous swelling of the cheek.

membrum virile the penis (L., 'the male part', 'masculine member').

menarche the commencing of the menstrual function or cycle in a young girl.

mendacity the quality or state of being false or lying. Deceitfulness.

mendosus false or incomplete.

menidrosis (menhidrosis) bleeding from the skin occurring as a form of vicarious menstruation.

Meniere's disease (auditory vertigo) an affection characterized clinically by vertigo, nausea, vomiting, tinnitus, and progressive deafness. First described by the French physician P. Meniere (1799-1862).

meninges (sing. meninx) the membranous coverings of the brain and spinal cord.

meningism a condition of irritation of the brain or spinal cord in which the symptoms simulate a meningitis but in which no actual inflammation of the membranes is present.

meningitis (cerebro-spinal fever) inflammation of the membranes of the brain or spinal cord.

meningitis basilaria inflammation of the meninges at the base of the brain.

meninx (pl. meninges) one of the membraneous coverings of the brain and spinal cord.

menochesia feeble menstruation or the retention or inhibition of menses.

menophania the first appearance of the menstrual period.

menoposis (menopause) cessation of the menses in a middle-aged woman.

menoplania (vicarious menstruation) 1) bleeding from other parts of the body rather than the uterus during the menstrual cycle. 2) the tendency of a woman's menstrual cycle to coincide with that of other women with whom she lives or works closely.

menorrhagia an intensified and prolonged menstrual flow.

menostasia a suppression of the menstrual flow.

menstrual nisus a condition in which the menstrual period is labored, difficult, an effort or struggle (L. *nisus,* 'effort, struggle, labor pain').

mentagra (sycosis) an eruption about the chin, caused by inflammation of the hair follicles of the beard.

mental symptoms see entry under SYMPTOMS.

meralgia sciatica or pain in the thigh.

Merc. iod. Mercurius proto-iodatus.

mercurial 1) a medical or chemical preparation containing mercury. 2) being quick or changeable in character, as in 'he has a mercurial temperament'.

mercury a metallic element which is employed in many forms as a homeopathic remedy: Mercury = *Mercurius vivus* = *Mercurius solubilis* = *Mercurius Hahnemannian. Merc. sol.*, the mercury of Hahnemann, is a combination of mercuric nitrate and ammonium. All four are considered the same and have like symptoms. *Merc. dulcis* (Hg_2Cl_2) or calomel acts primarily on the Eustachian tube. *Cinnabaris* (the sulfur salt of mercury) acts on the eye, sinus, and skin. *Merc. corrosivus* ($HgCl_2$, corrosive sublimate of Mercury) is comparable to *Merc. sol.* in symptoms except it may be said that its symptoms are more acute and intense. *Merc. cyanatus* ($HgCN_2$), *Merc. biiodatus flavus* (HgI_2) and *Merc. protoiodatus* (Hg_2I_2) have actions centered on the mouth, throat, and pharyngeal mucosa. *Merc.-i.-flavus* and *Merc-i.-ruber* are used for right-sided and left-sided sore throats, respectively.

meridian complexes homeopathic mixtures originally formulated many years ago by the German physician Helmut Schimmel and marketed by Kern Pharma. Each meridian complex has a combination of three homeopathic remedies, one each from the animal, plant, and mineral kingdoms. These mixtures effect energy flow through the organs associated with their corresponding acupuncture meridians, vessels, and chakras. The effect is to release and regulate blocked energy circulation in the patient.

Dr. Schimmel is the founder of the VEGATEST, an EAV test method as well as the co-author of *Functional Medicine, Vol. 1, The Origin and Treatment of Chronic Diseases* (Schimmel/Penzer, 1996, Haug). See EAV, FUNCTIONAL MEDICINE, KERN MERIDIAN COMPLEXES.

meridrosis a perspiration in local or specific spots.

mesenteric referring to the mesentery, a double layer of peritoneum (membranous folds) attached to the abdominal wall and enclosing in its folds a portion or all of the abdominal viscera (organs), conveying to it its vessels and nerves. Simply, the peritoneal attachment of the small intestine.

mesmerize to hypnotize, to overcome by suggestion, massage or touching. From the 18th century German physician F.A. Mesmer (1734-1815), who was also interested in astrology, believing starry emanations could influence man. He tried to connect those emanations with electricity and magnetism and established a therapeutic method of stroking ill persons with magnets. Mesmerism and 'animal magnetism' became synonymous terms. Mesmer first started treating patients in 1773.

Following the studies of Mesmer, the Puysegur brothers (*Du Magnetisme Animal*, 1807), particularly Mesmer's pupil the Marquis de Puysegur, developed a cult following in this field. They used animal magnetism in the fashion of the Druids and performed rituals in the dense forests. Carl A.F. Kluge, a German mesmerist, did much to spread Mesmer's theories. His book, *Versuch einer Darstellung des Animalischen Magnestismus als Heilmittel* (1811), is said to have been reprinted as many times as Virchow's book on cellular pathology. P.P. Quimby (1802-1866) an American mystic, practiced mesmerism and mental healing (mind-cure). It is postulated that Quimby laid the foundations for Christian Science. His theories, along with F.W. Evans and the Dressers', formed what was called 'New Thought', which basically means the importance of the mind in the healing process. Mary Baker G. Eddy, a patient of Quimby's, further developed all of this into what is now termed Christian Science, which states that 'illness is non-existent and that to maintain health one needs to rely solely on God.' Hahnemann briefly mentions mesmerism/animal magnetism in his Organon. Od is the supposed force responsible for mesmerism.

Robert Rohland wrote about magnetism, mesmerism, and the Od-force in his treatise, *Od, or odo-magnetic force, an explanation of its influence on homeopathic medicines...* (translated from the German, 1871, 39 pp.). Another homeopath, Carl Caspari (1798-1828), wrote *Dr. Caspari's Homeopathic Domestic Physician* (edited by F. Hartmann, preface by C. Hering) which contained a chapter on magnetism and mesmerism. By 1826, Caspari had 'Mesmerismus' (a potency of mesmerized water) for sale in his pharmacy (Hausapotheke), and Boenninghausen mentions Mesmerism as a cure for nerve diseases. Provings on 'Mesmerismus' were conducted in the mid 1800s in Europe.

It was left to James Braid to coin the terms 'hypnotism' and 'hypnosis' in his *Neurypnology; or, the Rationale of Nervous Sleep, considered in relation with Animal Magnetism* (1843). This extensive treatise and his researches changed his life and determined to some extent the development of psychology and psychiatry. For a while, before he coined those two terms, hypnotism was called 'Braidism'.

Hahnemann first mentions magnetismus, Mesmer and his theories in his doctoral dissertation (8-10-1779). It is also mentioned in his *Organon*. Mesmer and Hahnemann, in addition to mundane similarities (both lived in Paris at the height of their careers, both had lawyers/jurists as loyal adherents, and both were persecuted relentlessly), had more important similarities in that both believed in a dynamis/vital force theory and each suggested or proposed a worsening of symptoms (aggravation/crisis) before disease resolution. Mesmerism, hydrotherapy and dietetics are the only non-homeopathic treatments mentioned in a positive way in the *Organon*.

meta-analysis a higher order or higher level of analysis. A way of examination which is more than just analysis but engenders introspection. A systematic analysis of previous research which uses a specific method to compare the results of various trials. A meta-analysis of 107 controlled trials of homeopathic remedies was published in the *British Medical Journal* (302: 316-323).

metacarpal pertaining to the metacarpus. See METACARPUS.

metacarpus that part of the hand that includes the five bones between the phalanges (fingers) and the carpus (wrist).

metachysis transfusion.

metamorphosis transformation; a change in form.

metaphorical naturalism a term coined by Greg Bedayn, RSHoм (NA) which refers to the metaphorical relationship between the natural characteristics of a remedy and the characteristics of the patient who is cured by or responds to that remedy. It can be likened to an expanded Doctrine of Signatures. For instance, consider a vibrant flower blossom that wilts from lack of water or proper nutrition. The similar patient whose normal 'effervescence' has gone flat may also need that similar vibrational medicine, *Phosphorus*. It is interesting to note that phosphorus is the primary ingredient in fertilizer for blossoming plants and is an essential component of carbonated beverages. This same person may show a common, yet unlisted, symptom of being ameliorated by water (bathing, swimming, drinking, playing, etc.) The element phosphorus must be stored submerged in water or it will diffuse into the air.

"Anacardium is a nut from the mountains of Eastern India. It has an external coating of an oil which is black, caustic and 'bad', but the heart of the nut is sweet. The personality [of the patient] may be called malicious, but with a sweet heart. Dissociation, splitness and separation up to the extreme of schizophrenia are part of its characteristic proving picture. A symptom mentioned in its proving and clinically typical, is a sense of two wills, one bad, one good." - E.C. Whitmont ('Alchemy, homeopathy and the treatment of borderline cases' *(Journal of Analytical Psychology,* 1996, 41, p. 382)

This type of pondering is no substitute for repertory and materia medica work, but it does help the practitioner gain added insights into his patient.

metastasis the spread of a disease from the primary focus or site of origin to a distant part of the body.

metastasize to spread by metastasis, as in 'the cancer has metastasized'.

metasyphilis the constitutional state due to hereditary or congenital syphilis but without skin symptoms.

metatarsus the middle part of the foot. The five bones between the toes and the tarsus (heel) that form the instep.

meteorism gas and/or feces expelled from the anus with explosive force. 'Meteorismus' is an extreme inflation of the intestines.

meteorosensitivity a sensitivity to the changes in the weather.

metralgia uterine pain.

metrectopia (metrectopy) a displacement of the uterus.

metritis (hysteritis, uteritis) inflammation of the uterus.

metrodynia uterine pain.

metromania insanity associated with uterine complaints.

metroptosis a displacement or prolapse of the uterus.

metrorrhagia irregular, acyclic bleeding from the uterus. Profuse flow of blood from the uterus at any time other than that of the menstrual period.

miasm/miasmatic a noxious influence. 'Miasm' as defined by Hahnemann is the infectious principle, or virus, which, when taken into the organism, may set up a specific disease. Other texts of the mid 1800s defined 'miasms' as 'peculiar effluvia or emanations from swampy grounds'. The principle miasms are psora, sycosis, syphilis and tuberculinism (which is theorized to be a combination of psora and syphilis). Miasms may be inherited, acquired, or acute. It is said that cancer is a combination of the three major miasms.

The miasmatic keynotes are as follows: for psora, hypersensitivity, periodicity, skin symptoms, anxiety, > cold, > night, energy-giving; for sycosis, hypertrophy, water retention, warty growths, obsessions, < cold damp weather, < night, repugnant sort of energy; for syphilis, destruction, degeneration, severe phobias/anxieties, insomnia, deformities, < night, energy-taking.

Miasms and miasmatic theory are too complicated to be discussed in this setting; there are a number of books devoted to this subject. Vithoulkas' *The Science of Homeopathy* is a good place to start. Also helpful may be: P.S. Ortega, *Notes on the Miasms,* H.Choudhury, *Indications of Miasm*, H.C. Allen, *Materia Medica of the Nosodes*, and S.C.F. Hahnemann, *Chronic Diseases.* For a non homeopathic treatment of the subject consult *Miasmas and Disease* (Carlo M. Cipolla).

miasmata (miasmas) plural of 'miasm'.

mickles great or much. A great sum or amount. To a great degree.

micropus an individual with very small feet (Gr. *micro-,* 'small', and *pus,* 'foot').

microsomia dwarfishness or smallness of the body.

microsporia (Gruby's disease) a form of alopecia caused by *Microsporon audouini,* as first described by D. Gruby (1810-1898), a Parisian doctor.

micturition urination.

mictus cruentis a bloody urination.

miliaria (sudamina, prickly heat, heat rash, strophulus, lichen tropicus, miliaria rubra) a disorder of the sweat glands with obstruction of their ducts. An acute inflammatory skin disease, the lesions consisting of vesicles and papules, accompanied by a pricking or tingling sensation. It occurs especially in summer and in the tropics, often in the folds of the skin. From the Latin *miliarius,* 'of millet', referring to the millet seed. 'Miliaria' may also refer to miliary fever, which is a fever accompanied by an eruption of small, isolated, red pimples which resemble a millet seed.

miliary resembling a millet seed in size (1-2mm). Marked by the presence of nodules the size of millet seeds.

miliary tuberculosis an acute form of tuberculosis characterized by very small tubercles spread throughout the body caused by the dissemination of tubercle bacilli through the blood stream.

milieu the environment or surroundings.

milium a skin disease characterized by formation of small, pearly, non-inflammatory elevations or globoid masses situated on the face or genitalia. They may become hard and persist for years.

milk crust (cradle cap) see CRUSTA LACTEA.

milk fever a slight rise in the mother's temperature once her milk begins to flow, which may involve an increased pulse rate, malaise, and breast tenderness and distension.

   The term was formerly applied to all febrile conditions following childbirth; thus it may or may not be synonymous with child-bed or puerperal fever, depending on the context. See PUERPERAL FEVER.

milk leg (phlebitis, phlegmasia alba dolens) inflammation of a vein, especially a vein of the lower limbs. See PHLEGMASIA ALBA DOLENS. It is an archaic term but so coined because it was thought that the varicosed condition of the woman's leg was due to a 'disease' in her milk, hence the association.

milk pox see AMAAS.

milk punch a preparation made by adding rum, whiskey, or brandy to milk in proportions of 1:4 or 1:6 (spirits:milk), flavored with nutmeg, cinnamon and sugar, once considered nutritious.

milk sugar see LACTOSE.

Millar's asthma (laryngismus stridulus, Kopp's asthma, Wichmann's asthma) differs from true croup in that it has no membrane and no concurrent flu or cold symptoms. It usually attacks children suddenly, usually in the middle of the night, producing difficulty of breathing, hoarse cough, a deep, harsh-sounding voice, great anxiety, and apparent suffocation. Fits of vomiting, sneezing or coughing may occur, then the child may sleep briefly only to reawaken with a recurrence of symptoms.

milliards billions.

milt the spleen *(archaic; in modern usage, reproductive exudate of the male fish)*.

miner's asthma (miner's tuberculosis, miner's phthisis, anthracosis) shortness of breath due to anthracosis, a black pigmentation of the lungs associated with inflammation due to inhalation of coal/carbon dust.

miner's tuberculosis (miner's phthisis, anthracosis) see MINER'S ASTHMA.

minim a measurement of liquid equivalent to approximately 1 drop. 16.23 minims = 1cc.

minister naturae 'nature's servant/attendant' or 'tool/instrument of nature' (Latin).

mirbane nitrobenzol, a substance used in perfumery with a very sweet taste and an odor resembling that of bitter almonds. (*'Mirbane'*, as in 'essence of mirbane, oil of mirbane', is a French word of obscure origin).

misanthrophy hatred or distrust of mankind.

miseriae poverty (L., 'miseries, troubles').

miserere spasmodic (copremesis) the spasmodic vomiting of fecal matter.

mistura a mixture.

mithridatism the phenomenon whereby the toxic effect of a poison is decreased if a low concentration of that poison is given before or after that poison is administered.

mitral bicuspid (pertaining to the atrioventricular valve on the left side of the heart).

mixology (combination homeopathy, complex homeopathy) the prescription of more than one remedy at a time. See POLYPHARMACY.

mixologists practitioners who "mix allopathic and homeopathic remedies either in the same dose (!) or in the same treatment, or those who combine several remedies in one bottle as a specific for certain ailments."— T. Borghardt (*Homoeopathic Links,* 2/93, p. 7)

MK an abbreviation for the 1000C Korsakovian potency (M standing for one thousand).

mnemonical delineation a memorization device for a remedy picture. For instance, **"THYROIDINUM**: **T** = temperamental disturbances of adolescence: iritability, whimsical moods, etc. **H** = hyperthyroidism. **Y** = yields wonderfully to icterus and chronic vomiting. **R** = rachitic, thin, scrawny, cachectic, with mental retardation, is the characteristic appearance. **O** = oedema of the face and extremities, yet emaciated, anaemic subjects. Also, = obesity with oedema associated with anaemia**. I** = infantile convulsion withut fever or trauma (esp. born of mothers suffering from eclampsia or of parents suffering from various nervous and metabolic disorders). **D** = diabetes mellitus: when symptoms appear with great rapidity, accompanied by weakness. **I** = infantile eczema during dentition esp. in elbow and knee is characteristic. Also exfoliation of skin from palms and soles. **N** = nodular goitres. **U** = uterine fibroids. **M** = mixed miasmatic with strong tubercular preponderance. Myxodema and cretinism; one of our sheet-anchors. Manias: irritable, impatient, suicidal tendences, fear of being arrested."—S.K. Banerjee (*Homoeopathic Links*, 2/93, p.17).

modality a condition that makes the ill person or a particular symptom better or worse; a circumstance giving rise to an increase or decrease of a symptom. For instance, the patient is worse (<) from wet weather, after midnight and from cold drinks; or he is better (>) from heat, elevating the head and from warm/hot drinks. Modalities are helpful in choosing the correct remedy.

"Modalities are conditions which influence or modify drug action. The main group are time, temperature, weather, motion, menstruation, position, perspiration, eating and emotion. A practical point also is that there are two types of modalities: 1) those that apply to the person as a whole, 2) those that apply to a person's particular complaint or involve an organ."—*Principles of Homoeopathy* (G. Boericke).

One must learn to differentiate between modalities. For example, if the patient says, "I am better with company," this must be distinguished among four rubrics: Company amel. (p. 61), thinking of complaints agg. (p. 350), diversion amel. (p. 90), conversation amel. (p. 64).—R. Sankaran (*Homoeopathic Links*, 2/93, p. 34).

modus medendi 'way of healing' (Latin).

mogigraphia writer's cramp.

molecular pathology a theory of disease developed by Schade and Busse-Grawitz in 1946, centered on infection and actual physico-chemical alterations in the cells and tissues. This theory is supplemented by pharmacological research concentrating on the direct effects which drugs have on subcellular aspects such as enzymatic cycles, metabolic pathways, and neurotransmission. It is this area in which H.H. Reckeweg, founder of homotoxicology, concentrated his therapeutic efforts by developing theories of homotoxins, homotoxones, detoxification, the Greater-Defense System, vicariation of disease, retoxification, and his Table of Homotoxicosis. From this came his therapeutic approach utilizing combinations of nosodes, homeopathics, intermediary catalysts, organotherapies, auto-sanguis dilution therapy, potency chords, etc. See HOMOTOXICOLOGY.

molimen an effort. The laborious performance of a normal function, as in an effort to establish the menstrual flow. The unpleasant symptoms, feeling of weight in the pelvis, nervous and circulatory disturbances, etc., experienced during the menstrual period (Latin, 'great effort, exertion').

mollities ossium (osteomalacia) softening of bone with the development of deformities.

molluscum a chronic disease marked by the occurrence of soft rounded tumors of the skin.

mongrel a term applied to a homeopath who strayed from classical homeopathy to blend other therapies into his so-called homeopathic practice. It was generally used in a derogatory sense.

monocular amblyopia a dimness of vision or partial loss of sight of one eye without discoverable lesion in the eye structures or the optic nerve.

monomania insanity in relation to a single idea or subject. An unreasonable pursuit of one idea.

mononucleosis see GLANDULAR FEVER.

monorrhagia a term peculiar to homotoxicology which means the discharge of a homotoxin.

mons veneris (mons pubis) pubic mound; the prominence or eminence caused by a pad of fatty tissue over the pubic bone covered with hair in women after puberty (Latin, 'mount of Venus').

Monsel's salt (persulfate of iron, ferric subsulfate) a substance which acts as a styptic when made into a solution.

MORA therapy a bioresonance therapy. Here the instrument, using the patient's electromagnetic frequency, cancels pathological information in the body, while intensifying the healthy frequencies. Saliva, blood, urine, medications and other substances can be homeopathically potentized, amplified and then transferred back into the patient. Allergies and geopathic disturbances can also be diagnosed and treated. From Morell-Rasche, the two researchers who collaborated on this theory and instrumentation. See EAV.

morbid diseased, unhealthy; mentally unwholesome, gloomy.

morbific pathogenic, disease-producing, generating a sickly state.

morbilli measles, hence *Morbillinum* is the measles nosode.

morbus an old term for 'disease'. 'M. divinus' (epilepsy), 'm. gallicus' (syphilis).

morbus animi a general term for 'mental disease' (L., 'illness of the mind/soul/spirit').

morbus Bechterew chronic arthritis of unknown origin with progressive deformity, stiffness, and bony fusion of the vertebrae. From the Russian neurologist V.M. Bekhterev (1856-1927).

morbus caducus epilepsy (L., 'falling sickness').

morbus coeruleus (blue disease) cyanosis of the newborn. See CYANOSIS.

morbus coxarius (morbus coxae) hip disease. Tuberculous inflammation of the hip (coxitis).

morbus divinus epilepsy (L., 'divine illness')

morbus niger (meloena, black jaundice, morbus niger hippocratis, melena) vomiting of black blood or a blackish discharge from the rectum. Black vomit. (L., 'black disease').

morbus regius see JAUNDICE.

morbus sacer epilepsy (L., 'sacred illness').

morbus sudatorius excessive or foul smelling sweat (L., 'sweating disease').

moria foolishness, dullness of comprehension. A mental condition marked by frivolity and continued tendency to make fun or jest of everything and being unable to take anything seriously.

moribund dying or at the point of death.

moron an archaic term used to describe a person with a retarded mental development having a mental age between 7-12 years according to Binet or an IQ of between 50-75. See BINET TEST.

morose gloomy, melancholic, ill-humored.

morphinism (from Morpheus, the god of dreams or of sleep) effects caused by the habitual use of morphine; morphine addiction. A morbid state induced by excessive use of opium marked particularly by lethargy, lassitude, and chronic depression. In 1805, the German pharmacist Frederick

Serturner (1784-1841) isolated morphine, the chief narcotic principle of opium. His paper, 'Morphis, a New Salt-forming Substance, and Meconic Acid, as the chief constituents of Opium', ushered in a new era of development in organic plant chemistry. This was soon followed by the isolation of narcotine by Robiquet and strychnine by Pelletier and Caventou.

morphoea (morphea, circumscribed scleroderma, Addison's keloid) a skin disease marked by the presence of indurated patches of a whitish or yellowish white color surrounded by a pinkish or purplish border.

morphology science of the form and structure of organisms.

mors death (Latin).

mortification gangrene; as in m. of tissues. Also humiliation or indignation.

morsus a bite.

Morvan's disease (analgesic panaris) analgesic paralysis with whitlow, a progressive paralysis and atrophy of the forearms and hands with analgesia and the formation of painless whitlows; probably the same as syringomyelia. First described by the French physician Morvan (1819-1897). See WHITLOW.

motes minute particles or specks, as in 'dust motes' (specks of dust).

moth patch liver spot. See CHLOASMA.

mother tincture (M.T. or f, the Greek letter *phi*) the starting alcoholic liquid from which homeopathic potencies are made. This tincture may also be used therapeutically in material doses (drop doses), either internally or topically. See MATERIAL DOSES.

mottled resembling a pattern with spots or streaks of different shades or colors.

mountain sickness (veta, mountain fever) a condition marked by giddiness, dyspnea, nausea, rapid pulse, and headache due to lack of oxygen in the rarefied air at high altitudes.

mountebank a charlatan. One who sells quack medicines.

moxa a cone of cotton or wool mixed with an herb (usually aiye-mugwort, or *Artemisia vulgaris*), placed on the skin and then ignited to produce counter-irritation and/or stimulate an acupuncture point, in order to treat an ailment. It works by balancing bodily *chi*. This is the direct method of moxabustion, while the indirect method involves placing an agent between the moxa and skin. Ginger, garlic, aconite or salt are often used as this medium. Sometimes a stick of moxa will be placed on the top of the acupuncture needle and lit. It is a treatment with Yang properties, in other words, adding heat to the body. See ACUPUNCTURE.

mucopurulent referring to an exudate which contains chiefly pus but also mucous material.

mucopus a discharge made up of mucus and pus.

multicord a potency chord including remedies from different potency scales (x, c, LM). See POTENCY CHORD.

multifarious having a great diversity or variety. Manifold.

multiple sclerosis (Charcot's disease, disseminated multiple sclerosis, MS) a progressive degenerative disease of the central nervous system (CNS) in which hardening of tissue (demyelination of nerve tissue) occurs throughout the brain and/or spinal cord. First signs are abnormal sensations in the extremities, muscle weakness, vertigo, and visual disturbances. As the disease progresses, symptoms include difficulty in urination, ataxia, abnormal reflexes, emotional instability. The disease cycles through severe and less severe periods or episodes. Charcot (1825-1893) was one of the greatest neurologists of all time, describing many neurological diseases.

mumps (epidemic parotitis, parotiditis) inflammation of the parotid gland. It is characterized by swelling of the parotid and salivary glands as well as the pancreas, ovaries, and testes. It begins with fever, pain below the ear, and swelling of the parotid gland. The swelling subsides in about a week. One attack usually confers immunity.

murias magnesia magnesium chloride (Latin *murias,* 'chloride', as in *Natrum muriaticum,* sodium chloride).

muqueses (Spanish) mucous or referring to mucus.

muscae volitantes (floaters) an appearance as of moving spots before the eyes. (Latin, 'flies that are flying around').

musty having a stale or moldy odor or taste.

mutinism (mutism) dumbness, absence of the faculty of speech.

mutisia the flowering heads of *Mutisia vicioefolia,* a Bolivian plant used as an expectorant in tuberculosis and as a sedative in chronic diseases of the heart.

mutton sheep or lamb meat.

mycosis the presence of parasitic fungi in the body, as well as the disease caused by them.

mydriasis dilation of the pupil of the eye. 'Myosis' is constriction of the pupil.

myelalgia pain in the spinal cord or its membranes.

myelitis inflammation of muscle tissue. Also, depending on the context, an inflammation of the spinal marrow.

myelon the spinal cord.

myelopathy a disease or disorder of the spinal cord.

myocardial of or relating to the heart muscle.

myocarditis inflammation of the heart muscle itself.

myodynia (myalgia) muscular pain.

myogelosis a firm mass or nodule within the muscle tissue. It may be formed of muscular or tumor-like tissue.

myoma (pl. myomata) tumor of a muscle.

myoma uteri (fibroid) a benign tumor of the uterus.

myomectomy removal of a fibroid tumor from the uterus.

myonosus (myopathy) any disease of the muscular tissues.

myopia nearsightedness. The ability to see objects when held close to the eyes.

myopic astigmia (nearsighted astigmatism) astigmatism in which the images are focused in front of the retina. Objects held close to the eye are seen more clearly than distant ones, but still fuzzy.

myosis (miosis) constriction of the pupil of the eye (the pupil getting smaller). 'Mydriasis' is dilation of the pupil (the pupil getting larger).

myositis ossificans a rare disease characterized by progressive hardening of the muscles. A non-inflammatory ossification of the muscles.

myotonia congenita see THOMSEN'S DISEASE.

myringitis inflammation of the tympanic membrane (the ear drum).

myxoedema (myxedema) a disease caused by decreased activity of the thyroid gland in adults, and characterized by dry skin, swellings around the lips and nose, mental deterioration, and a subnormal basal metabolic rate.

N

Nabothian cyst a cyst of the Nabothian glands. The Nabothian glands or follicles (from Martin Naboth, a Leipzig anatomist and physician, 1675-1721) are located in the cervix and secrete mucus. When these glands become obstructed, cysts are formed. The discharge of thin mucus from the pregnant uterus, which accumulates as the result of excessive secretion of the uterine glands, is known as Nabothian menorrhagia.

naevus (nevus) (plural 'naevi') a birthmark. A congenital mark or discolored patch of the skin due to pigmentation or to hyperplasia of the blood-vessels. A beauty mark or mole.

nanism dwarfishness.

nape back of the neck.

naprapathy a system devoted to the correct alignment of the skeletal system. Here, manipulation of the spinal, thoracic and pelvic ligaments are made in order to improve bodily alignment and general health. "Naprapathy relies primarily on specific connective tissue manipulative therapy to relieve neurovascular interference, which may generate circulatory congestion and nerve irritation."—Bulletin of Chicago National College of

Naprapathy (the only school of naprapathy, located at 3330 N. Milwaukee Ave., Chicago, IL 60641).

Oakley Smith founded the science of naprapathy in 1905 and directed the college for many years until his death in 1970. Though not the same, myopractic is a very similar technique.

Naprapathy is a licensed health care specialty in Illinois.

narcolepsy an uncontrollable tendency to have attacks of deep sleep of short duration at any time.

narcosis deep unconsciousness, usually caused by a drug.

narcotic a medicine which produces stupor or complete insensibility. 'Narcotism' is stupor produced by narcotics or other drugs. Also addiction to habit-forming drugs.

nares the nostrils.

nasitis inflammation of the nose.

nasus nose.

nates the buttocks.

naturopathy (naturopathic medicine) a system of therapeutic medical science comprising many natural healing techniques. It is a 'drugless' system and employs herbology, spinal and soft tissue adjustments or manipulations, homeopathy, botanical medicines, hydrotherapy (see HYDROTHERAPY*)*, acupuncture, nutritional guidance, and supplements (vitamins, glandular extracts, enzymes, etc.). Naturopaths (indicated by N.D. after the name) are licensed to practice medicine in about twelve states. There are four naturopathic schools in North America. For more information contact the American Association of Naturopathic Physicians, 601 Valley St., Ste #105, Seattle, WA 98102.

naupathia seasickness.

naus a dwarf.

ne plus ultra the ultimate, the best (Latin, 'nothing better than').

neats' tongue tongue of cattle or oxen.

necrobiotic referring to death or killing of life. A gradual degeneration and death of a part, usually referring to that which occurs in old age; spontaneous dying of a living part.

necrosis local death; the death, more or less, of extensive groups of cells with degenerative changes in the intercellular substance. Death of tissue may be assigned three grades of intensity: local ischemia, local asphyxia and local gangrene.

neonatorum of newborns, referring to the newborn infant.

neoplasia the disease or pathological process which results in cancer. Neoplasm means an abnormal new and proliferative growth of tissue; a cancer.

nephralgia kidney pain.

nephritis inflammation of the kidney.

nephrolithiasis the formation of kidney stones or the diseased state that leads to their formation.

nephrorhaphy to suture a wound in a kidney. To attach a floating kidney to the side or posterior wall of the abdomen.

nephrosclerosis a hardening of the kidney from overgrowth and contraction of the interstitial connective tissue.

nervous affections of cigar makers see NICOTINISM.

nether underneath, below.

nettle rash urticaria.

Nauheim baths see SCHOTT TREATMENT.

neural analysis see EAV.

neural therapy the injection of local anesthetics (primarily lidocaine and procaine) into points of the body to relieve pain, functional, circulatory, rheumatic and orthopedic disorders. A prominent aspect of neural therapy is the concept that the cause of a problem may be found at a distant site on/in the body. For example, a woman who had broken her wrist two years ago was still unable to have normal ROM (range of motion) yet alone move it without discomfort. A scar from a trauma she had received to her thigh many years ago was discovered and injected with procaine. Immediately her wrist got better. This is an example of Huneke's flash phenomenon/lightning reaction which often, though not always, occurs with this type of therapy. Usually if the neural therapy is successful the patient will notice benefits which will last from 8-20 hours. Then intervals between treatments should increase until the patient's complaint completely disappears.

This therapy may be likened to acupuncture and, according to one practitioner, good results can also be seen without the use of anesthetics. However, it must also be mentioned that the injected anesthetic carries a slight electrical charge of 290 millivolts. The resulting removal of this blockage in the field of disturbance (the scar) promotes the restoration of normal bodily functions.

First described in 1925, this method has cured or greatly ameliorated a variety of chronic problems. The definitive text in this area is P. Dosch's *Manual of Neural Therapy According to Huneke* (1984). Also, by the same author, *Facts About Neural Therapy According to Huneke* (1985).

Surprisingly, an allopathic medical journal published, in 1956, two installments of a paper entitled 'Neural Therapy', written by K.E. Kretzschmar, M.D. (*Medical Times*, 84:5, p. 516 and 84:6, p. 635).

neuralgia nerve pain. Pain of a severe, throbbing or stabbing character in the course or distribution of a nerve.

neurasthenia nervous prostration; a nervous exhaustion characterized by abnormal tiredness. See BEARD'S DISEASE.

neuritis degeneration or inflammation of a nerve/s. Symptoms include pain, lost reflexes, hypersensitivity, anesthesia or paresthesia, paralysis, and muscular atrophy.

neuritis a frigori an inflammation of nerves which causes a sensation of coldness in the part (Latin, 'neuritis from cold').

neurodermatitis inflammation of the skin of a nervous origin.

neurodynia nerve pain. See NEURALGIA.

neuroma a nerve tumor. A fibroma on a nerve.

neurosis a nervous disease, especially a functional nervous disease (such as one characterized by obsessions, compulsions, anxieties or phobias) or one which is dependent upon no evident lesion. A peculiar state of tension or irritability of the nervous system; any form of nervousness[*archaic*].

nevus (naevus, mole) birthmark. 'Naevus maternus' (congenital naevus), birthmark.

New Code Sect in the late 19th century, a way of referring to the homeopaths by the allopaths. 'New School' was also used. See OLD SCHOOL.

new science topics and phenomena which can't be explained by traditional/orthodox science, yet which may have a potential for significant benefit for the health and conditions of humanity and Earth as a whole.

new symptom see entry under SYMPTOMS.

nicotinism chronic tobacco poisoning characterized by stimulation and subsequent depression of the central and autonomic nervous system, with death due to respiratory paralysis.

nictalopia spasms of the eyelids.

nictitatio (nictation, nictitation) a twinkling or fluttering of the eyelids.

nidus a focal point (L., 'nest').

night blindness see NYCTALOPIA.

night terrors (night cry, pavor nocturnus) similar to nightmare but more common in children. The child awakens screaming with fright which gradually subsides but persists for a short period of time during a state of semi-consciousness. The child is still asleep yet sits up eyes wide open, tearing at the bedding and clothes. It may often begin after a shock or repeated little frights.

night-sweat profuse sweating at night, traditionally associated with pulmonary tuberculosis. Frequently accompanies diurnal fevers (fevers which recur every 24 hours).

night-watching 1) an inability to sleep which causes the person to remain alert at night, constantly moving and looking about, restless and aimless. 2) staying up at night to care for a loved one who is ill..

nil nothing. Of no account, worthless.

nil desperandum 'giving up nothing' 'giving up no hope' (Latin).

nisus an effort or struggle. Also, the contraction of the diaphragm and abdominal muscles for the expulsion of feces or the urine.

noctambulation night-walking, sleep-walking; somnambulism.

nocturnal at night.

node a knob or circumscribed swelling, such as a lymph node.

nodosity bump, knot-like swelling.

nodus a bony tumor coming out from a bone.

nodular characterized by the presence of nodules (small masses of solid tissue that can be felt).

nodule a lump deeply set in the skin, less than or equal to 1cm in diameter.

noli-me-tangere (ulcus exedens, rodent ulcer, Jacob's ulcer) a form of malignant epithelial ulcer that can be found in many tissues and bones, most commonly on the face. It is fragile in nature and breaks down or erodes easily. (Latin, 'do not touch me').

noma (cancrum oris, gangrena oris, gangrenous stomatitis) an often fatal stomatitis in debilitated children during convalescence from disease (usually an exanthemous disease). A noma is a progressive gangrenous ulcer beginning on the mucous membrane and spreading to the surrounding skin. 'Noma pudendi', a noma involving the external genitalia of the woman.

non compos mentis 'of unsound mind'. Mentally incapable of managing one's affairs.

non inutilis vixi 'I have not lived in vain' (Hahnemann's epitaph).

non plus ultra there is 'nothing better than'.

non sequitur an inference that does not follow from the premise.

nootropic supportive or nourishing to the mind. For example, the ginkgo leaf, especially the phytochemical EGb 761, has nootropic effects.

nos hoc facimus 'we do this' (Latin).

nocebo negative outcomes result because the patient or individual in the study believes the outcome will be negative. See PLACEBO.

nosocomium (nosocomion) a hospital or facility which cares for ill persons. 'Nosocomial infection' is an infection acquired during a patient's stay in the hospital.

nosode (Gr. *nosos*, 'disease', *eidos*, 'from') the potentized homeopathic remedy prepared from diseased tissue or the product of disease. It can be used to prevent or treat a miasm or the associated disease of the tissue material or a miasm, as well as for many other uses. *Pyrogenium, Psorinum,* and *Syphilinum* are examples. See MIASM, BOWEL NOSODES.

"Hahnemann was the first man to conceive that the products of disease could be used in the cure of diseases. His preparation, *Psorinum*, was the first vaccine to be made."—T.T.M. Dishington (1928).

"Had Hahnemann been with us today, he would undoubtedly have been first and foremost in the field of 'nosodes'—'vaccines'—whatever you choose to call them. We *know* it, for he was already there some eighty years ago, in the first volume of his *Chronic Diseases*. Lux, Hahnemann, Hering, Swan, Burnett, Heath, were always years ahead, sometimes half a century, of Pasteur, Koch and Wright."—M.L. Tyler.

"What do homoeopaths want immunizing substances for? We have got much better agents which have been used clinically and proved many years before immunization was even thought of. We call them nosodes."—*More Magic of the Minimum Dose* (D. Shepherd).

nosogeny pathogenesis; the origin and progress of a disease.

nosology the classification of diseases.

nostalgia homesickness; the longing to return to one's home or previous place of residence, or to a previous time in one's life.

nostrum a quack medicine. A medicine with little if any effectiveness.

notalgia pain in the loins or lower back.

nucha the nape of the neck, back of the neck.

nullipara never having borne children.

numquam pars pro toto 'do not generalise; always individualize' (L., 'never a part for the whole').

nun's murmur (*bruit de diable,* French: 'devil's noise') a buzzing venous or heart murmur. A venous hum heard over the veins at the base of the neck especially in anemic persons.

nutmeg liver (cirrhotic liver, cirrhosis, Laennec's cirrhosis) a chronic disease of the liver marked by progressive destruction and regeneration of liver cells and increased connective tissue formation which may result in liver structure changes, congested liver, high blood pressure, liver failure, jaundice and ascites. It is often associated with alcoholics but it is uncertain whether the alcohol itself, nutritional deficencies or a combination of the two is the cause.

nutmeg mottled in appearance, like a nutmeg.

nutraceuticals (nutriceuticals) food-based agents such as ascorbic acid, flavonoids, and carotenoids, etc. that help maintain, enhance, or promote health. This term was first coined by S.L. DeFelice. Allied terms are 'phytomedicines' and 'neuroceuticals'.

nyctalgia night-pain; especially the bone pains of syphilis occurring at night.

nyctalopia (day blindness) a disease of the eye in which the patient can see well in faint light or at twilight, but is unable to see during the day or in strong light. A related term is 'moonblink' which is a temporary blindness, or impairment of sight, said to be caused by sleeping in the moonlight. Compare HEMERALOPIA.

nyctobasis (nyctobadia, nyctobatesis) sleep-walking, somnambulism.

nycturia nocturnal enuresis or bed-wetting.

nymphs (labia minora) the two membranous folds, situated within the labia majora at the sides of the entrance of the vagina.

nymphomania abnormally strong and uncontrollable sexual desire in the woman.

nynaism a system of maintaining healthfulness of the body. It encompassed nine areas: administrativeness, activeness, agreeableness, alimentation, aeration, appeasement, accoutrement, ablution, and actinism. A nynaist is one who practices nynaism or the 'simple habits of regularity of life, cleanliness and carefulness of person' which mean so much for health. Nynaism was mildly popular in the late 1800s.

nystagmus an involuntary, rapid oscillation of the eyeballs. Rhythmical oscillation of the eyeballs, either horizontal, rotary, or vertical.

$$\text{o} \ \text{O} \ \text{O} \ \text{O} \ \text{O} \ \text{O} \ \text{o}$$

o tempora o mores 'oh the times, oh the customs' (Latin).

0/LM the 50-millesimal potency. See POTENCY.

objective symptom see entry under SYMPTOMS.

obloquy abusive or detractive language.

obnubilation dizziness or giddiness. A beclouded mental state.

obstacle to cure/recovery something which hinders or prevents cure or recovery from an illness or injury.

obstipatio constipation.

obstructio alvi constipation.

obstupefaction the state of being senseless or stupefied.

obtuseness dullness, stupidity. Lacking sensibility.

occipital referring to the occiput, the back of the head.

ochre an orange yellow color.

octana an intermittent fever which returns every eighth day.

octavo (8⁰, 8vo, eightvo) a book approximately 5" x 8" to 6" x 9.5". There are duodecimo (12⁰, 12vo, 12mo, twelvemo), 5" x 7.75"; sextodecimo (16⁰, 16mo, sixteenmo), 4.5" x 6.825"; octodecimo (18⁰, 18mo, eighteenmo), 4" x 6.5", quarto (4⁰, 4to), 7" x 10", etc. A broadside (1⁰) is a large piece of paper printed on one side.

oculus leporinus see LAGOPHTHALMUS.

odious loathsome

odium a strong dislike, contempt or aversion.

odontalgia tooth pain; toothache.

oesophagectasia (esophagectasia) a dilatation of the esophagus of unknown origin.

oesophagus see esophagus.

ogival vault-shaped, referring to the shape of the roof of the mouth. The shape of the cavity above the tongue.

oil of cade (oleum cadinum, juniper tar oil) a reddish, dark brown liquid with a tarry odor used in the treatment of a variety of chronic skin diseases.

ol. olivarum olive oil, sweet oil.

Old School (heroic treatment) a term homeopaths gave, in the 19th century, to their allopathic colleagues, the homeopaths themselves being of the New School.

old symptom see entry under SYMPTOMS.

oleaginous oily, greasy.

olecranon the tip or point of the elbow.

oleum animale (Dippel's Oil, Aethereum, rectified oil of hartshorn) a colorless or slightly yellow oily liquid which was first prepared in 1711 by J.C. Dippel from stags' horns then further rectified (purified). (Latin, 'animal oil').

oleum jecoris (oleum morrhuae, oleum jecoris aselli) cod-liver oil.

olfaction administering a homeopathic remedy by smelling it rather than dissolving it in the mouth. To quote Hahnemann, "Olfaction is performed by opening a small bottle containing an ounce of alcohol or brandy where one globule is dissolved and inhaled for an instant or two."

Hahnemann used olfaction as early as 1813/15 and on the majority of his patients between 1832-33. (In 1835 Hahnemann also began to advise dissolving the remedy in water and then drinking the water.) Boenninghausen used olfaction as early as 1829 in his practice. In the 4th Ed. of the *Organon*, Para. 283, Hahnemann wrote, "After the sniffing, the vial is closed with a cork and saved and, if necessary, it can be used many times over for many years without any noticeable loss of its medicinal effect."

"In the last years of his practice, Hahnemann seemed to have devoted essentially all his skill to lowering ever more the doses of his prescriptions. This is why he frequently resorted to olfaction during his last years."— Gypser, *Bonninghausens Kleine Medizinische Schriften,* 1984.

In Hahnemann's later years, he used olfaction (using 30C in water/alcohol or brandy) more so than the Q potencies. However, he only briefly mentioned it in the 6th Ed. (Para. 248, 284). No one really knows the extent to which Hahnemann used olfaction from 1829-42, nor why it received only passing comments in the 6th *Organon*. After 1844, Boenninghausen quietly dropped references to olfaction, too. "It would be advisable to collect and publish current experiences with olfaction in order to become acquainted with this procedure praised so highly by Hahnemann and Boenninghausen."—A. Waldecker in *Classical Homeopathic Quarterly*, 4:2, 1991, p. 78-79.

Much experimentation has been conducted on the best way to administer remedies, some of it by Hering. He suggested that remedies be dissolved in water and then given: "I have discovered the law that the larger the mass of the vehicle, the milder is the action of the medicine."— *Townsend Letter for Doctors and Patients* (10/1996, p. 108)

olfactory pertaining to or contributing to the sense of smell.

oligemia a diminished quantity of blood.

oligodynamic active in very small quantities.

oliguria a deficient excretion of urine.

oligotherapy a method of therapy using homeopathic potencies of the trace elements (oligoelements) found in the body. The approach here is to bring equilibrium back to a deranged metabolism since the trace elements are essential catalysts in enzymatic and metabolic pathways.

omagra a gouty inflammation of the shoulder joint.

omalgia (omodynia) pain in the shoulder joint.

omarthritis inflammation of the shoulder joint.

omentum (caul) a fold of the peritoneum connecting the abdominal organs with the stomach.

omphalitis inflammation of the navel and surrounding tissue.

onanism incomplete coition. During sexual intercourse the man withdraws his penis just prior to ejaculation. Onan, the son of Judah (Genesis 38:9), spilled his seed on the ground in this manner (a form of birth control?). In the older medical literature, onanism means masturbation in men.

oneirism relating to dreams or a dream-like state, or interpreting dreams.

oneirogmus (wet dream) the emission of semen while asleep, often related to erotic dreams.

one-sided disease/case (mute case, partial disease/case, defective case) a case with a paucity of symptoms which does not allow the practitioner to see the case clearly. Karl Robinson, M.D. would prefer to term this a 'scanty case'.

Here one must make the best use of a few symptoms, perhaps one or two, by paying keen attention to the modalities. Thus a general symptom may become a characteristic symptom, which in turn leads to the correct remedy. For example, in dysentery, tenesmus is a diagnostic/common symptom which cannot be used to select the remedy. If tenesmus is accompanied with the modality 'ceases with stool', it points to *Nux v.* rather than

Merc. ('tenesmus continues after stool').

One must also consider the 'inability of the observer to observe accurately enough'. That is perhaps the greatest dilemma of homeopathy—the ability to understand specific trees and yet to grasp the forest as a whole, to understand the remedies of the materia medica, yet to comprehend the materia medica as a whole.

For example, it is not good enough to 'know' *Hyos.* If you 'know' the related group, *Hyos., Verat, Stram.,* and *Bell.* then and only then do you really understand *Hyos.* A. Lippe understood and grasped the entire materia medica so well that he did very little, if any, repertory work. Obviously this is a rare talent and one which comes after many years of study. Refer to *Organon* (Para. 172,-184 6th Ed.)

ontogeny (ontogenesis) the development of the individual. Cf. 'phylogenesis', the evolutionary development of the species.

onychauxis excessive nail growth. Enlargement of the nails of fingers or toes.

onychia inflammation of the nail bed with suppuration and shedding or loss of the nail.

onychogryposis deformed, brittle, thickened nails.

onychomadesis a loosening and shedding of the nails.

onychomycosis any parasitic fungal disease of the nails.

onychophagy nail biting.

onychorrhexis abnormal brittleness of the nails with splitting of the free edges.

onyx an abscess or collection of pus between the lamellae of the cornea of the eye. Called so because of its resemblance to the gem stone.

onyxis an ingrowing toe-nail.

oophoritis (oothecitis) inflammation of an ovary.

op. cit. (abbrev. for 'opus citatum') Latin, 'cited work' (used in a bibliography to avoid repeating the title of a work already cited).

opacity a lack of transparency; an opaque or non-transparent area.

ophthalmia inflammation of the eye especially where the conjunctiva is involved. A severe and often purulent conjunctivitis. Any inflammation of the deeper structures of the eye.

ophthalmia neonatorum (blennorrhea neonatorum) gonococcal conjunctivitis in the newborn infant.

opisthotonos (emprosthotonos) a condition in which, from a tetanic spasm of the back muscles, the head and lower limbs are bent backward and the trunk arched forward. The body rests on the head and the heels. (Gr. *opisthen,* 'behind, in the rear', and *tonos,* 'stretch').

opodeldoc a liniment made of soap in alcohol with camphor or other aromatics being added.

opotherapy the therapeutic use of sarcodes. See SARCODES.

opprobrium the disgrace which follows a wrongdoing, e.g., 'o. medicorum', medical disgrace/wrongdoing.

opsonic pertaining to opsonins. See OPSONINS.

opsonins substances existing in the bodily fluids can render bacteria more susceptible to phagocytosis (devouring and digestion of bacteria by the phagocytes or scavengers of the body). Opsonins occur normally and may be increased by immunization and certain homeopathic remedies.

orbicularis palpebrarum the muscle that closes the eye.

orbicularis palpebrarum ophthalmias onyx the presence of pus between the layers of the cornea or involving the muscle that closes the eye. See ONYX.

orbit the cavity formed by the bones around the eyes and eyebrows.

orchitis inflammation of the testicle(s).

organic disease a disease which alters the structure of the affected organ or area (as opposed to functional disease, in which the function of the organ changes but not necessarily its structure). See FUNCTIONAL DISEASE.

organon an organ or system. A group of logical requirements for scientific inquiry or demonstation. 'Organon' also means any major work of an author which sets down many fundamental principles in that specific topic. Hahnemann's *Organon of Medicine* (*Organon der Rationellen Heilkunde*) is often referred to as simply 'The Organon'.

Hahnemann's *Organon* went through six editions (1810, 19, 24, 29, 33, 42). His 1842 edition was not published until 1921! The *Organon* is divided into two broad sections: *Basic Principles,* containing definitions of fundamental ideas, the law of similars, and demonstration that the homeopathic method is the only one to achieve cure, and *Study Plan and Study of the Disease,* containing study of the disease, study of the remedies, and application of the remedies to the diseases. Also included are sections on how to conduct the treatment and how to prepare the remedies.

Hahnemann's *Organon* was first published in America in 1836 under the title of *Organon of Homoeopathic Medicine.* It was based on the 4th German edition.

To be precise, the first edition of the *Organon* was titled *Organon of Rational Medical Doctrine* (*Organon der Rationellen Heilkunde*). Later editions were titled *Organon of Medical Art* (*Organon der Heilkunst*).

organotherapy the treatment of diseases by administering small quantities of organ extracts derived from healthy animals. This stimulates the diseased organ to function in a normal or healthier way. Organotherapy may have had its origin with Louis Hallion (1862-1940), a French biologist. His idea was formulated into Hallion's Law: 'extracts of an organ have a stimulating effect on that organ'.

orgasm a rush, as in an orgasm of blood to a part. The culmination of the sexual act: 'the crisis of the venereal passion'.

orifice an opening.

orificial relating to an orifice.

ornithosis see PSITTACOSIS.

orthopnea a condition in which the breathing is difficult and requires the person to sit up or take an erect posture in order to breathe better.

os a bone; also an opening or mouth, such as an opening into a hollow organ or canal, especially one with thick, fleshy edges.

os calcis the calcaneus or heel bone.

os coccygis the coccyx or tail bone.

os externum (os tincae, os uterus) the external opening of the uterus. The mouth of the womb. (Womb is the same as uterus).

os hyoides the hyoid or lingual bone, located at the root of the tongue.

os pubis the pubic bone.

os tincae (os externum). The mouth of the womb, the opening of the cervix into the vagina.

os uterus the mouth or opening of the uterus or cervix. 'Os uterus' and 'os externum' to some people are one and the same.

oscheocele (oscheoncus, oscheoma) a scrotal hernia; a tumor of the scrotum.

osmidrosis the secretion of malodorous perspiration.

ossicles (ossicula auditoria) the small bones of the ear which are responsible for detecting sound.

ossifluent marked by or causing a softening of bone.

ossify to change into bone, to harden; also, to become rigid, callous or hardened in one's ideas.

ostealgia (osteodynia, osteocope) pain in a bone.

osteitis (ostitis) inflammation of the bone.

osteochrondrosis/osteochrondritis inflammation involving bone and cartilage. These terms are technically not interchangeable as '-osis' is the degeneration and regeneration of bone (particularly of the epiphyses), while '-itis' is the inflammation.

osteocopi a violent and deep seated bone pain, occasionally associated with syphilis.

osteomalacia the softening of bone with the development of deformities; from loss of calcium salts, usually due to vitamin D deficiency. The bones gradually soften and bend easily with more or less severe pain; it is more common in women than men and often begins during a pregnancy.

osteomyelitis inflammation of the bone marrow and adjacent bone cartilage.

osteopathy (osteopathic medicine) a form of therapy originally based on manipulations of the spine and joints as a means to improve health and cure disease without drugs. Founded by Andrew T. Still (1828-1917) in the late 19th century (the American Osteopathic Assoc. was founded in 1897; 1892 saw the founding of the first American osteopathic school, the American School of Osteopathy, in Kirksville, MO).

Today osteopathic doctors (D.O.) are virtually no different from medical doctors (M.D.). Fewer and fewer osteopathic doctors do manipulations. For an interesting account of the history of this profession consult N. Gevitz's *The D.O.'s* as well as his *Other Healers*. An outstanding book dealing with cranial osteopathy is R.R. McCatty's *Essentials of Craniosacral Osteopathy*. As you probably know, chiropractors also perform manipulations. Though techniques between the two groups may differ slightly, their pathological theories are further removed: traditionally, osteopaths have maintained that manipulations improve blood supply, while chiropractors maintain that they improve nerve functioning. Manipulations no doubt do both.

osteophytosis a condition characterized by bony outgrowths from bone.

osteoporosis a reduction in the quantity of bone mass; skeletal atrophy. The loss of bony substance results in brittleness or softness of the bones.

osteosarcoma a sarcomatous tumor (a tumor consisting of connective tissue) growing from the bone.

ostitis see OSTEITIS.

otalgia (otodynia) ear pain, earache.

otheromatous (atheromatosis) referring to a sebaceous cyst.

otitis inflammation of the ear, usually referring to otitis media (ear infections commonly seen in children).

otodynia ear pain.

otorrhea a mucopurulent discharge from the ear.

otosclerosis a hardening of tissues in the inner ear (that part of the ear responsible for hearing and balance).

oturia a discharge from the ear which resembles urine.

ovaralgia ovarian pain or pain in the ovarian region.

ovariotomy removal of an ovary; oophorectomy.

The first successful ovariotomy was performed on Christmas Day in 1809. Ephraim McDowell removed a cystic ovary weighing 22.5 pounds from a woman. This achievement was the birth of abdominal surgery.

overweening pride a boastful conceit or arrogance, an excessive sense of self-importance. It is normal for one to have a sense of pride, but it can become exaggerated and overbearing as in the case of *Gratiola*.

oxaluria presence of oxalic acid or oxalates in the urine.

oxidology see BIO-OXIDATIVE THERAPIES.

oxygenoid one of the three constitutions delineated by Edward von Grauvogl (1811-1877). It is characterized by an excess of oxygen or its influence on the body and corresponds to the syphilitic miasm of Hahnemann. The two other Grauvogl constitutions are CARBO-NITROGENOID (psoric) and HYDROGENOID (sycotic).

oxyhemoglobinemia the presence of oxidized hemoglobin in arterial blood.

oxyopia (oxyblepsia) an extreme acuteness of vision.

oxytocin a hormone causing uterine contractions and as a result hastening childbirth; also involved in the flow of milk during nursing.

oxyuris (pinworm, threadworm, ascaris) a genus of nematode, *O. vermicularis*. A small white worm, 3-10mm in length, inhabiting the ileum and cecum, and frequently at night wandering to the anus, where it causes intense itching; it sometimes causes reflex symptoms of a convulsive nature.

oxyurosis having worms of the genus *Ascaride* (threadworm).

ozaena (ozena) a foul odor present in certain cases of atrophic, syphilitic, and other forms of chronic rhinitis. A fetid nasal ulceration and discharge. A malignant ulcer in the nostrils.

ozena atrophica sicca (atrophic rhinitis) chronic inflammation of the nasal mucous membrane with thinning of the membranes, crust formation and a foul-smelling discharge.

ozone therapy often mentioned in homeopathic circles, this therapy uses ozone (O_3) to kill or inactivate viruses. Some practitioners withdraw blood from the patient to treat it with ozone and return it to the body. The return of killed viruses is hypothesized to stimulate the immune system. R. Viebahn's *The Use of Ozone in Medicine* (1987) is a good text, as is *Ozone: The Eternal Purifier of the Earth and Cleanser of All Livings Beings* (HE Satori, MD) which is available from Medicina Biologica, 2937 NE Flanders St., Portland, OR 97232.

ozostomia bad breath; a foul odor from the mouth.

P P P P P P P

pabulum 1) food, any nutrient. In the old literature it is often referred to oatmeal. 2) nonsense, meaningless utterances.

Pablum was a trademark name for a specific infants' cereal. 'Old Fashioned Quaker Oats', introduced in 1877, is considered pabulum, although the company would not like referring to it as such. They would much rather you recall that Henry Seymour, a partner in Quaker Oats, read an article about Quakers in an encyclopedia and decided that his product should reflect the same qualities of integrity, honesty, and purity. An older picture of the Quaker had him holding a scroll with the word 'pure' printed on it.

pachaemia (pachyemia) an extreme thickening of the blood.

pachydermia see ELEPHANTIASIS.

Paget's disease 1) disease of the mammary areola preceding cancer of the breast. An eponym from Sir James Paget (1814-1890), who first described it. 2) osteitis deformans, a chronic progressive disturbance in bone metabolism. Here, an initial phase of decalcification and softening is followed by calcium deposition with resultant thickening and deformity of the skeletal system.

Pagot's Law see PAJOT'S LAW.

pains unpleasant, uncomfortable sensations which occur in varying degrees of severity.

boring dull and advancing steadily, burrowing.

cutting sharply penetrating, shearing or piercing.

darting rapid, sudden and swift, with or without changing direction.

digging forcefully thrusting against.

drawing pulling or stiffening up.

fulgurating lightning-like; sudden and excruciating.

gnawing chewing or eroding in a persistent manner.

lancinating piercing, stabbing, or sharply cutting.

rending tearing, splitting, bursting, or coming apart.

shooting passing through swiftly, rapidly or suddenly.

sticking pricking (similar to stitches).

stitching sudden sharp tearing, pricking, usually of momentary duration.

painter's colic (colica saturnina, lead colic) a colic caused by the toxic agent lead. Colic is a paroxysmal abdominal pain due to spasms of the stomach. See COLIC.

Pajot's law (may be seen as Pagot's law) the principle that a solid body contained within another body having smooth walls will tend to conform to the shape of those walls (e.g. the fetus in utero). From C. Pajot (1816-1896), a Parisian obstetrician.

palate (palatine) the roof of the mouth.

palatitis (uranisconitis) inflammation of the palate of the mouth.

palatoglossal relating to the palate and tongue.

palilalia (paliphrasia) the involuntary repetition of words or sentences.

palliative 1) tending to lessen or reduce pain or sickness when cure is no longer possible (although homeopathy can and does sometimes revive a case previously declared incurable). In a terminally ill patient, homeopathy can be used to ease the patient's suffering. 2) reduction of a portion of the symptom picture without curing the entire picture, which can happen if the remedy is not the simillimum yet is similar enough: "There is no extinction of the natural illness, but at best there will be a temporary suppression or displacement, which Hahnemann calls palliation."—*Classical Homoeopathy Quarterly* 4, 1991, p. 123. (From 'palliate', to conceal, hide, disguise or cover; L. *pallium*, 'cloak').

pallid pale, lacking color.

pallor pale.

pallor virginum (pallor luteus) see CHLOROSIS.

palma cristi the castor-oil plant.

palmar referring to the palm of the hand.

palpable able to be felt.

palpebral relating to the eyebrows.

palpitation a fluttering or throbbing, especially referring to the heart.

palpitatis/o cordis palpitation of the heart.

palsy a loss of muscle function or of sensation caused by injury to nerves or by destruction of neurons. Sometimes used synonymously with paralysis, but palsy is usually just a slight loss of function. 'Writer's palsy' (writer's cramp) thus would be a palsy affecting the hands.

paludism see MALARIA.

pan-ophthalmitis an inflammation of the eyeball and all its parts.

panacea (Gr. *pan*, 'all', *akeisthai*, 'to heal') a cure-all, remedy claimed to be curative for all diseases. From Panacea, the daughter of Aesculapius (Greek god of medicine). She could cure all ailments.

panada a thick seasoned sauce or paste. Milk and bread crumbs served with meat, a sort of stuffing.

panaris an inflammation around the nail. See PANARITIUM.

panaritium (panaris, whitlow, paronychia, felon) an inflammation of the structures in the far end of a finger or a toe, either those surrounding the nail or the bone itself.

pancreopathy any disease of the pancreas.

pandemic an epidemic of widespread proportions which may even spread across oceans to other continents.

pandiculation (chasma) the act of stretching as when one wakes up or yawns.

panna a pannus.

pannus (pannis) a corneal vascularization and opacity. A patch of greyish, membrane-like vascularized tissue covering the upper half of (sometimes the entire) cornea.

panphobia (pantophobia, panophobia) fear of everything. A state of general anxiety.

panus an inflamed, nonsuppurating lymph node.

papescent of a soft consistency. 'Pap' is a food of soft consistency, like that of bread crumbs soaked in milk or water.

papillae small, nipple-like projections.

papillo-retinal referring to the infiltration of papillae into the retina of the eye.

papilloma a benign, circumscribed skin tumor projecting from the surrounding surface. A growth of hypertrophied papillae of the skin.

pappy mushy, pulpy.

papular/pustular resembling papules.

papule a small, circumscribed solid elevation of the skin, varying in size from a pinpoint to split pea.

parablepsis a general term for any perversion of the vision, such as double vision or nyctalopia. 'P. illusoria' would mean 'seeing illusions'.

Paracelsus 'next to or beyond Celsus', the name given to Philippus Theophrastus Bombastus von Hohenheim (c. 1493-1541) by friends who saw in him a genius 'next to', or even 'surpassing' Celsus, a famous Greek physician of the first century ACE. He was born in Swabia, now Switzerland, and was educated at Basel, where he later worked as town physician and university professor. His unconventional ideas and teachings did not endear him to his colleagues, so he spent the greater portion of his adult life as an itinerant chemist, physician, philosopher, theologian, and alchemist.

In clinical medicine he was usually in advance of his time, attracting many followers. His influence on the 1500s and 1600s was profound. He was a prolific author but few of his works were published during his lifetime. His ideas sparkled of astrology and alchemy, and writings ensnarled in mysticism made them difficult to comprehend. He was a forerunner of Hahnemann, used the simillimum principle, and found specific relationships between plant and mineral remedies and disease symptoms. "Nature is the first doctor, man is the second," and "The more modest the body of a drug the greater the drug's virtues" are quotes attributed to Paracelsus. His medical and philosophical writings were collected into one massive volume and edited by F. Bitiskius called *Opera Omnia Medico-Chemico-Chirurgica* (1658, Vol. 1 & 2). "Paracelsus has been called the last of the alchemists and astrologers. . . . He probably did as much as any to end the era of superstition and magic by sound medical and pharmaceutical practice."—Dibner, *Heralds of Science*.

Paracelsus was the first to write on miners' diseases, to establish the relationship between cretinism and endemic goitre, and to understand the geographical differences of diseases.

Osler said that Paracelsus was "the Luther of medicine, for when authority was paramount he stood out for independent study."

Lazare Meyssonnier was another character of interest. A physician of Lyon, he wrote a number of works including the *Pentagonum Philosoph.- Medicum* (1639) with a strong emphasis on astrological medicine, chiromancy, and physiognomy. He was a proponent of the powder of sympathy (see SYMPATHETIC POWDER) and relied primarily on herbs in his medical practice.

paracentesis puncture; especially the puncture or tapping of the wall of a cavity by means of a hollow needle to draw off the contained fluid.

paracusis illusoria 1) tinnitus. 2) unusual sounds heard by a person but no others.

paradentosis (pariodontosis) a degenerative disturbance of the periodontium (the supporting tissues surrounding the tooth, i.e. the periodontal membrane, gingiva and alveolar bone), which may be accompanied by pockets of pus and eventual loss of teeth.

paraesthesia an abnormal sensation of tingling, crawling, or burning of the skin.

paralalia any defect in speech, especially in which one letter is continually substituted for another.

paralysis agitans shaking palsy. See PARKINSON'S DISEASE.

paramenia any disorder in the menstrual period.

paraphimosis constriction of the glans penis by the foreskin, in which the foreskin has retracted behind the corona and cannot be drawn forward. (Another definition, albeit a rare one, is a retraction of the lid behind a protruding eyeball).

paraplegia paralysis of the lower limbs.

paratyphoid fever an acute disease caused by the *Salmonella* genus of bacteria (paratyphoid bacteria). The symptomatology resembles typhoid fever but of a less severe nature. Cf. TYPHOID FEVER.

parenchyma the specialized part of an organ as distinguished from the supporting connective tissue, interstitial connective tissue or stroma. Cf. STROMA.

parenchymatous relating to the parenchyma.

paresis (paretic) a slackening or weakness. A slight, partial, or even general paralysis.

paresthesia see PARAESTHESIA.

pareunia coitus; sexual intercourse. Thus 'dyspareunia', difficult or painful intercourse.

parietes walls, as of the thorax and abdomen.

Parkinson's disease (paralysis agitans, shaking palsy) so named by the English physician, J. Parkinson (1755-1824). A progressive nervous disease of the later years, characterized by muscular tremor, slowing of movement, partial facial paralysis, peculiarity of gait and posture, and weakness.

parodynia (dystocia) labor pains. An abnormal or difficult labor.

paronychia (whitlow, felon, panaritium) an inflammation around the nail. If mycotic, it is usually associated with *Candida albicans*.

The term, years ago, was considered synonymous with whitlow, felon, panaritium, but today has a different meaning. Here the fold of the nail is damaged and the cuticle is lost. Bacteria, yeasts, etc. can enter the pocket between the nail fold and nail plate, producing chronic infections such as *Candida albicans*. The area is tender. Malformations and hyperpigmentation of the nail can occur.

parosmia a perversion of the sense of smell.

parotid fistula an abnormal passage coming out of the parotid (salivary) gland.

parotids referring to the parotid glands which are situated near the ear.

parotitis (parotiditis) inflammation of the parotid gland, as in mumps; inflammation of the lymph node overlying the parotid.

parotitis gangrenosa inflammation and gangrene of the parotid glands.

parovarian near or beside the ovary. Relating to the parovarium (Organ of Rosenmuller or epoophoron, a collection of rudimentary tubules in the area of the ligament between the ovary and the fallopian tube).

paroxysm sharp spasm or convulsion. The sudden onset of a disease or of any symptoms, especially if they are recurrent, as in malaria. 'Paroxysmal', spasmodic or convulsive.

Parrish's food (Parrish's syrup) a compound syrup of ferrous phosphate. A tonic developed in 1845 by the century pharmacist Edward Parrish. It contains therapeutic amounts not only of iron but also of calcium. It was a very popular product in the U.S. and England, too.

According to the British Pharmacopoeia (1949) it consists of phosphates of iron, calcium, potassium, and sodium with cochineal (a red coloring agent made from the same beetle as the remedy *Coccus cacti*) and orange-flower water in syrup, given in 1/2 to 2 teaspoonful doses.

parrot fever see PSITTACOSIS.

parsimony stinginess or excessive saving; avarice. The Law of Parsimony is the concept that the simplest explanation is often the best. Ockham's Razor, after the medieval philosopher Wm. of Ockham, states: "Entities should not be unnecessarily multiplied."

partial case see ONE-SIDED CASE.

particular symptom a symptom relating to a part of the body or area, e.g., a pounding pain in the head, sharp pains in the shoulder. See entry under SYMPTOMS.

parturients agents or substances designed to aid in childbirth.

parturition childbirth, labor, giving birth to a child.

parulis see GUM BOIL.

parvule a small pill. Pillule, pellet, granule.

Pascoe complexes complex homeopathic formulae developed by the German firm Pascoe and Dr. H. Schimmel. Determining 'key nosodes' which the ill person requires is one aspect which this therapy addresses. See EAV, BEV, RADIONICS.

passio hystericus see HYSTERIA.

passio iliaca (ileus) pain in the abdomen, fecal vomiting, and spasms of the abdominal muscles.

patches circumscribed discolorations with the characteristics of macules but larger (greater that 1cm in diameter), e.g., vitiligo, senile freckles and measles rash.

patella (rotula) the kneecap. 'Patellar', referring to the kneecap.

pathema any diseased condition.

pathogenic disease-causing.

pathogenesis (nosogenesis) the origin and progress of a disease.

pathogenetic symptoms the symptoms surrounding the onset or evolution of the disease.

pathognomonic something which is characteristic of a disease and distinguishing it from other diseases. A pathognomonic symptom is a symptom indicative of a disease. See listing under SYMPTOM.

pathological prescribing the administration of remedies based on the pathology of the disease, adapting the remedy to a disease rather than to the individual patient. For example, for a patient with liver disease the practitioner might immediately review remedies known to have liver affinities/actions and choose a remedy based on his findings.

patulous open or spreading.

pavor fear or terror. 'Pavor nocturnus', a nightmare, especially as seen in children. See NIGHT TERRORS.

peccans sinful, full of sin. Wicked.

pectoral referring to the chest or the chest muscles.

pediculated (pedunculate) having a peduncle, stalk, or stem, such as a wart.

pediculosis lousiness, phtheiriasis. The state of being infested with pediculi (lice).

pediluvium a bath for the feet.

pedum referring to the feet.

pedunculated having a support, stalk or stem, as a pedunculated tumor.

peevish annoying, discontented, ill-tempered, resentful.

pelioma (pelidnoma, peliosis) see PURPURA.

pellagra (erythema endemicum, Lombardy leprosy, elephantiasis, italica, maidism) an affection characterized by gastrointestinal disturbances, erythema followed by desquamation, and nervous and mental disorders. It was formerly believed to be an intoxication caused by eating diseased corn, but is now known to be caused by a lack of niacin in the diet.

pellet (globule) see GLOBULE.

pellicle a film or scum on the surface of a liquid.

pelopathy the treatment of disease with mud therapy.

pelvic calculitis (wombstone) a calcified, hardened tumor composed of muscular tissue of the uterus. A uterine myoma.

pelvis of the kidney the basin-like or cup-shaped cavity in the kidney which serves to collect and direct fluids from the kidney into the ureter. Structures anterior to this area are the renal papilla and renal sinuses.

pemphigus (morbus phlyctenoides, morbus vesicularis) an acute or chronic skin disease characterized by the appearance of blisters (bullae) which develop in crops or in continuous succession.

pemphigus foliaceus a form of pemphigus in which the lesions persist and rupture, leaving denuded surfaces exuding a seropurulent fluid which dries on the surface; nearly the entire body may finally become involved and the buccal mucous membrane is often affected as well; it may cause death from exhaustion.

pendulous hanging loosely or freely.

penitis (phallitis, priapitis) inflammation of the penis.

penurious frugal, stinting, miserly due to necessity.

penury destitution or extreme poverty.

pepper-pot any highly seasoned dish or soup. A seasoned soup containing meat, vegetables, and dumplings.

pepsin the main digestive substance of the gastric juice as it breaks down proteins. It is therapeutically employed as a digestive aid.

per os by mouth; often abbreviated p.o. or just PO (referring to the administration of medications), as contrasted with IV (intravenous), IM (intramuscular), SQ (subcutaneous), etc.

periarthritis inflammation of the parts surrounding a joint.

pericarditis inflammation of the membranous sac enveloping the heart.

perichondritis inflammation of the tissue which covers cartilage.

perineal referring to the perineum.

perineal tears hardened lumps in the perineum.

perinephritis inflammation of the tissues around the kidney.

perineum the pelvic floor and the associated structures of the pelvic orifices; the external surface or base of the perineal body, lying between the vulva and the anus in the female and the scrotum and the anus in the male.

periodic recurring at regular intervals as in a disease with regularly recurring exacerbations or paroxysms.

periosteal referring to the periosteum, the thick fibrous membrane covering the surfaces of bone.

periosteum the thick fibrous membrane covering the entire surface of a bone except its articular cartilage. It consists of two layers: an inner which is osteogenic (forms new bone tissue), and an outer connective-tissue layer conveying the blood vessels and nerves supplying the bone.

periostitis an inflammation of the periosteum (the lining of the bones).

peripheral outermost part or region. The area immediately beyond a precise boundary. Also, relatively unimportant, not central (e.g. symptoms peripheral to solving the case).

peripneumonia inflammation of the lungs.

peristalsis the worm-like movement of the intestine or other tubular structure; a wave of alternate circular contraction and relaxation of the tube by which the contents are propelled onward.

perityphlitis an inflammation of the peritoneum surrounding the cecum and appendix area. This term was used in the late 1800s to refer to inflammation around the intestines. When doctors and anatomists found the exact location, the appendix, they changed the name to appendicitis.

periungual surrounding a nail; involving the nail folds.

Perkinism a form of magnet healing developed in 1796 by Dr. Perkins of Norwich, CT. It involved the repeated movement of two 'metal tractors' over the wound or affected area for a short period of time (twenty minutes or so). The tractors were three-inch pieces of metal (one iron, one brass) blunt at one end and pointed at the other. Before its demise, in 1835, Perkinism became popular in England and Denmark.

pernicious tending to cause death or serious injury; deadly. Causing great harm, destructive.

pernicious anemia (Addison's a., Biermer's disease, primary a., essential a., idiopathic a.) a severe and life-threatening anemia (hence the term pernicious) generally of older adults (after the fifth decade) and thought to result from a defect of the stomach, with atrophy and an associated lack of the 'intrinsic factor' necessary to absorb vitamin B_{12}. It is characterized by numbness and tingling, weakness, and a sore smooth tongue, shortness of breath, faintness, pallor of the skin and mucous membranes, anorexia, diarrhea, and frequently hemorrhages either into the skin (petechia) or from the mucous membranes.

pernio (pl. perniones) see CHILBLAIN.

pertinacity persistence; holding firmly or tenaciously to some purpose, belief, or opinion.

pertussis (morbus cucullaris) see WHOOPING COUGH.

peruvian bark see CINCHONA, CINCHONISM.

pessary a vaginal suppository, or something placed in the vagina to keep the womb (uterus) in place.

petechia (pin-point hemorrhage) a minute hemorrhagic spot in the skin, of

petechia (pin-point hemorrhage) a minute hemorrhagic spot in the skin, of pinpoint to pin-head size. Petechiae are red or purple in color but later may turn to a blue or yellow.

petit mal a form of epilepsy which causes very short lapses of consciousness and a sudden momentary pause in conversation or movement rarely lasting more than thirty seconds.

petrous stony, hard, rocky; resembling rock.

petulant unreasonably irritable or ill-tempered; peevish.

Peyer's gland (P. patch) an aggregation of lymphatic nodules closely packed in the mucous membranes of the ileum opposite its mesenteric attachment. Named for J.C. Peyer (1653-1712), a Swiss naturalist and anatomist.

Pfeiffer's disease (mononucleosis) see GLANDULAR FEVER.

phagadena a rapidly spreading destructive ulceration of soft tissues. A sloughing and widely spreading ulcer.

phalanges the bones of the fingers and toes.

phallus the penis.

phalanx (pl. 'phalanges') any bone of a finger or toe.

phanera the skin.

phantasma an illusion or hallucination, product of a morbid imagination.

pharmacopoeia see DISPENSATORY.

pharyngalgia (pharyngodynia) pain in the pharynx.

pharyngitis inflammation of the pharynx and associated tissues at the back of the throat and mouth. Painful swallowing, soreness, and redness are the common symptoms.

pharyngitis sicca inflammation of the pharynx characterized by dry mucous membranes (Latin *sicca,* 'dry, desiccated').

pharynx that space in the back of the mouth often referred to as the throat. This space extends upward to the roof of the mouth, forward to the opening of the mouth, and back and downward to the esophagus. Since this area is so large and non-specific it is often specified in the following way: laryngeal p. (the pharyngeal area near the larynx) or nasal p. (nasalopharynx, rhinopharynx; the pharyngeal area bordering the sinuses), etc. (Gr. *pharynx,* 'throat').

phenomenology H.A. Roberts, M.D. in his *Art of Cure by Homoeopathy,* quotes the philosopher O.L. Reiser: "a study of that which exhibits or displays itself: it is the descriptive point of view obtained by viewing the thing as a whole. Much of the trouble . . . comes from an overemphasis upon microscopic details. Thus it comes about that we can no longer see the forest for the trees." "This is another way of saying that the homoeopathic concept of disease and cure is from the phenomenological viewpoint in that it considers the broad outlines of the whole rather than some of the minute divisions compassed by microscopic vision, and at the same time embraces the meaning of which the microscopic vision demonstrates but a part."—H.A. Roberts, M.D.

The 'phenomenon' is upmost in the homeopath's mind—in other words, the homeopath is concerned with the phenomenon of the patient, e.g., you cough only when you go outside, the cough is better with hot drinks, the cough only comes on during warm, rainy days. To the allopath these phenomena are more often than not meaningless.

phial vial.

philoprogenitiveness producing many offspring. Prolific.

phimosis tightness of the foreskin of the penis such that it cannot be retracted back over the head of the penis. See PARAPHIMOSIS.

phlebitis inflammation of the veins. It may be superficial or more general and deeper. Redness, tenderness, swelling, throbbing, and pain are the common symptoms.

phlegm a viscid, stringy mucus, secreted by the mucosa of the upper air passages. One of the four humors of humoral theory of medicine. See HUMORS.

phlegmasia an angry-appearing inflammation. An inflammation of the veins (phlebitis), especially when acute and severe.

phlegmasia alba dolens (milk-leg) an extreme edematous swelling of the mother's leg following childbirth, due to thrombosis/thrombitis of the veins which drain the part.

phlegmasia malabarica see ELEPHANTIASIS.

phlegmatic 1) having a slow, sluggish, apathetic temperament; unemotional. Referring to a calm, apathetic, or unexcitable situation or person. 2) pertaining to phlegm, a stringy, thick mucus secreted by the respiratory tract. Relating to the heaviest of the four humors. See LEUCO-PHLEGMATIC.

phlegmon acute suppurative inflammation of the subcutaneous connective tissue.

phlegmonous relating to PHLEGMON *(see above)*.

phlogistic inflammatory. 'Phlogosis', inflammation.

phlyctenotherapy (phlyctenular autotherapy, artificial phlyctenular autotherapy) see PHLYCTENULAR AUTOTHERAPY.

phlyctenula (pl. phlyctenulae) a minute vesicle or blister. It may refer to an inflammatory vesicle, pimple or blister upon the conjuctiva or cornea of the eye.

phlyctenular authotherapy (phlyctenotherapy, artificial phlyctenular autotherapy) a form of auto-isopathy/isopathy developed by French physicians C. Rousson and Fortier-Bernoville. Here a blister is created on the skin of the deltoid muscle by applying dry ice or cantharidin paste. In 24-48 hours a blister forms containing serous fluid. Some of this fluid is collected, then potentized and administered to the patient as a remedy. Good results have supposedly been obtained in treating migraine, herpes zoster, multiple sclerosis, etc. in this manner.

phlyctenular conjunctivitis inflammation of the conjunctiva accompanied by the formation of small red nodules of lymphoid tissue (phlyctenulae) on the conjunctiva.

phonation the act of speaking with the voice. The production of a vocal sound.

phonophoresis the use of therapeutic ultrasound to drive topical applications deep into the tissues. This usually improves the clinical effect of either the topical agent or the ultrasound alone. It is possible to cause deep penetration (up to 2 inches) of not only ions but entire molecules.

phosphaturia a condition in which an excess of phosphates is present in the urine.

phosphorescent shining or glowing.

photomania an insane desire for light or insanity caused by prolonged exposure to intense light.

photophobia an unusual intolerance or insensitivity to light. Morbid fear of light.

photopsia sparks or flashes of light occurring in the field of vision.

phrenitis inflammation of the brain. Brain fever.

phrenology a study or philosophy which deals with the dilemma of why people are different from one another, how man can be understood and developed, and why people have different human characteristics.

At the end of the 18th century Franz J. Gall, a German physician, developed organology, or the theory of reading a person's character by observing the contours of the skull called 'organology'. He charted the skull into 26 areas or faculties to which his followers added many more over the course of the next century when phrenology came into vogue. The term 'phrenology' was popularized by J.C. Spurzheim (1776-1832). Later Gall and Spurzheim collaborated, writing *Anatomie et Physiologie du Systeme Nerveux* (1810-1819). Gall was ridiculed as Dr. Galimartias or Dr. Nonsense.

This system was based on the theory that human faculties, personality, and attitudes originate in certain parts of the brain's surface and these patterns can be detected as they appear on the skull. A forerunner, Robert Thidd, attempted to synthesize similarities between the human head and the 'celestial world' and show how those energies or influences enter the cranium. Ehrenberg and Luigi Ferrarese were two other influential individuals in this field. The latter wrote *Memorie Risguardanti La Dottrina Frenologica* (1836-8), which was one of the fundamental 19th century works in the field.

Systems of phrenology were also created by J.G. Lavater (1741-1801; *Von der Physiognomik*, 1772) in collaboration with Goethe. According to Lavater, the face is sectioned into three worlds; the forehead is the divine world; the psychical world is formed by the nose, eyes, mouth and forehead; the jaw and chin constitute the physical world. His physiognomy differed from others in that he paid particular attention to the structure of the forehead. Interestingly enough, Lavater's work influenced artists of that period especially in portraiture.

Phreno-somnambulism and phreno-magnetism are discussed in *Artificial Somnambulism, hitherto called mesmerism or animal magnetism* (1869), by a homeopath, W.B. Fahnestock.

phrensical pertaining to the mind. Thus 'phrenalgia' and 'psychalgia' mean 'mind-pain', 'soul-pain'. However, it may also refer to the diaphragm, as *phren-* is Greek for 'diaphragm' or 'heart'—the seat of the emotions. 2) referring to distress attending a mental effort, noted especially in melancholia.

phtheiriasis see PEDICULOSIS and PHTHIRIASIS.

phthiriasis (morbus pedicularis, pediculosis pubis) infestation by the pubic louse. *Phthirius* is a genus of lice.

phthisis (pulmonalis) a wasting away of the body. An old term for pulmonary tuberculosis, with subsequent emaciation and loss of strength. Tuberculosis, specifically tuberculosis of the lungs, consumption.

phthisis florida acute tuberculosis, galloping consumption. An active case of tuberculosis or consumption of the lungs.

phylsis see WHITLOW or PANARITIUM.

physconia a distension of the abdomen.

physiatric relating to natural medicine therapies.

physic 1) a cathartic or laxative. 2) of or relating to the practice of medicine. The art of medicine. To treat with medicine. To administer medicines to relieve, heal, or cure. May be spelled as 'physick' or 'physicke'.

One of the earliest books on the general practice of medicine in English was *The General Practise of Physicke* (1617). It was originally published in German in 1568 as *Artzney Buch* by Christopher Wirtzung. "Throw physic to the dogs."—Shakespeare.

physiognomy the 'science' of determining character by a study of the face. The art of discovering temperament and character from outward appearance. The divination by facial features is based on the assumption that there is a connection between the human body (microcosm) and the universe (macrocosm). Cesare Lombroso's *L'Uomo Delinquente* stated that criminals were the products of heredity and could be recognized by features like small restless eyes (thieves) or bright eyes and cracked voices like sex criminals. Though many were involved in this mid-18th century pseudo-science, perhaps the most noteworthy was Jean Gaspard Lavater, who wrote the definitive book on physiognomy entitled *Essai sur la Physiognomonie* (1781-1803, Vols. 1-4). This work figures prominently in the history and development of psychiatry.

Sir Samp: Has he not a rogue's face? Speak, brother you understand physiognomy; a hanging look to me. He has a damn'd Tyburn-face, without the benefit o' the clergy.

Fore: Hum—truly I don't care to discourage a young man. He has a violent death in his face; but I hope, no danger of hanging.

—Wm. Congreve, *Love For Love* (1698)

physiological prescribing prescribing remedies according to their known physiological affinities. For example, *Stannum, Chelidonium, Carduus* and *Hepar sulph.* have an affinity to the liver, thus they may be prescribed to support the functioning of the liver.

physiomedicalism (neo-Thomsonianism, independent Thomsonianism, botanico-medicalism) a system of herbalism founded by Alva Curtis (1797-1881). It utilized a larger botanical materia medica than Thomsonianism, eliminated the use of toxic substances in any form, and believed strongly in scientific education. Curtis established his school, the Literary and Botanico-Medical Institute of Ohio, in Columbus in 1839. He later moved it to Cincinnati. Physiomedicalism survives to this day in England. See ECLECTIC, THOMSONIANISM.

physiosis abdominal distension.

physiotherapy the art and science of physical treatment and diagnosis by means of heat, cold, water, electricity, sound radiations, massage, therapeutic exercises, etc.

physometra gas in the uterus. Distention of the uterine cavity with air or gas.

phytonutrients nutrients helpful to the body and derived from plants (such as indoles from the brassica vegetables like broccoli and cauliflower, lycopenes from tomatoes, phytoestrogens from soy, and lignins from rye).

phytotherapy (phytomedicine) a general term for the scientific use of purified, standardized extracts from medicinal plants in the treatment of diseases (as distinct from herbal medicine, which uses the whole plants). Once the extract is confirmed in the clinical setting, dosages are established and standardized products are then formulated. This then allows for a more accurate prediction of the clinical response.

Also, research into manufacturing techniques may yield products which can then be formulated into more bioavailable ones. Phytotherapy or phytomedicine has five advantages over traditional herbal medicine: 1) a standard dosing schedule, 2) a basis in clinical research, 3) widely used by the medical community, 4) tested for toxicity, and 5) consistent quality.

'Phytopharmacon' is an allied term. H. Leclerc, M.D. (1870-1955), is the father of modern phytotherapy. R.F. Weiss, M.D., introduced phytotherapy into medical practice and is the author of *Herbal Medicine*, one of the best references for those interested in the medical application of herbs. "The art of healing does not lie before us in the gray mysteries and doctrines of the future, but far behind us in the past of the green, original life of nature."—J.H. Rausse (1805-1848).

An example of a phytochemical is the antioxidant pycnogenol or proanthocyanidin. This phytochemical is derived from pine bark, used by the Canadian Indians as a tea which could prevent scurvy in the 1500s. A University of Bordeau researcher, Jack Masquelier, developed the process of extracting pycnogenol from pine bark in 1964. It is now available in pill form and in standardized doses. Sulforaphane is a phytochemical found in broccoli. As an aside, the ancestors of Albert R. Broccoli, the producer of the 007 James Bond films, created this vegetable when they crossed cauliflower with Italian rabe!

pian see FRAMBOESIA.

pica 1) a desire for unusual or strange foods. 2) the recurrence in later life of the infantile tendency to bring everything to the mouth.

piety a pious act or thought. Devotion and reverence to parents or family or God.

pigeon chest (pectus carinatum, chicken breast) a chest which is flat on either side with a forward projection of the sternum.

pileous hairy.

piles hemorrhoids.

pinna (auricle) the external ear.

piquant stimulating; pleasantly sharp to the taste.

pisiform pear-shaped or pea-sized (L. *pisum,* 'pea').

pituita phlegm or viscid mucus.

pituitous asthma (humid asthma) a productive asthma. An asthma which has a discharge of mucus with it.

pityriasis a skin disease characterized by the shedding of fine, flaky scales, like bran.

pityriasis capitis dandruff (Latin *capitis,* 'of the head').

pityriasis pilaris (p. rubra pilaris, keratosis pilaris) an eruption of papules surrounding the hair follicles, each papule pierced by a hair, and tipped with a horny, more or less greasy, scale.

pityriasis versicolor see TINEA VERSICOLOR.

placebo an inert drug or substance given to satisfy patients, or as the control in a research study. From the Latin, 'I shall please'.

In 1830, Isaac Jennings, M.D. wrote *The No Medicine Approach to Medicine.* In this book, Dr. Jennings described his treatment of thousands of patients with nothing but pills made of bread and colored water. His 'experiment' showed that people got well in the same or less time as if they had used other therapies available at that time. A similar situation occurred around the turn of the 20th century when Emile Coue (1857-1926), by mistake, gave distilled water in place of medicine to the patient. Nonetheless, the patient recovered, and impressed Emile with the power of the mind. He lectured widely on the subject of positive thinking (Coue autosuggestion) and is credited with creating the phrase, "Day by day, in every way, I am growing better and better."

"A positive healing effect resulting from the use of any healing intervention, and is presumed to be mediated by the symbolic effect of the intervention upon the patient."—Complementary and Alternative Medicine at the NIH (4:1, p. 3). See NOCEBO.

placenta praevia a placenta which has superimposed itself upon and around the internal opening of the vagina (os), causing serious bleeding during labor.

plague usually refers to bubonic plague, but non-specifically it refers to any disease of wide prevalence or of excessive mortality. See BUBONIC PLAGUE.

plantar referring to the sole of the foot, as in 'plantar wart'.

plasmapheresis see AUTOHEMIC THERAPY.

plasson an albuminous or gelatinous (jelly-like) substance.

plastic celluloid, as in 'plastic exudation'. An exudation occurring on a wounded area and acting as a healing agent.

Platt's chlorides a solution containing chloride salts of aluminum, sodium, zinc, and calcium, used in the treatment of diphtheria. A cloth is soaked in an equal solution of water and Platt's chlorides and placed over the mouth and nose for 10 minutes at a time every 1/2 to 1 hour.

pledget a small piece or tuft of cotton, wool, or lint.

pleno full.

Pleo remedies see SANUM REMEDIES.

pleomorphism the (as yet unproven) theory that microbes in the body can pass through different stages of development to evolve into bacteria which are hostile to the body and cause serious diseases. In other words, certain bacteria can take on multiple forms within a single life-cycle and become the cause of disease. However, during pleomorphism DNA does not change.

The German physician, bacteriologist, and zoologist G. Enderlein (1872-1968) developed this hypothesis in his book, *The Life Cycle of Bacteria* (*Bakterien Cyclogenie*, 1925) and in a sense continued the work of Bechamp. Bechamp and Pasteur in the latter part of the 19th century disagreed on the origin of bacteria and thus ultimately of disease. Enderlein's researches not only outlined bacterial evolution in the body but also focused on treatment (Sanum remedies, or homeopathic remedies of dried cell wall fragments of fungus, such as *Candida albicans*) to re-establish balance in the ill. This subject is too vast to be discussed in this setting. You may wish to consult *Hidden Killers* (M. Sheenan and E. Enby), *Cell Wall Deficient Forms: Stealth Pathogens* (L.H. Mattman), 'Studies Upon the Life Cycles of the Bacteria' (F. Lohnis, *Mem. Natl. Acad. Sci.*, 16, 1-335, 1921), *Die Blut-Mykose* (B. Haefeli, 1987), and *Bechamp or Pasteur* (E.D. Hume, 1925). See SANUM REMEDIES.

Another researcher in this area, Gaston Naessens, calls his work 'somati–dian orthobiology'. Royal Raymond Rife (1888-1977) and Wilhelm Reich also had interesting theories about pleomorphism. 'Endobionit', 'protit', 'microzymas', and 'somatid' are synonymous terms.

plethora an overabundance or excess. General congestion, fullness of blood. A 'plethoric' appearance would mean a red, robust complexion, as though the blood and flesh could burst through the skin. Excessive in style, over-burdened, turgid. An excess of blood in the circulatory system or in an organ. Fullness of the vessels; a redundance of blood. The following from R. Hughes, *The Principles and Practice of Homeopathy*, p. 505, may help with your understanding. "More frequently according to my experience, the delay of the venous current is on the hither side of the portal vein. This is the 'abdominal plethora' of the old writers, showing itself by weight, fullness and heat in the bowels, with slow digestion delayed stools and scanty and pale urine."

plethoric full and robust, full of blood, ruddy.

pleura the membrane enveloping the lungs and chest cavity.

pleurisy (pleuritis) inflammation of the pleura, the membrane enveloping the lungs and lining the walls of the chest cavity.

pleuritic referring to the lung or pleurisy or pleuritis, i.e., pleuritic effusion would mean a loss of fluids from the lung into the pleural cavity.

pleurodynia (false pleurisy) pain in the lungs or chest.

pleurothotonos a tonic muscular spasm which curves the body to one side.

plica polonica a matted condition of the hair caused by filth and neglect. Verminous matting of the hair.

It was first described by Tobias Cohn (1652-1729), a Jewish physician, in his opus *Maaseh Tobiyyah* (1707). This medical text, unlike others, contains the following diverse sections: 1) theology, 2) anatomy, 3) medicine, 4) hygiene, 5) syphilitic maladies, 6) botany, 7) cosmography, 8) essay on the four elements, and a Turkish-Latin-Spanish dictionary.

plumbism (saturnism) lead poisoning, or the symptoms of lead poisoning. The classic work on lead poisoning was done by Louis Tanquerel des Planches in his *Traite des Maladies de Plomb* (1838). "Reporting on 1200 cases of lead poisoning, Tanquerel's studies were so complete that later studies added little knowledge of the symptoms and signs of that disease."—G. Morton.

plussing a method, of which there are several variations, to slightly increase the potency or quantity of a remedy administered in water. It is especially useful for the prescriber who wants the patient to be gently pushed in the direction of cure on a daily or more frequent basis. 1) Here the patient is instructed to dissolve the remedy in a glass of water and take a dose. For the next dose the patient discards the remaining water, and without cleaning the glass, adds fresh water then stirs it. This produces the next dose but in a slightly higher potency. 2) a method of extending a Q potency in a remedy solution bottle, by filling the bottle with water again when it is almost empty (only one teaspoon remains) then stirring or shaking gently. 3) administering an acute remedy in a bottle filled with water, which is succussed 100 times between frequent repetitions (as described in C. Coulter, *Portraits of Homeopathic Medicines,* Vol. 2).

pneumoconiosis (pneumonoconiosis) dust disease of the lung. A hardening of the lungs due to irritation caused by dust inhalation.

pneumogastric nerve (10th cranial nerve, vagus nerve) the 10th and longest of the cranial nerves, originating on the sides of the medulla oblongata and passing through the neck and thorax into the abdomen. It supplies sensation to the pharynx and larynx, part of the ear, motor impulses to the vocal cords, and motor and secretory impulses to the thoracic and abdominal organs (lungs, heart, esophagus, stomach, etc.).

PNI psychoneuroimmunology.

PNIE psychoneuroimmunoendocrinology.

pock a pustule on the skin containing eruptive matter. A pustule of small-pox.

podagra gout, especially of the large toe or joints of the foot.

podalgia (tarsalgia, pododynia) pain in the foot.

podarthrocace abscess of the ankle-joint.

polioencephalitis inflammation of the grey matter of the brain, an acute infectious disease marked at the onset by fever, headache, convulsions, or stupor, followed by ocular palsies, aphasia, etc.

poliomyelitis ('polio') inflammation of the grey matter of the spinal cord. Most common in children, producing a paralysis of certain muscle groups or of an entire limb. Onset is sudden, with fever, gastrointestinal complaints, and pain in the affected muscles with extensive paralysis. The muscles atrophy, the reflexes are lost, and contractions of antagonistic muscles cause deformities later in life. Some cases do not show paralysis. In older homeopathic literature it may have been referred to as infantile paralysis.

pollex the thumb or first finger.

pollution (defilement) seminal emission outside of intercourse (i.e. in masturbation, a wet dream, etc.) 'Self-pollution' or 'self-abuse': masturbation.

polyarthritis arthritis affecting many areas (Gr. *poly*, 'many').

polychrest (polycrest) a remedy whose provings and clinical applications show that it has many widespread uses, covering a wide variety of mental, emotional and physical symptomatology. For example, compare the uses of *Nux vomica*, a polychrest, with *Selenium*. Other well-known polychrests include *Sulphur, Phosphorus, Arsenicum, Lachesis* and *Natrum muriaticum*.

"A polycrest is a remedy which affects all or nearly all the tissues of the body, has a wide variation in symptoms and its curative power reaches deep into the anatomy ... is equally useful in acute and chronic disorders, but in chronic work may prove curative or ameliorative when all other methods fail."—J.V. Allen, Jr., *Journal of the AIH*.

From his introduction to *Nux vomica* in his *Materia Medica Pura*, Hahnemann defines polychrest: "There are a few remedies in which the majority of symptoms corresponds in similarity to some common disease, and which can therefore often be effectively applied homoeopathically. We could call these remedies polychrests." In this definition of a polychrest a remedy is prescribed on the more or less common symptoms of frequently observed ailments and not primarily on unique symptoms.—Kees Dam, *Homoeopathic Links* (3/95, p. 42).

polycythemia a condition characterized by an increase in the number of red blood cells.

polymorphonuclear neutrophils one of the five types of white blood cells, making up 62% of the total. They protect the body against invading organisms by ingesting them, via phagocytosis.

polymyelitis inflammation of many muscles.

polyneuritis (multiple neuritis) simultaneous involvement of several nerves, usually symmetrical. Often results from ingestion or topical exposure to poisons. Diseases such as diphtheria, typhoid and syphilis may be a cause.

polypharmacy (mixology, combination/complex homeopathy) the administration of more than one remedy at a time either through giving a number of single remedies at the same time or giving a combination homeopathic product.

This method of administering homeopathic remedies, a hotly debated topic now, was argued about even during the infancy of homeopathy. Hahnemann warned against the use of mixtures of medicines on many occasions (in particular P. 273 *Organon*, 6th Ed.). "The question now arises: Is it good to mix various kinds of medicine in a prescription? The human mind never understands more than one thing at a time and can hardly determine accurately the causes resulting from two simultaneous forces acting on one object. How can medicine attain a higher degree of certainty, when the doctor seems to be intent only on allowing a number of miscellaneous forces to be exerted at the same time on a pathological state? ... I take it upon myself to avow that of two and two medicines put together, no single one will exert its own particular effect on the human body, but almost always an effect quite different from that of the two separately. This is a middle effect, a neutral effect, if I may borrow the expression of chemical compounds."—*Aesculapius in the Balance*, 1805 (as quoted in *Resonance,* Ju/Aug. 1996, p. 4).

"Boenninghausen, in a letter written March 25, 1865, to Carroll Dunham, M.D. of N.Y. states: 'It is true that during the years 1832 to 1833 at the insistence of Dr. Aegidi, I made some experiments with combined remedies, that the results were sometimes surprising, and that I spoke of the circumstance to Hahnemann who, after some experiments made by himself had entertained for a while the idea of alluding to the matter in the fifth edition of the *Organon*, which he was preparing in 1833. But this novelty appeared too dangerous for the new method of cure, and it was I who induced Hahnemann to express his disapproval of it in the fifth edition of the *Organon* in a note to P. 272. Since this period, neither Hahnemann nor myself have made further use of these combined remedies. Dr. Aegidi was not long in abandoning this method, which resembles too closely the procedures of allopathy, opening the way to a falling away from the precious law of simplicity, a method, too, which is becoming everyday more entirely superfluous owing to the increased wealth of our remedies. If consequently in our day, a homeopathician takes it into his head to act according to experiments made thirty years ago, when our science was still in its infancy, and which were subsequently condemned by a unanimous vote, he clearly walks backwards, like a crab, and shows that he has neither kept up with nor followed the progress of science."—*Resonance,* Ju/Aug, 1996, p. 4.

"Patent medicines [*which consist of several substances*] are more dangerous than these simple drugs [*meaning the single homeopathic remedy*], because they are usually a throwing together of a number of remedies to cover a very large range of symptoms, and hence are more injurious because of a greater disturbance of the vital force."—W.A. Yingling.

"Homoeopaths do not follow the objectionable practice of mixing several drugs together, trusting to the discriminating powers of the stomach to discard the unsuitable and appropriate the suitable one. They endeavour to prescribe with precision, by administering one medicine only at a time."— E.H. Ruddock, *The Lady's Manual.*

polypous/polypoid polyp-like. A growth or mass or tumor protruding from a mucous membrane, e.g., nasal p., rectal p., ear p.

polysarca (lipomatosis) obesity, corpulence.

polyuria large amounts of urine.

pomatum (pomade) an externally used preparation, especially used for the hair, like an ointment but of thinner consistency and usually scented. The common pomatum used in the 1860s and '70s was made of lard, suet, and lemon essence.

pompholyx see PEMPHIGUS.

Poncet-Lericke's rheumatism an inflammatory condition of the joints or fibrous tissues caused by the toxins of tuberculosis.

popliteal relating to the posterior surface of the knee, the area behind the knee on the back of the leg.

porrigo any scurfy disease of the skin, such as ringworm, favus, or eczema.

porrigo capitis porrigo of the scalp.

porrigo cervalis milk crust; milk-scab. See CRUSTA LACTEA.

porrigo decalvans see TINEA.

porrigo larvalis eczema of the scalp.

porrigo scutulata ringworm of the scalp.

portal stasis decreased flow of blood through the liver. A damming of blood in the liver.

portal 1) a doorway or entrance. 2) a communicating part or area of an organism; a point of entrance, as of disease into the body. 3) referring to a large vein such as the portal vein. 4) relating to the liver.

posology the science of the dosages of medicines.

posterior in anatomy, situated behind or to the back of a part.

posthitis inflammation of the prepuce of the penis.

post-prandial after a meal.

post tenebras lux L., 'after darkness there is light'.

potash potassium carbonate, *Kali c.*

potatorum L., 'of drinkers or drunkards', a term used to describe symptoms or a syndrome caused by the abuse of alcohol, e.g., hepatocirrhosis potatorum.

potency the power, vitality, strength, or dynamis which a homeopathic remedy possesses, often represented as a number attached to the remedy name, either immediately before or after. The potency of the remedy comes as a result of the succussion step in the remedy preparation process. See POTENTIZE.

For substances readily soluble in alcohol and water the mother tincture is prepared and then potencies made from it. Insoluble substances, i.e., metals, must first be triturated to the 3C level before the liquid potentization process can begin.

The centesimal scale (1:100) is the scale which Hahnemann first developed. These potencies are made in the following way: 1 part of the mother tincture is mixed with 99 parts of 87% alcohol and succussed (shaken) yielding the 1C potency. Taking 1 part of that potency (the 1C),99 parts of 87% alcohol is added and succussed to yield the 2C. This can be continued until very dilute yet highly potentized remedies are created. If this is done using a fresh vial at each step the potencies are termed CH (Centesimal Hahnemann, e.g., 30CH, 200CH, etc.).

Since this takes a lot of vials, Korsakoff, a Russian physician in the 1820s, suggested to Hahnemann using one vial and allowing the solution left clinging to the walls of the vial to be considered 1 part, adding the required amount of 87% alcohol and succussing in the usual manner. This is, in fact, how potencies are made above the 30C level as it saves vials and has no effect on remedy effectiveness. This method is called CK (Centesimal Korsakovian) or Korsakovian potency. If a potency has a K attached to it, it means it was prepared according to the Korsakovian method, e.g., 200K, 200CK, 10MK. (10M is the same as 10,000C, the M serving as the Roman numeral designation for *mille*, 1000. Thus, 1M is 1000C, 5M is 5000C, and CM and DM are 100,000C and 500,000C, respectively).

As mentioned, centesimal potencies were Hahnemann's original discovery, and as a result (or out of convention) one often refers to them, either in print or verbally, as simply the number. "I gave the 30th" or "I gave the 200th potency", means the person gave the 30C and 200C potencies, respectively.

As vials are not reusable, many vials are saved using this method, but what about alcohol? For potencies up to 30C not a great deal of alcohol is used, but to go to 200C, 1M, 10M, etc. great quantities of alcohol would be required. Through experimentation it was found that just water could be used. Thus for potencies 31C and higher, purified water is the vehicle. For example, in the preparation of the 200C potency, water would be used until the 196th potency. Then dispensing alcohol (87%) is used to make the 197th, 198th, 199th (called 'back potencies'), to make the 200th and higher. In other words, potencies 31C-196C are discarded and enough of the three back potencies are retained in order to continue making higher potencies. This also saves on storage space.

The decimal scale (1 to 10 dilution ratio, X, D; namely, 10X = D10, 200X = D200; D is widely used in Europe) is a scale introduced by Samuel Dubs, a Philadelphia doctor, in 1838. It is unsure whether or not Dubs knew of Hering's earlier work or not because one reference says Constantine Hering, the father of American homeopathy, suggested the decimal potencies and Hahnemann approved of it. As early as 1833, Dr. Hering wrote of his experiments with the decimal scale. At about the same time (1835) it was introduced by Vehsemeyer in Germany. Decimal potencies are less powerful than centesimals (1x is less powerful than 1c, 2x less than 2c, 3x less than 3c, etc.) The decimal process is a method for obtaining intermediary potencies, i.e., potencies between centesimal levels (5x is between 2C and 3C in dilution). They are prepared just like centesimal potencies, but in a 1:9 ratio. While 6x and 3c are equivalent in dilution, it is not known at this time how they differ qualitatively, as the 6x has received more succussions than the 3c. Without some sort of exacting methodological research it can only be assumed that 6x and 3c, or 30x and 15c, are equivalent potencies producing equivalent healings.

Trituration is used to prepare centesimal and decimal potencies in solid or powder form: 1 part medicinal substance to 9 or 99 parts of lactose is gouind ('triturated') in a mortar using a pestle for approximately 30 minutes yields the first level of potency ... then 1 part of this mixture to 9 or 99 parts lactose, triturated, yields the second level. This can be carried out, *ad infinitum,* just as with liquids. This is inconvenient and less efficient but homeopathic remedies can and are made this way but once the 3c or 6x level is reached, all substances (soluble and insoluble) can be further diluted and succussed in the liquid medium. Making high potencies of homeopathic remedies is a long and intensive process, as you may well imagine. This problem was solved in several ways: B. Fincke, M.D. (1821-1906) believed that succussion was not as important as the dilution process in the making of a remedy. Dr. Fincke developed a machine which allowed water to flow into a vial which contained 1 drop of the 30th potency. The vial held 1 dram (about 3.5 ml). Fincke believed that for every dram of water which flowed through the vial (approx. 1 dram per minute) the potency was raised one level. To make the 10M potency he would start with a drop of the 30th, let 9969 drams of water flow through the vial (now the 9999 potency), empty the vial, fill it with alcohol, and shake it 180 times. The result is the 10,000 potency or 10M or 10MFincke or 10MF or 10M(F). These are called Fincke Fluxion Potencies or *continuous fluxion* potency. He maintained that his potencies were not the same as potencies prepared other ways. Fincke sold very few of his potencies but rather gave them as gifts to his friends.

Thomas Skinner, M.D., developed a machine which measured 99 drops into a vial which was then emptied and refilled with 99 drops. This would be repeated over and over again until very high potencies resulted. No true succussion takes place and this method is called *intermittent (discontinuous) fluxion.* High potency remedies are made with this machine starting with the 30th potency. It is a reliable method and is still in use today. SK (S̲k̲inner) appearing after the numeral indicates it was made in this manner. Samuel Swan, M.D. developed an apparatus similar to that of Fincke, but it makes intermittent fluxion potencies.

Another machine, made by M. Deschere, M.D., also used the intermittent fluxion process. Kent and H.C. Allen made their own potentizing machines. Carroll Dunham also made potencies, indicated by a notation such as 200C(D). Michael Quinn, R.Ph., the pharmacist at the Hahnemann Clinic in Albany, California, developed a machine which makes Korsakovian potencies.

Lock of South America and Muntz of Austria make continuous fluxion potencies in which the solutions are stirred very vigorously (2,400 to 15,000 rpms) in order to potentize them. In addition, Muntz creates his remedies at a controlled temperature, 98.6^0 F and measures the dilution steps precisely. "Using this [Muntz's] potentising machine 15 potency levels can be reached in one minute or 21,600 in a 24 hour operation (compared with Lock's method of 432,000 levels in 24 hours)."- *Homoeopathic Links* (1997, 10:2, p. 86). See JENICHEN.

The most commonly prescribed potencies are 3x, 6x, 12x, 24x, 30x, 3c, 6c, 12c, 30c, 200c, 1000c or 1M, 10M, 50M, 100M (or CM), 500M (or DM), and 1000M (or MM).

Q (quinquaginta millesimal, 50-millesimal potencies, LM, 0/LM) potencies, sometimes erroneously referred to as LM potencies, are the last potencies which Hahnemann used (from 1837 to 1843), and discussed in the 6th edition of his *Organon* (1842). He began experimenting to find a method of remedy preparation to avoid aggravations. Hahnemann described the preparation and guidelines for use of this scale in paragraphs 246-248, 270, 271, and 278 of the 6th edition. Because this edition was not published for some 80 years (in 1921), this information surprised the homeopathic community but was given little attention. Slowly in the 1940s and 1950s with R. Flury and Pierre Schmidt, M. Dorcsi, and later H. Farrington, Charles Pahud, S.M. Battercherjee and still later with Robert Schore, H. Choudhury, Kunzli V. Fimelsberg, R.P. Patel, Sheilagh Creasy, Tomlinson and others, research and clinical trials were carried out using this latest potency method of Hahnemann.

The inspiration for the Q potencies may have come from Hering in a letter to the editor he wrote for a journal *Archiv fur die Homoopathische Heilkunst* to then editor and long time student of Hahnemann, Ernst Stapf. Today Q potencies are growing in popularity because of their advantages (virtually no aggravations, administration may be repeated frequently, they work faster and are gentler in their action than the high centesimal potencies, treatment may be initiated using any Q potency-level, and they are indicated for acute and chronic disease.) Though it is theoretically possible to go beyond Q30, the potencies currently available are Q1, 2, 3 ... 30 (Q 0/1, Q 0/2, ... or 0/Q1, 0/Q2, with the 0 indicating that the medicine is on poppyseed-sized pellets, or simply 0/1, 0/2, 0/5).

The preparation process of these potencies is complex and different than the centesimal and decimal methods. The dilutions are in a 50,000 to 1 ratio, or LM (from the Roman numerals L, 'fifty' and M, 'thousand', because each succeeding potency contains one 50,000th of the preceding one). Q1 is prepared in the following way: first a 3c potency is made by trituration, even if the original remedy substance is alcohol and water soluble. Then one grain (65mg) of the 3C potency of the desired substance is dissolved in 500 drops of diluent (1:4 ratio of 95% alcohol and distilled water, respectively). One drop of this solution is added to 2 ml of 95% alcohol and succussed 100 times, yielding the Q1 dilution. 1 drop of this solution is added to and mixed with 500 pellets (size #10, poppyseed). Now all the 500 pellets are at the Q1 level of dilution. To go to Q2 one pellet of Q1 is dissolved in 2 ml of 95% alcohol and succussed 100 times, yielding the Q2. One drop of it can then be added to and mixed with 500 pellets to yield Q2 pellets. This can be continued to Q30. While conceivably possible to go further it has not been found necessary to do so.

The administration of these Q potencies is complicated as there is no standardized method within the homeopathic community. For instance, some physicians have the patient dissolve 1 pellet of the chosen Q in approx. 5 oz. of distilled water to which a small amount of grain alcohol has been added. This becomes the stock solution from which the patient takes doses. Some physicians have the patient place the dry Q pellet directly onto the tongue or first dissolved in water then swished in the mouth. Then, according to the physician's instructions, the patient takes varying dosages of the remedy in addition to diluting it further and stirring it with a spoon or succussing the bottle (potentizing it further) between dosages. Q potency administration, as mentioned, can become quite complicated.

In the sixth edition of the *Organon* (para. 247-248), Hahnemann recommended dissolving a single pellet of the appropriate Q potency in a vial of water, succussing the vial 8 to 12 times between doses, and giving one teaspoon to the patient every day or every other day in chronic cases, or as often as every two to six hours in acute cases. The vial could hold as much as 40 tablespoons; or, to avoid the inconvenience of a large initial vial, the pellet could be dissolved in 7 or 8 tablespoons of water in the vial, then each teaspoonful dose further dissolved in another 7 or 8 spoonfuls of water and the patient given a teaspoonful from this further diluted mixture.

Some authorities say that Q1 is approximately equivalent in dilution to 10X or 11X, with Q30 being approximately 150X. Though rather modest when compared to 200C or 1M, etc., it should be emphasized that the uniqueness of these potencies does not depend on dilution but rather on their total composition. It is somewhere between Q2 and Q3 (probably closer to Q3) that Avogadro's number is surpassed and no molecules of the starting substance will be found in the dilution.

For further information on Q-potencies consult: H. Choudhury, *50 Millesimal Potency in Theory and Practice,* Robert Barker's *LM Potencies,* and R.P. Patel's *My Experiments with 50 Millesimal Scale Potencies.* Hahnemann had this to say about his Q-potencies: "My new method produces medicines of the highest power and the mildest action." (Paragraph 270 of the *Organon)*

"Generally each patient has an ideal potency—a potency which they respond to best."—R. Moskowitz

potency chord (potency accord, PC, homeochord, potency complexes, multi-attenuations) several potencies of a substance(s) mixed to form one medicinal entity, e.g., Echinacea PC is a homeopathic product containing *Echinacea purpurea* 6x, 12x, 30x, 200x and *Echinacea angustifolia* 6x, 12x, 30x, 200x. Though not popular until the 1970s, early work was done by Cahis of Barcelona, who presented his findings at the International Homeopathic Congress in London in 1911. He likened such mixtures to musical melodies or chords and believed the sum total therapeutic effect to be quite different from the individual potencies themselves. Others who did research in this area were Kroner, Nebel, Reckeweg, Zimmerman, Fuhry, Sunder, Junker, Kolisko, Konig, and Vosgerau. A 'multicord' is a potency chord which includes remedies from different potency scales (x, c, LM).

potentization (dynamization) the process of preparing a homeopathic remedy by repeated dilution with succussion (shaking). It may be said that potentization involves the transfer of information from one substance to another. See POTENCY.

Pott's disease (tuberculous spondylitis, Pott's caries, spinal caries) weakness and collapse of the spinal vertebrae because of an infiltration of tubercular bacteria, *Mycobacterium tuberculosis,* resulting in kyphosis (hunchback). If untreated, severe kyphosis may be produced, causing a destruction of nerve trunks and paraplegia. Dr. P. Pott (1713-1788), an English surgeon, first described this condition but did not realize tuberculosis to be the cause.

poultice (cataplasm) a soft mixture applied to a sore or inflamed part of the body. A moist, warm, pasty mass folded inside a thin cloth and laid on inflamed skin to reduce inflammations, draw out infection or act as a counter-irritant. It promotes local circulation, causing collected pus and serum to be either absorbed into the system or brought to a head to discharge outwardly, thus giving relief.

Poupart's ligament a ligament in the groin extending from the top of the ilium to the spine of the pubis, first described by F. Poupart (1616-1708), a French surgeon to the court of Louis XIV.

pouting a protrusion of the lips in an expression of displeasure or sulkiness.

Showing displeasure or disappointment; sulking.

pox 1) an archaic term for syphilis. 2) a general term for any exanthemic disease characterized by purulent skin eruptions which have a tendency to cause vesicles and pustules. 3) misfortune. 4) the pit-like scars of small-pox.

praecordial (precordial) that area of the chest where the diaphragm is located. That region of the chest in front of the heart (L. *prae*, 'before/in front of', and *cordis*, 'the heart').

praecordial distress pain, anxiety or tense feeling of an area of the chest overlying the heart.

praeputialis of or pertaining to the prepuce of the penis.

prairie itch (grain itch) an eruption due to *Pediculoides ventricosus*, acquired by contact with grain or straw which harbors the parasite.

prattle to babble. To talk idly or meaninglessly.

precocity characterized by unusually early development or maturity, especially in mental aptitude; also inappropriate behavior for the age level, as in 'precocious' sexual behavior in a child.

premonitory forewarning; giving an indication of what is to follow. 'Premonition', anticipation or prophesying.

prepuce the foreskin of the penis; the loose fold of skin that covers the head (glans) of the penis.

presbyophrenia (Wernicke's syndrome) one of the mental disorders of old age marked by loss of memory, disorientation, and confabulation, with, however, a relative integrity of judgment.

presbyopia (hypermetropia, old-sightedness) farsightedness, the inability of the eye to focus sharply on nearby objects, resulting from a hardening of the crystalline lens with advancing age.

From the Greek *presby-*, 'old', from the same root as *presbyteros*, 'elder', as in the Presbyterian Church, which was founded on a principle of government by a council of elders rather than a church hierarchy.

presenescence pre-senility. The state of growing old. The beginning of old age.

priapism (from Priapus, the god of procreation) a persistent abnormal painful and tender erection of the penis especially when due to disease and not provoked by sexual desire.

prima causa morbi L., 'the primary cause of illness'.

primae viae the stomach and intestinal tube. The digestive tract (L., 'first or primary way').

primary action of drugs "...many drugs [in material doses], in the first or primary stage of their action produce one group of symptoms, and in the second stage a directly opposite set of phenomena; as when the deep sleep of the primary action of Opium is followed by a much longer lasting wakefulness; or where the diarrhea induced by a cathartic is followed by a longer lasting constipation." -*The Genius of Homoeopathy* (S. Close, p. 184-5)

primigravida a woman who is pregnant for the first time.

primum non nocere 'first do no harm' (L., from the Hippocratic Oath).

Pringle's disease (sebaceous adenoma, Pringle's type of adenoma) from the English dermatologist J.J. Pringle (1855-1922) who described small, translucent tumors, usually multiple and occurring on the face, originating in the sebaceous glands.

prn L. *pro re nata*, 'as circumstances require' (lit. 'as the thing is born' or 'as things unfold'). If necessary, if needed (referring to the administration of a medication): "take as needed."

pro tem. (pro tempore) L., 'for the time being'.

probiotic referring to treatment which supports, stimulates or encourages the natural healing abilities of the body, as in 'probiotic therapy', as opposed to antibiotics which kill the supposed pathological source rather than supporting the body's own curative powers. Thus probiotic therapies would include homeopathy, botanicals, massage, acupuncture, proper diet, etc.

procidentia a prolapse or sinking down of an organ or part.

proclivity a natural tendency or inclination. A predispostion.

proctagra a sudden pain in the anus.

proctalgia pain in the anus or rectum.

proctitis inflammation of the anus or rectum.

prodromal relating to the initial stage of a disease, as in 'prodromal symptom' (a symptom indicating the imminent start of a disease; a forewarning).

prognosis the foretelling of the probable course of a disease; a forecast of the outcome of a disease.

progressive muscular atrophy "A chronic wasting and degeneration of the muscular tissue, more especially of the muscles of the extremities, in consequence of which there is a corresponding loss of motor power."— C.P. Hart, *Therapeutics of Nervous Diseases.*

prolapse (prolapsus) the falling downward or displacement downward of a part or organ (commonly seen with the rectum or uterus/womb).

prolapsed womb the dropping down of the womb or uterus into the vagina. In the healthy non-pregnant woman the womb is 3–4 inches in length, weighs 30–90 grams, and resembles an upside-down pear in shape. The lower part opens into the vagina at the cervix, and the upper part opens into the fallopian tubes. There are three degrees of severity of this condition, with the first being a slight displacement and the third being the most severe, as the womb protrudes beyond the vulva. Related conditions include cystocele (bladder bulges into the front wall of the vagina), urethrocele (the urethra bulges into the front wall of the vagina), and rectocele (the rectal wall bulges into the back wall of the vagina). These three conditions are due to a sagging of the vaginal walls and their surrounding supporting tissues. Though they can occur on their own, they always occur with a prolapsed womb. A prolapsed womb is usually caused when the ligaments supporting it become overstretched, e.g., during childbirth or in very obese women. Often there are no symptoms, though some women do experience a 'dragging' feeling in the pelvis, or a sensation that something is being forced downward.

prolapsus ani (proctoptosia) the falling downward or displacement downward of the anus. Similar terms which may be found include prolapsus recti (rectum) and prolapsus uteri (uterus).

pronation downward rotation of the palm or rotation of the instep inwards.

prone lying face downward.

prosopalgia (prosopalgia fothergilli, tic douloureux, facial neuralgia) nerve pain in the trigeminal nerve region. See FACEACHE.

prostatorrhea a thin urethral discharge coming from the penis, originating from the prostate.

prostration extreme exhaustion.

proud flesh exuberant granulations; a fungous growth from a granulating surface which shows no tendency toward scar tissue formation. Warts, figwarts.

proving (Ger. *Prüfung*, hyganthropharmacology) the process of determining the medicinal/curative properties of a substance. This process involves the administration of substances either in crude form or in potency to healthy human subjects in order to observe and record symptoms. A test of the action of a drug upon the healthy body, and a record of the unusual sensations/ symptoms produced and/or alterations from the normal health experienced by one taking the drug.

"All our progress as a school depends on the right view of the symptoms obtained by proving with *Camphor* and *Opium*."—Hering. "Symptoms appearing last in a proving have the highest value."—Hering.

"It is a well-known fact that Hahnemann reasoned from the working definition that drugs do not have healing powers, but that they are impulses of illness. A drug proving produces an illness called pathogenesis or pathopoiesis. This artificial illness is also transmitted to the patient. It is stronger than the natural illness which it replaces and causes to vanish. ... The healing occurs because the artificial drug disease that replaces the natural illness is stronger, yet of much shorter duration and soon after having distinguished the natural illness, it disappears on its own."—G. von Keller, 'On Q Potencies', *Classical Homoeopathy Quarterly* 4, 1991, p. 123.

Hahnemann's *Materia Medica Pura*, based on provings, was published in Dresden in six parts from 1811-21. Approximately fifty people assisted Hahnemann in conducting his provings.

Consult *The Dynamics and Methodology of Homoeopathic Provings* (Jeremy Sherr)

Prüfung Ger. 'test'or 'examination'. See PROVING.

prurient characterized by lascivious or lustful thoughts and desires. Having a restless desire or longing (L. *pruriens,* 'itching').

pruriginous relating to or suffering from prurigo.

prurigo a chronic inflammatory disease of the skin characterized by small, pale papules and severe itching. The papules are deeply seated and most prominent on the extensor surfaces of the limbs. The disease usually begins in early life. It has two forms: a mild form, p. mitis and a severe form, p. ageia or p. ferox.

pruritis a sensation of itching, not necessarily associated with visible skin disease.

pruritis ani itching of the anus.

pruritis pudendi itching in the pudendum (genital area, especially female).

pruritis senilis the itching of the aged, probably caused by a lack of oil in the skin; accompanies the atrophy of the skin in old age.

pseudocyesis false or spurious pregnancy. A state in which some of the signs of pregnancy are present but no conception has taken place.

pseudo-croup (catarrhal croup) see LARYNGISMUS STRIDULUS.

pseudo-hypertrophic paralysis (Duchenne's disease) a disease of childhood, marked by progressive muscular atrophy and paralysis in which there is a deceptive appearance of hypertrophy because fat is deposited, taking the place of the wasted muscles.

pseudo-plethora a deceptive resemblance to plethora. The person may look plethoric (robust) but in reality is not.

pseudopia (pseudopsia) a visual hallucination or error in visual perception.

pseudoplasma a neoplasm (malignant tumor).

pseudopsora the tubercular diathesis/miasm, commonly considered a result of the hereditary bonding of psora and syphilis.

psilosis falling out of the hair. Also may refer to sprue, an afebrile, chronic disease characterized by the passage of voluminous, mushy, and often frothy stools, weakness, emaciation, changes in the tongue and anemia. It is common in Caucasians living in S.E. Asia, East Indies, Sri Lanka, and the West Indies. Originally the disease was thought to be caused by *Monilia psilosis,* but researchers now seem to think it is a deficiency disease, or a defective absorption of nutrients.

psittacosis (parrot disease, parrot fever) an infectious disease of birds once thought to be caused by a virus but now known to be caused by *Chlamy-*

dia psittaci, a parasite. It can be transmitted to man, causing such symptoms as headache, nausea, bronchopneumonia, nosebleeds, constipation and fever preceded by a chill.

psoas either of two internal muscles of the loin, stretching from the lumbar vertebrae to the brim of the pelvis or the femur.

psoitis an inflammation of the psoas muscle. See PSOAS.

psora (from the Hebrew *tsorat* , 'blemish, taint, dirt, stigma') scabies, the itch. A genus of contagious disease appearing first on the wrists and between the fingers in small pustules with watery heads. This definition is one found in a medical dictionary of 1801. In that same dictionary 'psoriasis' is defined as a species of itch which affects the scrotum. 'Psora', or 'itch dyscrasia', is also one of the three major miasms as described by Hahnemann. He said it was the parent of all chronic diseases and developed as a result of suppression of the 'itch' or scabies infection and is the root of many of our present chronic diseases. Unlike the other two miasms, syphilis and sycosis, psora does not produce major destruction or gross malformations or alteration of tissue, but expresses itself more in skin symptoms and functional and mental symptoms. It is best to consult other reference works (see MIASM) for a more detailed explanation. See SCABIES.

"Psora is that most ancient, most universal, most destructive, and yet most misapprehended chronic miasmatic disease which for many thousands of years has disfigured and tortured mankind, and which during the last centuries has become the mother of all the thousands of incredibly various (acute and) chronic (non-venereal) diseases by which the whole civilized human race on the inhabited globe is being more and more afflicted."—*Chronic Diseases* (Hahnemann).

psoriasis (scaly tetter, lepra graecorum) a chronic, noncontagious skin disease characterized by inflammatory red, white or silvery scaly patches. The lesions occur primarily on elbows, knees, scalp and trunk. See PSORA.

psoriasis circinata (Willan's leprosy) see PSORIASIS LEPRA.

psoriasis diffusa a form of psoriasis with more or less coalescence of the lesions.

psoriasis gyrata psoriasis with a snake-like arrangement or appearance.

psoriasis inveterata a form of psoriasis in which the lesions are confluent, the affected skin being thickened, indurated and scaly.

psoriasis lepra (Willan's leprosy, psoriasis circinata) psoriasis which occurs in a circular pattern. This was first described in 1808 by the English dermatologist, Robert Willan (1756-1812).

psoriasis linguae (leucoplakia, smoker's tongue, buccal psoriasis, ichthyosis linguae) irregular white patches on the mucous membrane of the tongue. There is a thickening of the epithelium and the papillae may be hypertrophied. (L., 'psoriasis of the tongue').

psoriasis syphilitic this term may refer to the secondary stage of syphilis when skin symptoms predominate. Or it may refer to psoriasis caused by syphilis and the stress which that disease induces. The exact meaning is difficult to ascertain.

psoric referring to the miasm known as psora. See PSORA.

psorospermosis a diseased condition due to psorosperms (a type of parasitic sporozoa).

psychic relating to the mind or soul; mental. A person who is supposed to be endowed with the power of communicating with spirits; a spiritualistic medium. 'Psychic' symptoms would mean symptoms relating to the mind.

psychical referring to the emotions, mind, and/or spirit.

psyasthenia a mild psychosis or psychoneurosis marked especially by lack of self-control, in consequence of which the patient is dominated by morbid fears or doubts, impulses to do wrongful, foolish, unreasoning behavior, fixed ideas, etc., and feels a sense of unusualness or unreality in himself and his surroundings.

psysiatric medicine natural medicine. The use of natural medicine only to heal the ill.

pterygium/pterygion (wing-skin, web eye) a triangular patch of subconjunctival tissue extending towards the pupil from the inner canthus to the border of the cornea or beyond (Gr. *pteron,* wing).

ptilosis a loss of the eyelashes.

ptisan (tisane) a domestic decoction or 'tea', such as of pearl barley, which have nutritive value.

ptomaine a nitrogenous substance, sometimes poisonous, produced by the spoilage of protein, as in ptomaine poisoning.

ptosis prolapse or falling down of an organ or part, often referring to a drooping of the upper eyelid.

ptyalism salivation.

pubertal pertaining to puberty.

puberty the sequence of events by which a child is transformed into a young adult. The period at which the generative organs become capable of exercising the function of reproduction, signaled in the boy by a change of voice and discharge of semen, and in the girl by the onset of menses.

pubes pubic bones. See PUBIS.

pubis (pl. pubes) the forward portion of either of the hipbones, at the juncture forming the front arch of the pelvis.

puceau a deep red to dark greyish purple color.

pudendum (pl. pudenda) the external genitalia, especially of the woman (L.,'something to be modest or ashamed of').

puerile juvenile, immature, childish.

puerperal pertaining to childbirth. The period from childbirth to involution of the uterus, usually considered to last six weeks after delivery.

puerperal convulsions see ECLAMPSIA.

puerperal fever (childbed fever, puerperal sepsis) septicemia occurring within three weeks after abortion or childbirth. A febrile state caused by infection of the mother's bloodstream through the genital tract before, during, or following delivery. Symptoms include chills, abdominal tenderness and pain, rapid pulse and respiration, and fever.

Oliver Wendell Holmes, M.D. (1809-1894), one of the severest critics of homeopathy, arguably wrote one of the most important papers in 19th century American medicine, entitled 'Puerperal Fever as a Private Pestilence' (1855). In it, he demonstrated conclusively the contagious nature of childbed fever. He showed that this disease was carried by the unwashed hands of the physician from bed to bed and could be avoided by washing the hands before and after pelvic exams and after postmortem examinations. In this paper he also mentions the work of Ignac Fulop Semmelweis (1818-1865) who conducted seminal work before Holmes did.

Charles White (1728-1813) in 1773 wrote *A Treatise on the Management of Pregnant and Lying-in Women. . .* which was the first book in the modern period of medicine to help solve the etiology and management of puerperal fever. It maintains the necessity for hygiene in all facets of the care of the pregnant woman. To paraphrase historian Castiglioni: "If his recommendations had been adopted more generally, they would have largely prevented the horrible conditions in the maternity wards of the succeeding century."

puerperal mania (puerperal psychosis) the excessive excitement, passion, elevation of mood, and psychomotor overactivity of childbirth or labor.

puerperal metritis an inflammation of the uterus following childbirth.

pulmonary tuberculosis tuberculosis which affects the lungs wherein the bacteria form lesions in the lungs, causing the formation of mucus and obstruction of the air passages. See TUBERCULOSIS.

pultaceous macerated, pulpy, mushy, soft.

punctata albescens minute round spots, usually white, differing in color or otherwise in appearance from the surrounding tissues (L., 'a prick/puncture/point turning white').

punctum saliens a salient or important point (L., 'a point that leaps out').

pungent sharp or spicy; biting or penetrating.

pura/pure as it is found in *Materia Medica Pura* or in *Encyclopedia of Pure Materia Medica* means that the information found in that reference is solely based on provings and not on other sorts of data like toxicological or clinical symptomatology.

pure homeopathy the classical, pure homeopathy of Hahnemann, namely "...the single remedy, based on the totality of symptoms, in the minimum dose." -*Homeopathy Today,* (1997, 17:6, p. 2-3).

purgation (catharsis) purging, causing a bowel movement by cathartics.

purgative an agent which causes catharsis or movement of the bowels.

puriform having the form and appearance of pus (L. *puris,* 'of pus').

purist one who practices pure homeopathy. See pure homeopathy.

purpura an affection characterized by bleeding into the skin, the color being at first red, becoming gradually darker, then purple, fading to a brownish-yellow, and finally, in the course of two or three weeks, disappearing; it may result in a permanent pigmentation. These extravasations (leakages) may occur also into the mucous membranes and internal organs. Large petechiae.

purpura hemorrhagica (idiopathic thrombocytopenic purpura, land scurvy, morbus maculosus werlhoffii, Werlhof's disease) a disease characterized by extensive ecchymoses (bruising, bruises), bleeding from the mucous membranes, and great tiredness or prostration. A systemic disease with petechiae or large hemorrhages in the skin, usually appearing first in the extremities and then in successive crops over a larger area. There is a reduction in the number of platelets in the blood.

purpura miliaris (purple fever, roodvonk, scarlatina miliaris) a condition characterized by millet-sized (0.5-1mm) hemorrhages in the skin, larger than purpura petechiae but smaller than p. maculata. It is often found accompanying a fever and was mistaken for scarlet fever in the early 19th century.

purpura rheumatica (Schonlein's purpura) a form of purpura associated with acute arthritis. Here hemorrhages may be in the form of petechiae, macules or large patches. See PETECHIA.

purpura senilis the occurrence of petechiae and ecchymoses on the legs in aged and debilitated subjects (L. *senilis,* 'of old people').

purulent associated with or having the character of pus or forming pus.

pus a fluid product of inflammation consisting of a liquid portion (sera) containing leukocytes, and a colloidal portion containing dead cells and tissue elements. Cf. LAUDABLE.

pusillanimous cowardly and/or mean spirited.

pustule a small circumscribed elevation on the skin, containing pus, and less than 1cm in diameter. A pus-filled vesicle or bulla and tiny abscess in the skin that can vary in color (white, orange, yellow or green), depending somewhat on the infecting organism, e.g., acne pimples and boils.

putrefaction the state of being putrefied. A decomposition or decaying of organic material accompanied with foul odors. Rotting. To become fetid from decay.

putrescent becoming putrid or decaying. Pertaining to putrefaction (decomposition of organic matter).

putrillage putrid or rotten substance/matter.

pyaemia presence of pus in the blood, which is associated with fever and possibly septicemia. 'Pyaemic', relating to pyaemia.

pycnogenol (proanthocyanidin) see PHYTOMEDICINE.

pyelitis inflammation of the pelvis of the kidney (the basin-shaped area of the kidney).

pyelonephritis inflammation of the kidney and the pelvis of the kidney, often due to an infection ascending from the ureter.

pylephlebitis inflammation of the portal veins.

pyemesis the vomiting of pus.

pyloric relating to the pylorus or the lower part of the stomach.

pylorus the lower opening of the stomach into the small intestine.

pyodermia any pustular or other form of suppurative disease of the skin.

pyogenic pus-forming.

pyonex the instrument used in Baunscheidismus. See BAUNSCHEIDISMUS.

pyorrhea a purulent discharge.

pyorrhea alveolaris (Rigg's disease, Fauchard's disease, alveolar periostitis, pyorrhea alveolaris) see RIGG'S DISEASE.

pyrexia fever (Gr. *pyr*, 'fire').

pyrexial pertaining to fevers.

pyromania a mania for setting fire to things.

pyrophobia an extreme dread of fire.

pyrosis (waterbrash, heartburn) acidity of the stomach with eructations of sour, burning fluid from the stomach. May also include a sudden regurgitation of tasteless saliva.

pyuria pus in the urine.

Q

Q potency (quinquagintamillesimal) the 50-millesimal potency of Hahnemann as discussed in the 6th edition of the *Organon.* Commonly referred to as LM; the term is a misnomer, as LM is 50,000C. See POTENCY.

Q fever a rickettsial disease (see TYPHUS) which, unlike other diseases in this group, does not develop a skin eruption.

q.v. an abbreviation having two meanings, the more common being from the Latin *quod vide,* 'which see' or 'see which'. *Vide* means 'see' or 'look to'.

qualmishness a feeling of sickness, faintness or nausea. A sensation of doubt, misgiving, or uneasiness of conscience.

quartan recurring every three days, as in, for example, a malarial fever where the paroxysms recur every 72 hours. (Latin *quartus,* 'fourth', because the fever recurs every fourth day if the first day of occurrence is counted too, e.g. fever on Monday, again on Thursday).

quicksilver *Mercurius solubilis,* hydragyrum metallicum. See MERCURY.

quiescent dormant, still, or inactive.

quinine cachexia (malarial cachexia) chronic malaria. See CACHEXIA MALARIA.

Quincke's disease/edema (angioneurotic edema) an acute circumscribed edema of the skin, first described by H.I. Quinck, a German physician.

quinia quinine sulfate powder.

quininism see CINCHONISM.

quinsy acute inflammation of the tonsils and the surrounding tissue, often leading to the formation of an abscess. Inflammatory sore throat.

quintan recurring every four days, as in, for example, a malarial fever where the paroxysms recur every 96 hours. (Latin *quintus,* 'fifth', because the fever recurs every fifth day if the first day of occurrence is counted too, e.g. fever on Monday, again on Friday).

quintillionth the 15th centesimal level of dilution.

quo vadis 'whither goest thou?' 'where are you going' (Latin)

quotidian (amphemerous) daily recurrence, as a fever. Recurring every 24 hours.

quotient the number of times one amount is contained in another. The result of the process of division.

R

racemose resembling a bunch of grapes.

rachialgia spinal pain.

rachitis (rhachitis, rickets) see RICKETS. Inflammation of the vertebral column.

RADAR the acronym for a homeopathic computer software program, Rapid Aid to Drug Aimed Research.

Rademacherian referring to J.G. Rademacher (1772-1850), a physician who was influenced in great part by Paracelsus. He authored *Universal and Organ Remedies* and in that work developed his theory of organ and organ-system correspondences (remedies having affinities for certain parts of the body). He dealt more in the physical realm and did not emphasize mentals or modalities.

radiate to diverge from a common center. See EXTEND.

radiesthesia a method of diagnosing and treating disease by the use of devices that respond to vibrations. Consult *The Practice of Medical Radiesthesia* (Vernon D. Wethered, 1967). See RADIONICS.

radionics a system formed into a loose body of knowledge by Albert Abrams (1863-1924). His basic discoveries were: 1) all matter radiates, 2) this radiation differs in accordance with the molecular or atomic composition of the specimen, and 3) whatever its nature, this radiation can affect the human nervous system. Thus radionics could be considered the science and study of subtle vibrations/radiations which have effects on living systems.

Dowsing is a form of radionics in that these subtle energies can be tuned in upon and used to uncover information which otherwise is hidden. The dowser, after centering himself, uses one of a number of types of dowsing apparatus (rods, pendulums, etc.) to tune into and locate subtle vibrations associated with water, precious metals, oil, or even missing persons. It is even possible to dowse without using instruments or other specialized apparatus.

Edgar Cayce (1877-1945) was probably the most accomplished radionic diagnostician that ever lived. He could tune into vibrations just by touching objects or thinking about the subject in question. In addition, he could do this remotely (at a distance far removed from where the object or person was located).

The impact of the vast subject of radionics on homeopathy is in the work of Malcolm Rae (1913-1979). Mr. Rae, experimentor and inventor, combined his knowledge of radionics with homeopathy to establish a way of producing remedies using 'magnetically energised geometric patterns'. By inserting 'rate-cards', adjusting frequencies, and various controls on his instruments, energy is imparted into placebo pellets or liquids, thus 'making' a homeopathic remedy. What sparked his interest was his homeopathic cure of kidney and gall stones in 1959. He wrote a number of articles but no books.

Royal Raymond Rife (1888-1977), David V. Tansley (1934-1988), Ruth B. Drown, Guyon Richards, Curtis Upton, Wm. and George de la Warr, Thomas Galen Hieronymus, J. Cecil Maby, J.W. Wigglesworth, Georges Lakhovsky (inventor of the Lakhovsky Multiwave Oscillator), Riley H. Crabb, John Wilcox, Ted Serios, and Harold S. Burr are some of the important figures in radionic history. See *Report on Radionics* (E.W. Russell) as well as other volumes.

railway spine (Erichsen's disease) a form of traumatic neurosis following concussion of the spine produced in a railway accident (now commonly called whiplash). The symptoms are ill-defined and the pathology obscure.

A British physician, J.E. Ericksen, in his book *On Railway and Other Injuries of the Nervous System* (1867), first described injuries to the spine as a result of the increased speed of railway travel.

rake (wastrel) a lecherous, intemperate person, especially a man, who is recklessly wasteful; wildly extravagant. An idler or loafer.

rale abnormal sound arising within the lungs or air passages (Fr. *rale*, rattle).

ramollissement softening, as in the ramollissement of an organ or part.

ramus a branch of an organ, especially of a vein or an artery (L. 'branch').

rancid having a sharp disagreeable odor and taste, as in rancid butter.

ranine relating to the under surface of the tongue.

ranula (hypoglossis, frog tongue, hypoglottis) a cystic tumor of the floor of the mouth (under the tongue), due to obstruction of the duct of the sublingual glands. This obstruction in the mouth can, in turn, cause the person to sound like a frog (L. *ranula*, 'little frog').

raphania see RHAPHANIA.

raphe a seam, line, ridge, or crease. The line of union of two continuous and similar structures. For example, the raphe scroti is a central line, like a cord, running over the scrotum from the anus to the root of the penis (Gr. *raphe*, 'suture or seam').

raptus a sudden attack or seizure (L., 'seized, carried away').

rare remedy a remedy which is seldom called for in homeopathic practice. A symptom calling for its use very seldom arises in practice. A homeopath might use a rare remedy just a handful of times in his whole career, e.g.,

Pothos foetidus, Chloralum, Chromicum acidum, etc.

rasping harsh or grating (referring to a sound); scraping or grating (referring to a pain).

rationalist that approach in medical thought which views the living organism in mechanical or reductionist terms. Vital energies are largely ignored and symptomatology viewed as the disease rather than as curative expressions of the person's vital force.

This left brain/right brain duality can historically be seen in the conflict between allopaths and homeopaths. Even within the allopathic movement this divison can be seen, e.g., Koch and Ehrlich were mechanists whereas Pasteur and Metchnikoff were more vitalist in their approach. Koch saw vaccines as a way to treat disease, whereas Pasteur saw them as a preventative, a struggle of life versus life.

Compare this with empiricism, a vitalist approach, which says that practical interventions or treatments should be based on practical experience (in other words, a more vital approach). Thus homeopaths can be called empiricists, allopaths rationalists. For example, rationalists argue that the individual's resistance to disease is a result of physical or chemical aspects. The empiricists attribute a person's resistance to the quality of the individual's physiology and vitality.

raucedo (raucitas) hoarseness (L. *raucus,* 'hoarse, raucous').

Rayid see IRIDOLOGY.

Raynaud's disease a syndrome named after the French physician M. Raynaud who, in 1862, described this condition of vascular spasms in the fingers, which cause the fingers to become white and cold, then congested, and finally, in some cases, gangrenous; these changes are accompanied by neuralgic pains, tingling, burning, and other paresthesias.

Reclus's disease (ligneous phlegmon, woody phlegmon) multiple benign cystic growths in the mammary gland.

recrudescence an increase in the symptoms of a disease after a remission or a short intermission (from the Latin, 'becoming raw again').

rectal referring to the rectum.

recti interni the internal rectal muscles.

recumbent reclining, lying down.

red gum a red papular eruption of infants. Tiny red and sometimes white pimples on the face, neck, arms or even the entire body. Pimples contain no fluid, are hard and may bleed when scratched. See STROPHULUS.

rediscovery of homeopathy see SEHGAL'S HOMEOPATHIC METHOD.

redolent full of or diffusing a pervasive odor, especially one of an agreeable fragrance. More often used in a figurative manner, as in 'redolent of the past'.

reductionism the process of dividing a complex problem into smaller ones that can then be solved individually. Thus reductionists assume that it is possible to explain complex systems on the basis of molecular and elementary physical/chemical principles. Determinism is similar in that if initial conditions are known then it should be possible to predict the outcome of what follows.

These methods of looking at the world and life, however, are not useful in investigating the world-of-life coming into being. One needs to realize that "The theory of science says that the evolution of sciences is not the simple result of a growing body of knowledge and scientific advances but is essentially due to changes in theory. A change of paradigm, replacing established theoretical and methodological principles with new ones, may cause science to advance in leaps and bounds."—Andreas Goyent in *J. of Anthroposophical Medicine,* 10:1, 1993. This gives rise to chaos and its attendant theory of disorder and irregularity. The chaos theory attempts to address the 'processes that occur in time in the living world of nature'. See RATIONALISM.

related homeopathic remedies homeopathic drugs of the same origin which bring about similar therapeutic effects (are associated with a similar homeopathic drug picture). For example, *Bell.* and *Hyos.*

refractory obstinate, resistant; resistant to treatment, as in a disease.

Reiter's syndrome/disease a syndrome first described by German physician Hans Reiter (1881-1969), consisting of arthritic symptoms, urethritis (inflammation of the urethra), prostatitis, conjunctivitis, and uveitis (inflammation of the entire uveal tract—iris, ciliary body, and choroid). It was thought to be caused by a spirochete but is now commonly thought to result from an autoallergic hypersensitivity.

remedy as opposed to a drug or medicine, the homeopathic remedy does just that: it remedies a situation, causing symptoms (which are the expression of disease) to go away, leaving in their wake a more healthy functioning individual.

"What validates homeopathy is not so much that remedies work but that they exist as people."—R. Moskowitz.

As a sidelight, in the infancy of homeopathy in this country (1825-1835) remedies were mostly imported from Germany. In 1838 Dr. J. Tanner returned from a trip to Leipzig, Germany and opened the first homeopathic pharmacy in America, the United States Homeopathic Pharmacy in Philadelphia, PA. He imported the crude medicines and made the triturations and dilutions. In 1840 Otis Clapp opened another, and by 1851, there were twenty pharmacies. About 1845, the respected European pharmacist J.C. Jenichen sent his high potencies to Dr. C.J. Hempel (the 'great translator' of German homeopathic texts into English). Dr. Hempel advertised that anyone who wanted to try high potencies could purchase a set of 468 vials each containing 1200-1400 globules for $110.

By the way, up to the year 1850 there were 94 books published relating to homeopathy and 104 pamphlets. The first journal, *Correspondenzblatt*, was started in 1835-36, published in Allentown, PA (in German!) and edited by C. Hering. In that year there were 53 physicians practicing homeopathy in the U.S. By 1848 the number rose to 400-500; by 1899, ten thousand; by 1901, 14,000.

remedy epidemicus a remedy which has been determined to be curative in an epidemic disease for the vast majority so afflicted. See GENUS EPIDEMICUS.

remedy families remedies grouped according to similar characteristics and symptomatology they possess (often, but not always, based on botanical families). For example, the Solanaceae "*Dulcamara, Tabacum* and *Capsicum* have nothing to do with *Hyoscyamus* or *Stramonium*, while *Lyssinum* is quite similar to *Belladonna, Gallicum acidum*, and *Tanacetum*. This is the vertical level, as I said before. I arrrived at my point by cases where I gave for example *Belladonna* with some result, but the remedy that finally worked very well was *Tanacetum*."— M. Mangialavori, *Homoeopathic Links*, 4/96, p. 211.

Another example of a remedy family is *Rutacaea*, which consists of *Angustura, Jaborandi, Citrus vul., Citrus lim., Ptelea*, and *Xanthoxylum* among others. The snake venoms would include *Lachesis, Crotalus, Vipera*, etc.; the spiders, *Tarentula hisp.* and *cub., Lactrodectans*, etc.; the Natrum salts, *Nat. mur., Nat. sulph., Nat. carb.*, etc.; the Composite flowers, *Arnica, Bell. per., Millefolia*, etc.

remedy themes generally the prominent psychological aspects of a remedy. For example, the themes of *Causticum* revolve around injustice, grief, dictatorial (from a need to be in control), sympathetic and sensitive, fanatical, hysterical, and dramatic.

remittent a type of fever in which the symptoms temporarily lessen at regular intervals, but do not totally cease, e.g., malaria. 'Intermittent' refers to a disease with a fever which recurs at regular intervals.

renal colic see COLIC.

rending tearing apart or into pieces violently; splitting. Bursting, coming apart.

rennet wine an alcohol-based extract of rennet (the digestive enzyme in cows' stomachs) used to improve digestion, taken in teaspoonful doses in 4oz. of water after meals. Rennet wine is prepared in the following manner: Take the stomach of a freshly slaughtered calf, cut away the upper three inches, and slit the stomach lengthwise. Wipe clean with a cloth (to remove the mucus), cut into small pieces, and place in a bottle and fill with sherry. Allow this mixture to stand for three weeks, and decant.

repercussed driven in.

repercutient (repercussive) serving to repel harmful agents or reduce swelling. A repellent or substance that purges.

repertory a place/book where information is categorized so that it may be found easily or logically. A store or stock of things available. The homeopathic repertory is an index/library of symptoms derived from the materia medica and clinical/toxicological data. It is like an index to a book: instead of laboriously flipping through a book page by page to find information, one can look up the specific symptom in the index. By analogy, the materia medica is the white pages and the repertory is the yellow pages of the telephone book!

Most people are familiar with *Kent's Repertory* (1st ed. 1897, 2nd 1908, 3rd 1924), for it is the standard in the field. "Kent's legendary repertory is more systematic and readable than all its precursors and is still the popular choice today, being the standard text for all schools of homeopathy from strict Hahnemannianism, down. It is also the foundation for all 'new-and-more-complete repertories' and is currently the basis for all computerized repertorial programs. Kent's *Repertory* is structured after Swedenborg's scheme of 'from above downward', which simplified repertorizing by categorizing all symptoms as either Mental, General, or Particular."—*The American Homeopath* 2: p. 9, 1995. It lists approximately 55,000 symptoms and about 650 remedies. Kent based his repertory on the repertories of two greats who had gone before him, C. Lippe and E.J. Lee.

There are other repertories, other approaches to indexing and looking up symptoms. The *Symptom Register of T.F. Allen* (1879) is a huge twelve- volume collection of symptoms directly made from provings. At one time it was Kent's intention to include Allen's repertory in his, yet the inclusion was incomplete. It contains well over 100,000 symptoms with 880 associated remedies ... definitely more than Kent.

Boenninghausen's *Repertory* (1905) contains over 29,000 rubrics or symptoms and cites 500 remedies. This repertory, the one most commonly used by homeopaths before Kent, is quite helpful in cases with a paucity of mental symptoms, no strange, rare and peculiar (SRP) symptoms but in which modalities and concomitants abound. It is of special importance because of its concomitants, e.g., Boenninghausen would probably have the two symptoms 'pain in knee' and 'gout' together, while Kent would usually list the two separately.

Boenninghausen's *Repertory*, should not be confused with T.F. Allen's, *Boenninghausen's Therapeutic Pocketbook.* Allen's work is a condensed and consolidated version.

Herbert Roberts' *Sensations As If* (1937) is quite a useful repertory if a sensation symptom predominates. It is of help in finding peculiar symptoms.

Oscar Boericke's *Repertory* or simply *Boericke's Repertory* is helpful in finding small or lesser known remedies and finding specific pathological remedies. But since the total number of rubrics is quite small, and polychrests do not appear as often as they should, this repertory has limited use. It contains over 8,000 symptoms and cites about 1100 remedies.

The repertory compiled by Calvin Knerr, *Repertory to Hering's Guiding Symptoms* (1896) is huge, with 160,000 symptoms and 400 associated remedies. It is based on the work of C. Hering and is filled with very precise rubrics. It is very useful in finding a remedy fitting a precise symptom.

There are many other repertories, too, from the unique *Synoptic Key* (C.M. Boger), *Applied Repertory* (D. Aggarwal, 1990), *Synthetic Repertory* (Barthel & Klunker, 1982), *Kent's Repertorium Generale* (Kunzli), *A Pocket Manual or Repertory of Homeopathic Medicine* (J. Bryant), and *Ruoff's Repertory* (Ruoff), to the specific repertories, which deal with specific pathological conditions, of Wm. Guernsey, Kimball, Millspaugh, E.J. Lee, R. Gregg, etc., to the recently published (early 1990's) repertories: *Homeopathic Medical Repertory: A Modern Alphabetical Repertory* (Robin Murphy), *The Complete Repertory* (Roger van Zandvoort), and *Repertorium Homeopathicum Syntheticum*, or briefly, *Synthesis* (F. Schroyen), there is something for everyone! There is also Phatak's Repertory—*Concise Alphabetical Repertory*—which is based on Boger's *Synoptic Key*, but it contains many additions (rubrics, remedies), so that in effect it is an enlarged *Synoptic Key*. Boger blended Kent and Boenninghausen. S.R. Phatak also wrote a *Materia Medica*.

If that is not enough, peruse the computer repertories—Radar, Mac-Repertory, CARA, and Homeo21. Now there is no need to flip through hundreds and hundreds of pages of repertory texts. Just a half-dozen keystrokes and you are there!

How to Use the Repertory (G. Bidwell), *How to Find the Simillimum* (B. Desai), and *Encyclopedia of Repertories* (D'Castro) are three good books to help you learn how to repertorize (the process of matching the patient's symptom complex with the correct, curative remedy).

"I totally promise you it is good to repertorize."—Ben Hole, M.D. "You must learn your repertory by heart almost, and know where to search. Of course, I am searching this since the last 47 years, every day fifty times at least."—Pierre Schmidt. There are three main methods of repertorization: Kent, Boenninghausen and Boger's card method.

repetition of the dose "The only allowable exception for an immediate repetition of the same medicine is when the dose of a well-selected and in every way suitable and beneficial remedy has made some beginning toward an improvement, but its action ceases too quickly, its power is too soon exhausted, and the cure does not proceed any further. This is rare in chronic disease, but in acute diseases and in chronic diseases that rise into an acute state it is frequently the case."—*Chronic Diseases* (Hahnemann).

Rescue Remedy a Bach flower combination remedy available as a cream and an internal liquid. It consists of Cherry plum, Clematis, Impatients, Rock rose, and Ornithogalum. It is useful in injuries, accidents, shock, and physical/mental/emotional trauma in general. See BACH FLOWER REMEDIES.

resonance homeopathy that branch of homeopathy which is not classical but chooses the homeopathic remedy based on instrumental analysis which matches the biological resonance between the remedy and the disease or affected organ or disease.

The remedy chosen is not based upon the similia principle, but on resonance. For example, H.W. Schimmel, a prominent researcher in this emerging field, has found remedies which resonate with the liver, in particular *Carduus mar.* 6X and 12X (hepatic cells), *Chelidonium* 6X/12X (liver and bile capillaries) and *Vipera berus* 6X/12X (cell nuclei), *Vipera berus* 6X (cell plasma), *Vipera berus* 12X (cell membrane). Thus all patients with a generic liver dysfunction would receive a combination formula containing the three aforementioned remedies. Schimmel has written *Functional Medicine*, Vol. 1 & 2 (Haug Publishing Co, Heidelber, Germany, 1991, 1992)

It is said that resonance homeopathy and the bioresonance (BRT) and multiresonance therapies activate physiological oscillations and eliminate pathological oscillations. See MORA THERAPY, BIORESONANCE and MULTIRESONANCE THERAPY (BRT).

reticent characteristically silent in temperament. Restrained or reserved in style.

reticular net-like, resembling a net.

retinitis albuminurica an inflammation of the retina occurring in Bright's disease, marked by the presence of white spots on the retina.

retraction a shrinking or drawing back.

retro-bulbar behind the eye-ball.

retro-bulbar neuritis inflammation of the nerves behind the eyeball (the orbital portion of the optic nerve).

retrocedent going back; withdrawing, moving back, suppressed. When a disease that moves about from one part to another and is sometimes fixed, has been for some time in its more common situation and then changes, it is said to be retrocedent. 'Retrocedent gout' means an attack of gout in which the articular symptoms subside with subsequent involvement of some internal organ, such as the stomach.

retrocession withdrawal, a going back, a relapse. The cessation of the external symptoms of a disease followed by signs of involvement of some internal organ or part. The spreading of an eruption or tumor from the surface to the interior of the body. The noun form of RETROCEDENT *(see above)*.

retropharyngeal behind the pharynx.

retroversion a turning back. Often used in reference to the uterus (a condition in which the uterus is tilted backward without curvature of its axis).

rhachitis (rachitis) see RICKETS.

rhacoma an excoriation or chafing.

rhagades (fissures, chaps, rimae) linear cracks, fissures, or excoriations in the skin, especially as seen on the palms and soles of the feet, or of the mucocutaneous junctions (anus, lips). (Gr. *rhagades,* 'fissures, cracks')

rhaphania (ergotismus, raphania) a disease characterized by spasms of the limbs. (Gr. *rhaphanos,* 'radish', as the disease was attributed to a poisonous substance in the seeds of the wild radish, which became mixed with grain).

rheum 1) salt-like; referring to rhubarb and/or its properties (salty and purgative). 2) a mucous or watery discharge; catarrh.

rhigolene a petroleum distillate product with a boiling point of just 70⁰ F. Since it evaporates so quickly it was once used as a local anesthetic (sprayed onto the tissues which, as it cooled, would freeze or anesthetize the area).

rhinitis atrophica chronic inflammation of the nasal membranes with subsequent thinning of those membranes.

rhino-sclerma stony hard growths affecting the anterior nose and adjacent areas. The disease begins in the skin of the nose gradually forming flat nodules.

rhinopharyngeal pertaining to the nose and pharynx (naso-pharynx).

rhinophyma a tumor of the nose. See ACNE ROSACEA.

rhinorrhea a mucous discharge from the nose.

rhonchi (ronchi) a coarse snoring type of rale caused by secretions in the larger bronchi or in the trachea. They may be palpable ('fremitus' is the palpable vibration thus produced).

rhus poisoning being affected with poison-ivy.

rhyparia see SORDES.

rickets (morbus anglicus, rhachitis) a calcium deficiency disease, occurring mostly in infants and young children but also in adults. It is characterized by softening of the bones, enlargement of the liver and spleen, malnutrition, profuse sweating, and general tenderness of the body when touched.

Ricord's chancre a syphilitic chancre with a thin parchment-like base. From the Parisian surgeon Philippe Ricord (1800-1889).

Rigg's disease (Fauchard's disease, periodontoclasia, alveolar pyorrhea, periodontitis, alveolar periostitis, pyorrhea alveolaris) a disease of the tissues surrounding the teeth evidenced by inflammation of the gums, resorption of bone, and formation of pockets around the teeth. Described by the

American dentist J.M. Riggs (1810-1885), but actually first discovered by P. Fauchard, the father of dentistry, at the turn of the 18th century. Fauchard was also one of the founders of orthodontics.

right-sided remedy a remedy which is noted for being active, though not exclusively so, on the right side of the body. *Apis, Aurum, Bap., Bell., Bryonia, Calc c., Canth., Chelid., Colo., Crot., Lyco., Nux v., Puls.,* and *Sec.* are examples of right-sided remedies. *Cf.* LEFT-SIDED REMEDIES.

rigors coldness, attended by shivering.

Rilchinger water a mineral water commercially available in Germany.

rima glottidis (glottis vera, true glottis) the groove between the vocal cords. A 'rima' is a slit, fissure or groove between two symmetrical parts. (L., 'crack')

rimae see RHAGADES.

rinderpest a contagious, epizootic, viral disease affecting cattle, sheep, and goats. It causes fever and ulcerative, diphtheritic-like lesions of the intestinal tract.

risus a laugh; the facial grin of laughter.

risus sardonicus (canine spasm, cynic spasm) a peculiar grinning distortion of the face produced by spasms of the muscles around the mouth, often seen in tetanus. Involuntary spasmodic laughter.

rivo an exclamation used by persons engaged in drinking bouts.

roborantia (roborant) an invigorating or strengthening medicine or tonic.

rock fever Malta fever. See MEDITERRANEAN FEVER.

rock oil mineral oil, petroleum.

rodent ulcer see NOLI ME TANGERE.

Roemhold gastrocardiac syndrome (Roemheld's syndrome) a disturbance in the functioning of the heart due to an impaired functioning of the digestive system, particularly the stomach.

Roger's disease a congenital deformation of the heart allowing communication between the two ventricles. After H.L. Roger (1811-1892) a Parisian physician.

ROH rediscovery of homeopathy. See SEHGAL'S METHOD OF HOMEOPATHY.

ronchi see RHONCHI.

roodvonk see PURPURA MILIARIS.

rosacea vascular dilation involving the nose and sometimes the cheeks. Varies from mild involvement to extensive permanent thickening and hypertrophy of the tissues. Often seen in alcoholics.

rose-cold (June cold) hay fever occurring in the early summer.

roseola (rose-rash) any rose-colored eruption. Sometimes synonymous with 'rubella'.

rostrum any beak-shaped structure.

rotheln German measles.

rottlera tincture (kamala) tincture made from the hairs and glands of the capsules of a small evergreen tree (*Mallotus philippensis*), used as a cathartic and anthelmintic.

rotula (patella) the knee-cap (L, 'little wheel').

roup 1) hoarse, sore throat. 2) any of the various respiratory disorders of poultry.

rubefacient a medicine or substance which produces redness of the skin.

rubella (rotheln, German measles, epidemic rubeola, French measles) an acute, contagious, eruptive viral disease of short duration and of milder character than measles/rubeola. After a period of incubation (1-3 weeks), the disease starts with a sore throat and slight fever. The eruption consists of red maculopapular lesions, and disappears without desquamation in about 3 days. Enlargement of the superficial neck and posterior ear glands occurs.

rubeola see MEASLES.

rubigo rust or mildew.

rubor redness; one of the classical signs of inflammation.

rubric (rubrick) a short commentary or explanation covering a broad subject. Also, a name for a class or category or, in homeopathic circles, *a symptom*. The rubric is sort of an 'abbreviated symptom' and, in the repertory, is followed by a list of remedies that have been shown to produce this symptom in the healthy person or relieve this symptom in the ill. "A repertory is a collection of symptom-categories called rubrics. Each rubric is followed by a listing of all the remedies that have either brought out this symptom in a proving (pathogenic) or that have cured this symptom in a patient (clinical). This collection of rubrics has been arranged into some sort of structure in order to facilitate the finding of a specific rubric. ... One way of arranging the rubrics is by placing them in alphabetical order, as for instance in Phatak's repertory, in Allen's index, and more recently in Murphy's repertory. Kent has used the head-foot structure whereby the repertory is divided into several chapters (from Mind till Generalities) and where each chapter has its main rubrics arranged in alphabetical order."—'The Mind of the Repertory' by Kees Dam (*Homoeopathic Links,* 9:1, p. 18, 1996)

   sub-rubric a symptom listed below the main symptom which would be considered a modifier of that main rubric. For instance, 'Jealousy' (main rubric), 'as foolish as it is irresistible' (sub-rubric), or 'Lamenting' (main rubric), 'evening' (sub-rubric).

   super-rubric "a rubric that contains a collection of several rubrics with the same archetypical information, or a collection of various expressions of a same basic feeling. For instance, when someone is afraid of dogs we could look up 'Fear of dogs', but we know from experience that every remedy that has the archetype of dog in their subconscious will be afraid of dogs in one way or another. So we might also look up: 'Delusion, dogs, sees' and 'Dreams, dogs'. It would therefore be very useful to have a super-rubric in which all these rubrics were joined together (while still keeping the original rubrics where they are, or perhaps putting them as a sub-rubric under this super-rubic). The super rubric would then be named: 'Dogs'. The same could be done with snakes, mice, vermin, etc."—'The Mind of the Repertory' by Kees Dam (*Homoeopathic Links,* 9:1, p. 22, 1996)

ructus belching or eructation.

rudimentary undeveloped or not totally formed.

rufous a strong yellowish pink to moderate orange color.

rufa a wrinkle, fold, ridge or crease.

rumination (merycism) the raising of food from the stomach and rechewing it (chewing the cud). Also may refer to the act of pondering or meditating on one's thoughts.

run-around a superficial paronychia. See PANARITIUM.

rupia an eruption characterized by the formation of large, dirty-brown, layered cone-like crusts that resemble an oyster shell.

s S S S S S s

S an abbreviation for the repertory written by Schroyens, *Synthesis.*

saburral pertaining to a foul stomach, tongue or teeth. Affected with sordes (saburrae). See SORDES.

sabures see SORDES.

sac. lac. see SACCHARUM LACTIS.

saccharine relating to sugar; sweet.

saccharum lactis (SL, Sac. Lac., sl) lactose or milk sugar. It is used as a diluent in preparing triturations of homeopathic remedies. Some manufactures use pellets made of or partially made of lactose. The selected remedy dilution may be sprayed on to medicate them, or they may be used 'blank' (unmedicated) as placebos (thus 'giving a patient sac. lac.' means 'giving a placebo'.)

saccharum officinale sugar, as in table sugar, cane sugar. Sucrose.

sacralgia pain in the sacrum.

sacro-iliac symphysis the joining point where the sacrum and ileum meet.

saddlenose the flattened bridge of the nose.

saffron a deep-yellow or yellow-orange color.

sagacity quick and keen judgment. Having the quality of quick, sure decision. The ability to see promptly what should be done in a difficult situation.

sago a pearly starch made from the pith of the sago palm tree. It forms a light agreeable liquid recommended in febrile, phthisical and calculous disorders.

salacious lustful.

salivant an agent which increases the flow of saliva.

sallow having a pale, sickly yellow color, hue or complexion.

salpingitis inflammation of the fallopian tube or of the Eustachian tube depending upon the context.

salt rheum an eruption (variously considered eczema or ringworm) in children which appears on the palms of the hands or limbs and ending in an extensive exfoliation of the skin.

saltpeter a chemical, potassium nitrate, used in pickling and in the manufacture of explosives and fertilizers.

salutary healthful or wholesome. Good for the health.

salutatory an opening or welcoming address.

salvarsan (606, arsphenamine, sanluol, kharsivan) a yellow powder used, during the first half of the 20th century, to treat syphilis and relapsing fevers due to protozoans. It contains Arsenic, which is presumed to be the spirocheticide.

First discovered and prepared by Paul Ehrlich (1854-1915) in 1909, it required 606 trials before the correct formula was found that would destroy the syphilis spirochete (hence the name '606').

Salzborn's diet a way of eating recommended by practitioners of homotoxicology, especially advised in cases where bodily enzymatic systems have been compromised or damaged, e.g., cirrhosis of the liver. The patient eats very small amounts of food (a few tablespoonfuls of oatmeal, a few bites of meat, small portions of fruits and vegetables) frequently (every hour as the patient is hungry).

This sort of regimen continues for months until the patient regains health, then small increases in the diet can be made with an eventual return to normal dietary rhythms. Quantities of food, however, should still remain limited to just below satiety. Dr. Reckeweg, the founder of homotoxicology, maintained that even persons in robust health should never eat to satiation.

saneous (sanious) relating to sanies (a thin, fetid, greenish, sero-purulent fluid discharged from an ulcer, wound or fistula). Ichorous and blood-stained.

sanguine red, or of the color of blood. Having a warm and hopeful nature, confident. 'Sanguineous' relates to blood, bloody or plethoric. 'Sanguinolent' means blood-like.

sanious see SANEOUS.

santonine a chemical obtained from *Artemisia maritima* used as a vermifuge and especially effective against the round worm (*Ascaris lumbricoides*).

Sanum remedy complexes/therapy complex homeopathic formulae designed to fundamentally alter and bring back into balance the 'terrain' or 'soil' of the ill person. This lengthy therapy, which can last as long as a year, is based on Gunther Enderlein's (1872-1968) work on pleomorphism. These homeopathic formulae consists of remedies prepared from dried cell wall fragments of fungi, e.g., *Candida albicans, Mucor racemosus, Siphonospora polymorpha, Aspergillus niger, etc.* Sanum, a German company, makes about 100 preparations.

For example, "Mucokehl is *Mucos racemosus*, a fungus that regulates microorganisms affecting the thickness of blood. These remedies, injected around the tumor site, adjust the pH and cellular terrain and help the pathogenic microorganisms revert back to harmless forms. In effect, the Sanum remedies help the body restore the optimal cellular terrain for health." -*Definitive Guide to Cancer* (1997, p. 907). Pleo remedies are very similar to Sanum remedies. Some examples of their products are Pleo-Muc (Mucor racemosus), Pleo-Not (Penicillium notatum), and Pleo-Quent (Penicillium frequentans), etc. See EAV, PLEOMORPHISM, RADIONICS, BEV.

saphenous superficial, apparent. Generally refers to the two veins of the lower limb but may also refer to the nerves accompanying those veins.

sapient wise, manifesting wisdom. Having knowledge along with a keen discernment.

sapo domest (sapo animalis, curd soap) a soap made with soda and a purified animal fat. It was not a hard soap, but had the consistency of gelatin. It was popular in the late 19th century (L. *sapo*, 'soap').

saporific producing taste or flavor (L. *sapor*, 'taste', 'savor').

sapraemia the intoxication produced by absorption of the results of putrefaction (decay). Septic intoxication or blood poisoning.

sarcitis (myositis) muscular inflammation.

sarcocele a fleshy tumor of the testicle.

sarcode (iso-organotherapy, organotherapy) a healthy glandular or tissue extract made into a homeopathic remedy (cf. NOSODE, a remedy made from diseased tissue or discharges). When administered it acts to support and/ or restore normal functioning of the respective tissue or organ by stimulating its normal function. C.E. Brown-Sequard conducted seminal work in this field. Hering advocated the use of sarcodes as early as 1834. See ISOPATHY.

222

sarcognomy (Gr. *sarkos,* 'flesh', *gnomon,* 'indicator, discerner, pointer') a term used by J. Compton Burnett to relate certain cutaneous regions with internal organs. Dr. Burnett had several cases where a 'sternal patch' (a skin eruption covering the lower part of the sternum) co-existed with heart disease and liver inflammation. "I foretell that ... when the relations of the various cutaneous regions will be recognized as constituting the very base of medicine and diagnosis, this 'sternal patch' will be understood to indicate 'liver and heart' "—J.C. Burnett.

Perhaps Burnett was influenced in his thinking by Joseph R. Buchanan who wrote *Therapeutic Sarcognomy* in 1891. Buchanan coined the term in 1842: "Sarcognomy interpreted the character of the body, revealing its laws, connections, and sympathies to the physican. ... Diseases had mental as well as physical symptomatologies; in other words, the entire surface of the brain corresponded to the entire surface of the body." and "When an emotion or a passion of the soul (e.g., love or anger) worked through the brain, it expressed itself in the body by voice, action, and circulation of the blood. Similarly, the conditions of the body in health and disease acted upon the brain and soul."—*Medical Protestants: The Eclectics in American Medicine, 1825-1939* (J.S. Haller, Jr.).

sarcoma a cancerous tumor, usually highly malignant, of the connective tissue, e.g., Kaposi's sarcoma.

sarcomatous of the nature of, or resembling, a sarcoma.

sarcoma cutis a malignant tumor of the skin (L. *cutis,* 'of the skin').

sardonic sneering, bitterly sarcastic, derisive, scornful.

sartor resartus L., 'good health restored' (lit. 'good repair repaired again')

satiety the condition of being gratified beyond the point of satisfaction, especially with respect to hunger or thirst.

saturnine preparations containing lead. Of or relating to lead, or due to or symptomatic of lead-poisoning. 'Saturnine colic' is colic caused by the consumption of lead. 'Saturnism' is another term for lead poisoning. Lead is associated with the planet Saturn. See PLUMBISM.

satyriasis an excessive and often uncontrollable sexual desire in men.

Savill's disease an epidemic dermatitis followed by desquamation and accompanied with severe constitutional symptoms, conjunctivitis, pharyngitis, and enlargement of the cervical lymph glands. It may be fatal, especially in the elderly. T.D. Savill (1740-1779), a London physician, first described it.

scabies (itch, acarus itch, acarus scabiei seu sarcoptes hominis) the itch. An invasion of the epidermis by the acarus mite, *Sarcoptes scabiei.* Mites (0.4mm) are arachnids and are smaller than lice. Having scabies is characterized by egg-containing burrows (0.5-1cm) in the epidermis (stratum corneum) which are a source of constant irritation. The primary manifestation of psora. 'Scabies sicca' is a dry form of scabies. See PSORA.

scald head (scalled head, porrigo capitis) any crusted or scurfy disease of the scalp, such as favus or tinea capitis.

scales (squamae) shedding, epidermal flakes that may be dry or greasy, as in psoriasis, exfoliative dermatitis and atopic eczema.

scall scabby, scurfy. Also eczema capitis.

scalled head see SCALD HEAD.

scaphoid boat-shaped; hollowed out, as in a scaphoid abdomen (the sunken appearance of the belly seen in great emaciation) (Gr. *skaphe,* 'basin, bowl, small boat, skiff').

scapula either of two large, flat, triangular bones forming the back part of the shoulder. The shoulder blade (L., diminutive of *scapus,* 'shaft, beam').

scabrities roughness and scurfiness of the skin; also might refer to a chronic inflammatory granulation of the conjunctiva of the eyelids.

scarf-skin the epidermis or outer-layer of skin.

scarlatina (scarlet fever) scarlet fever or pertaining to scarlet fever. See SCARLET FEVER. 'S. anginosa' is scarlet fever with severe inflammation of the fauces (throat). It is one of the exanthematic fevers.

scarlet fever (scarlatina) an acute contagious disease commencing with vomiting or chill, followed by a high fever, rapid pulse, sore throat, swollen neck glands, and the appearance of a red rash, from 1-5 days after. The rash lasts for 5-6 days, fades and then flakes off. The tongue looks red like a strawberry. The kidneys are often involved. It is caused by hemolytic streptococci.

Hahnemann won some notoriety with his success in using *Belladonna* both as a prophylactic and cure in an epidemic of scarlet fever.

Scheurmann's disease (vertebral osteochondritis) the necrosis of the vertebral epiphyses in children described by Danish surgeon H.W. Scheuermann (1877-1960).

schism a division or separation, especially of an organized group or faith, based on differences in beliefs.

schizophrenia (dementia praecox) an acute or chronic mental illness, marked by a break from reality, delusions, anxiety, depression, emotional blunting (as seen in a mild to severe flattening of the facial expressions) and at times psychosis with feelings of unreality, hallucinations, and autism.

The term 'schizophrenic', meaning 'split mind', was first coined by Eugene Bleuler (1857-1939). It represents the postulated schism between thought, emotion and behavior. Schizophrenia affects 1% of the world's population, generally begins before the age of 25 and is usually lifelong. It affects men and women equally. There is a seasonality of birth in that more schizophrenics are found to be born in winter months (in both hemispheres) than at any other time of the year.

Schneiderian membrane that area of the nasal mucous membrane which secretes nasal mucus. Described in 1660 by the German anatomist C.V. Schneider (1614-1680).

Scholten's elemental approach an approach to prescribing and elucidating the actions of elements and combinations of elements (cations and anions, too) which may or may not have undergone homeopathic provings. This new field is based upon the vast researches of Jan Scholten, a Dutch homeopath. He has written *Homeopathy and the Minerals* and *Homeopathy and the Elements*.

Scholten divides the periodic table into series and stages: "The periodic system is a table of all existing elements, the atoms, from Hydrogen to Radon, and of the radioactive elements, such as Uranium and Plutonium. The table has rows and columns in which the elements are grouped. A theory is developed about the use of the periodic system in homoeopathy. This theory shows that every row and every column has a specific theme. The seven rows are called series. The first series, the Hydrogen series, has the theme of coming into being. The second series, the Carbon series has the theme of the development of the Ego. The third series, the Silicium series, shows the theme of relationships. The fourth series, the Iron series, covers the theme of work. The fifth series, the Silver series, has the theme of creativity. The sixth series, the Gold series, shows the theme of the king, the leader.

"Each series shows a development: the theme of the series is developed in eighteen stages. These stages, the columns, describe a development: starting a theme, rising, coming to a top, then declining again and in the end comes the loss.

"In this theory, every element can be described by the concepts of the series and the stage the element is in. A total picture is given of the periodic system as a spiral. Every wind of the spiral is a series or row. And every radiant is a stage or column. The spiral pictures the expanding consciousness: from the consciousness of the Ego in the beginning to that of a neighbourhood, a village, a city, a country and in the end the whole universe."—from Scholten's *Homoeopathy and the Elements* (1996).

Schott treatment the systematic application of short, warm, saline baths of precise strength and temperature in combination with a series of resistance movements to cure certain heart problems, kidney diseases, nervous affections, and rheumatism. This treatment was founded in Bad Nauheim, Germany, where the natural salt springs were located.

A good non-homeopathic source on the subject is Thorne W. Bezly's *The Schott Methods of the Treatment of Chronic Diseases of the Heart* (with an account of the Nauheim baths, and of the therapeutic exercises illustrated, 1902)

Schuessler a German homeopathic physician, W.H. Schuessler (1821-1896), who founded the Biochemic system as elaborated in his 1880 opus, *Twelve Tissue Remedies* (the full title being *Abridged Therapeutics, founded upon histology and cellular pathology with an appendix giving special directions for the application of the inorganic cell salts.* Translated by M. Docetti Walker, 1880, 199 pp.).

Schuessler's therapeutic method of biochemistry is based on the use of 12 cell salts (biochemic salts, tissue remedies, celloids, cell salts) which he determined to be essential to the healthy functioning of the body. Many of these cell salts were not used homeopathically at the time but have since become incorporated into the homeopathic materia medica. His premise is based upon a pathological theory and biochemistry (the restoration of cellular vitality and balance) and not necessarily upon provings. He maintained that his system was not homeopathy but rather a separate system based on biochemistry—yet he did potentize the salts.

"Biochemistry is not Homoeopathy. There is a wide difference between *similia similibus curantur* and supplying deficiencies with the exact material lacking. Symptomatology figures in the biochemic treatment only as calls for the lacking of inorganic workers, and not from the standpoint of similia." - *The Biochemic System of Medicine* (G.W. Carey, 1917, 18th Ed., p. 13). For example, "A child suffering with rickets shows a lack of phosphate of lime in the bones due to a disturbed molecular motion of the molecules of this salt. The quantity of phosphate of lime intended for the bones, but failing to reach its goal, would accumulate within the blood were it not excreted by the urine, for it is the office of the kidneys to maintain the proper composition of the blood, and, therefore, to cast out every foreign substance or surplus supply of any one consituent. Now after the normal molecular motion of the phosphate of lime molecules is again established within the involved nutritive soil by administering small doses of the same salt, the surplus can again enter the general circulation and the cure of the rachitis be brought about."—from the Boericke & Tafel pamphlet 'Cell Salts' (c. 1910).

The 12 salts with their astrological correspondences are *Silicea* (Sagitarrius), *Ferrum phosphoricum* (Pisces), *Natrum phosphoricum* (Libra), *Kali phosphoricum* (Aries), *Natrum sulphuricum* (Taurus), *Calcarea sulphuricum* (Scorpio), *Kali sulphuricum* (Virgo), *Natrum muriaticum* (Aquarius), *Kali muriaticum* (Gemini), *Calcarea phosphoricum* (Capricorn), *Calcarea fluoricum* (Cancer), and *Magnesia phosphoricum* (Leo). See BLACKMORE'S CELLOIDS.

sciatica (ischias nervosa) pain along the course of the sciatic nerve. There may be numbness, tingling and tenderness. Eventually the muscles innervated by it will waste away. In recent medical history, it was first described by D. Cotugno in *A Treatise on the Nervous Sciatica or Nervous Hip Gout* (1775). He differentiated it from arthritis and also gave the first detailed description of cerebrospinal fluid and the fact that it envelops the brain and spinal cord.

scintillation flickering; a spark or flash. A rapid variation in light.

scirrhus (scirrhous carcinoma) a cancer with a hard structure, fibrous cancer. A cancer in which induration has occurred through overgrowth of fibrous connective tissue in the stroma (the tissue forming the framework of the organ).

scirrhus ventriculi cancer of the stomach.

scission a fission or splitting.

sclera (sclerotica) the white of the eye.

sclerema sclerosis or hardening, especially of the skin.

sclerema neonatorum a disease of the newborn characterized by a hardening of the subcutaneous tissue, especially of the legs and feet. Dryness of the skin is marked, so that little fluid exudes on incision.

scleriasis see SCLERODERMA.

scleroderma (morphoea, scleriasis, dermatosclerosis, chorionitis) hidebound skin. Thickening of the skin caused by swelling and thickening of fibrous tissue with eventual wasting away of the skin.

sclerosis a hardening process. Induration or hardening of a chronic inflammatory nature.

sclerotic hard. Relating to the sclera of the eye.

sclerotica the sclera or white of the eye.

scoliosis a lateral curvature of the spine.

scorbiculus pit of the stomach.

scorbutic relating to or suffering from scurvy (scorbutus).

scotoma blind spot. An area of pathologically diminished vision within the visual field.

scrobiculis cordis the pit of the stomach; the point, normally a slight depression, just below the lower end of the sternum.

scrobiculum/us a pit or slight depression, or furrow. 'Anxiety felt in the scrobiculum' would refer to an anxious feeling in the pit of the stomach.

scrofula (King's evil, tuberculous lymphadenitis, tubercular adenitis) tuberculosis of the lymph glands. The word 'scrofula' is derived from *scrofa* meaning 'swine' or 'pig'. It was used because persons so afflicted resembled hogs, i.e., the lumps, masses, and swellings in the angle of the jaw and neck caused the person to appear hog-like. "Obsolete term for tuberculous cervical lymphadenitis"—B. Castro, *Encyclopedia of Repertories*, p. 206. "Scrofula is claimed by some writers to be nothing but hereditary syphilis."—E.P. Anshutz, *Sexual Ills and Diseases,* p. 64. "Sulphur is indicated in tuberculous lymphadenitis complicated by caseation, breakdown and multiple sinus formation with added secondary infection—a condition described as scrofula and met with in emaciated, shrivelled-looking children who are always voraciously hungry, also in older subjects where tuberculosis is rife."—D. Gibson, *Studies of Homeopathic Remedies,* p. 499.

A constitutional cachexia condition with a lack of resisting power of the tissues, a tendency to develop glandular tumors and tuberculosis. Lymphatism is present and there is a tendency to eczematous eruptions, ulceration, glandular swellings, respiratory catarrhs, and granular lids; tuberculosis of the glands, bones, or joints is common. Two types are recognized: the lymphatic/phlegmatic (torpid), in which there is a tendency to obesity with a coarse muddy complexion, thick lips, large head and neck, large belly, soft, flabby muscles, coarse hair, and stolid expression; and the sanguine (erethic), in which the skin is clear, changing readily from pale to pink, the eyes blue, and the hair fine and silky red lips and cheeks, thin and flabby muscles with spareness of figure, vivacity, and mental activity.

It was commonly referred to as 'King's evil' because it supposedly could be cured by the King's touch, e.g., Philip I (1061-1108), Louis VI (1108-1137), of France, Edward the Confessor (1002-1066), and Queen Anne of England. The practice has its origins in France when in 496 ACE King Clovis cured his favorite page. As he touched the boy's neck he said, "I touch thee, God heals thee." Supposedly as early as 300 BCE Pyrrhus, King of Epirus, cured diseases of the spleen with his touch. He used the great toe of his right foot! There was a bitter and extended controversy over who had the divine right, the French or British kings, yet the custom continued on both sides of the Channel. As late as 1824 Charles X revived the custom. For more on this, seek out Raymond Crawfurd's scholarly text.

scrofuloderma (cutaneous scrofula) skin lesions produced by the action of the tubercular bacillus beneath the skin, usually occurring on the neck from draining lymph nodes, resulting in ulceration, draining sinuses, and scar formation.

scrofulous ophthalmia (phlyctenular conjunctivitis) an inflammation of the conjunctiva of the eye accompanied by the formation of small red nodules of lymphoid tissue (phlyctenulae) on the conjunctiva. There is also an intolerance to light.

scrofulous suffering from scrofula (a constitutional state, occurring in the young, marked by a lack of resisting power of the tissues, predisposing to tuberculosis). Usually refers to tuberculous abscesses of the cervical lymph glands.

scurf dandruff; a branny desquamation.

scurfy like dandruff. Scaly or shredded dry skin.

scurvy (scorbutus) a disease caused by a lack of Vitamin C (ascorbic acid) in the diet which causes bleeding, spongy gums and a general weakness. Actually the gum symptoms are not the most characteristic feature of scurvy, but rather redness and bleeding around the hair follicles. In its more serious form, symptoms such as arthritis, edema of the lower extremities, and secondary infections are produced. It was quite common years ago, especially in the 18th century when seamen voyaged for long periods of time.

"Lind [James, 1716-1794], founder of naval hygiene in England, wrote a classic treatise on scurvy [*A Treatise on the Scurvy*, 1753], in which he described many important experiments he made on the disease. These experiments have been called 'the first deliberately planned controlled therapeutic trial ever undertaken'. Lind showed that in preserved form, citrus juices could be carried for long periods on board ship, and that, if administered properly, they would prevent the disease. The application of this knowledge by naval surgeons who followed Lind led to the eventual elimination of the disease from the British Navy."—Garrison-Morton, 3713.

scybala (sing. scybalum) hard, lumpy dried up feces (Gr. *skybalon,* 'excrement').

seat may be an abbreviation of seat-worm (pin-worms).

seaton see SETON.

seat-worms pin-worms. See OXYURIS.

sebaceous cyst (wen) a cyst filled with oily, fatty material.

sebaceous glands glands which secrete sebum, a whitish, waxy fat.

seborrhea a disease of the sebaceous glands characterized by an excessive secretion or disturbed quality of sebum which collects upon the skin in the form of an oily coating or of crusts or scales.

seborrhea oleosa a type of seborrhea characterized by an excessive oiliness of the skin, especially around the forehead and nose.

secondary action of drugs see PRIMARY ACTION OF DRUGS.

secondary to due to, or as a result of.

secondary syphilis the second of the three stages into which syphilis is clinically divided, characterized by cutaneous eruptions, sore throat, general enlargement of the lymph nodes, and a systemic toxemia.

sectarian belonging to a group which adheres to a distinctive doctrine or to a leader, as in 'sectarian medicine'. Thomsonianism, homeopathy, and chiropractic would be considered sects.

secundines the placenta and membranes discharged from the uterus after birth.

secundum artem 'according to the art'.

SEG segmentelectrography. See FUNCTIONAL MEDICINE.

Sehgal's homeopathic method (Dr. Sehgal's School for Revolutionised Homeopathy, Rediscovery of Homeopathy, ROH) a method of practicing homeopathy founded by Mandanlal L. Sehgal of Delhi, India. "He observes the way in which the patient presents his case to him, and from his expressions picks out the present, prominent and persistent symptoms and interprets them into rubrics (called king-pin rubrics) in Kent's Repertory, to arrive at the remedy. With the help of this new technique the mental symptoms are obtained in a short time. In this system the nature of the complaint (Particulars, Generals, or Modalities, etc.) is not taken into account" and "My method of homoeopathic prescribing is, as far as I know, new and unique. I prescribe on symptoms of the mind alone."— *Homoeopathic Links* 2/93, p. 18.

Dr. Sehgal came upon his unique method of homeopathic prescribing around 1970: "Dr. Sehgal believes that you only need the Mind symptoms to cure a patient. He completely ignores local and general symptoms, like food craving, sensitivity to temperature, desire for sex, etc. He considers the patient's physical complaints only to evaluate the improvement after the remedy has been given."—*Homoeopathic Links*, 2/94, p. 30.

Interestingly enough, Kent had similar thoughts: "The centre of man is Will and Understanding. Man's constitution exists of his will and thoughts, supported by his memory. This, in other words, is his mind. The mind is the most sensitive part of a human being. In case of disease or proving the mind is the first to react." Thus in this system one need not have much information about the patient's history or bother too much with physical symptoms.

Sehgal's system is detailed and is outlined in his four-part book, *Rediscovery of Homeopathy, I-IV.*

seminal vesiculitis inflammation of the small sacs which are responsible for secreting one of the components of semen.

semiology (semiotics) symptomatology; relating to the symptoms of a disease. The study of medical symptoms or disease symptoms.

semiotics 1) symptomatology. 2) the study of relationships between signs and symbols and what they represent.

senescence 1) senility. 2) aging, the state of becoming old.

senile dementia progressive mental deterioration with loss of memory, especially for recent events, and occasional intercurrent attacks of excitement, occurring in the aged.

senile gangrene (gangrene of the aged) dry gangrene of the extremities due to failure of the terminal circulation in elderly persons, especially those affected with arteriosclerosis.

sensitive crystallization test a cancer diagnostic test developed by anthroposophical physician and researcher E. Pfeiffer (1899 •) who presented his findings to the International Congress on Cancer in 1939. Here a homoeopathic dilution of the patients blood is mixed with copper chloride and allowed to evaporate. The pattern which formed is 'a picture of the whole being' and this pattern can show normality or abnormality. Pfeiffer worked at Hahnemann (Phil.) from 1936 to 1940 and found "...that if a drop of blood from an ill patient was mixed with this copper chloride solution and then the proper homoeopathic remedy was added to another dilution of the blood, that the ill pattern would become neutralized, and become normal again." - *The Layman Speaks,* 12:9, p. 296, 1959. He also developed a urine chromotography test to separate amino acids. This method, it was hypothesized, could show the effect of a homeopathic remedy on the excretion pattern of amino acids.

sentient sensitive, feeling, capable of sensation. A term applied to those parts of the body more susceptible to feeling than others (i.e., the extremities of the nerves).

sensorium a center for sensations. The complete sensing system of the body. That part of the brain which receives and combines impressions/ sensations which the individual sensory centers have received. How the individual receives and handles the information which the sense supplies.

septic having infection or toxins present.

septicemia blood poisoning. A systemic disease caused by the presence of microorganisms or their toxins in the circulating blood.

septum a dividing wall between cavities or spaces; a partition, e.g., gingival s. (the mucous membrane which projects into the area between two teeth), nasal s. (the wall separating the two nasal cavities), etc. (L. *saeptum,* 'wall')

sepulchral suggestive of the grave or burial vault. Funereal.

sequelae morbid/diseased conditions following as a consequence of another disease. Abnormal bodily states caused by a previous disease. After-effects or consequences of disease (pl. of L. *sequela,* 'follower, consequence').

"Sequelae, regardless of the disease which stirs them up, are psoric and crop out at the weakest time, which is the convalescent period. The better the acute disease is treated, the less likely there are to be any sequelae."— *Lectures on Homoeopathic Philosophy* (J.T. Kent).

sequential therapy a method of homeopathic treatment based on seminal work by Jean Elmiger, a Swiss homeopath. It was popularized in the Western hemisphere by Rudolf Verspoor and Patty Smith (*Homeopathy Renewed,* 1995).

By removing all trauma in a persons life 'sequentially' (in order), the person is brought back to health. In other words, all the traumas of the patient's life are treated in reverse order, eventually coming back to birth trauma, womb trauma, inherited miasms, and past lives, perhaps (?), to

231

finally arrive at the basic constitutional remedy. Each of these layers is treated with the appropriate remedy. According to Verspoor, once untreated trauma is past the acute stage, the individuality of it is lost and then generically treatable with a remedy widely known for its effectiveness in that realm (e.g., *Staphysagria* for repressed anger). Combination homeopathic therapy is often stressed.

sequestrum a piece of dead bone which has separated from the surrounding healthy bone.

seriatim one after another; serially. Point by point; in a regular order.

serotherapeutic isopathy see SEROTHERAPY.

serotherapy/serocytotherapy the use of low potency, homeopathically prepared anti-sera (usually administered parenterally or rectally) for use in the treatment of illness. For example, cells are taken from a cancerous liver and repeatedly injected into a host animal (horse or pig). After the animal developes antibodies, this anti-liver cancer serum would be potentized and then administered into a person suffering from cancer. It was developed by Jean Thomas, a Frenchman, in the mid-twentieth century.

serpiginous creeping, referring to an ulcer or other cutaneous lesion which extends gradually over the surface on one side while usually healing on the other. Resembling ringworm.

serpigo ringworm.

serrated having a notched or toothlike appearance.

serum a clear yellowish fluid obtained when whole blood is separated into its solid and liquid components.

serum flocculation test see HENSHAW FLOCCULATION TEST.

serum remedy sensitivity test see HENSHAW FLOCCULATION TEST.

serum sickness (serum disease) an anaphylatic reaction (urticaria, fever, edema, arthritis, prostration) following the injection of serum product, caused by foreign protein in the serum. It is rarely fatal and usually occurs after the second dose of the serum. 'Serum rash' is a related term.

seton a twist of horse-hairs, silk, or linen thread, drawn through the skin by a large needle and left to form an issue and act as a counter-irritant. An issue acts to allow fluids to drain away from an area. One of the methods related to bleeding which Hahnemann denounced in the *Organon*.

sewer gas as mentioned by Kent, a gas which emanates from sewers and consists of all sorts of poisonous substances which can inhibit the healthy functioning of the body. "Persons about to be made sick from bad habits should break off their bad habits, they should move from damp houses, they should plug their sewers or have traps put in if they are being poisoned by sewer gas."—J.T. Kent, Lecture 5, *Lectures on Homeopathic Philosophy.*

shadow dreams dreams which represent aspects of ourselves which need to be integrated into our lives but which we are, for some reason, avoiding. These aspects generally deal with depth psychology and carry profound weight and meaning for the psyche. C.G. Jung popularized this concept, feeling that this dream variety carries our emotional life and provides clues to what needs to be integrated and how to bring about this integration.

Sheehan's syndrome (thyrohypophysial syndrome) hypopituitarism arising from severe circulatory collapse post-partum, with resultant pituitary necrosis.

sheet anchor a person, concept or item which can be relied upon in times of need.

shibboleth a test-word or password. A phrase considered distinctive to a particular party or faction.

shingles see HERPES ZOSTER.

ship fever (putrid fever) see TYPHUS.

si modo essent 'if they were in the right manner or style.'

sialodochitis inflammation of the duct of a salivary gland.

sialogogue (ptyalogogue) stimulating the secretion of saliva. An agent which promotes the flow of saliva.

sialorrhea a profuse flow of saliva.

sibilant hissing or whistling in character. Referring to a type of rale, sibilus.

sic often written in parenthesis, and means 'thus' or 'so'. When written *(sic)* it indicates that the preceding unusual word, phrase, or fact was correctly quoted from the original and should be read as it stands.

sicca dry.

sideratio a sudden stroke; apoplexy.

siderosis (grinder's asthma, arc-welder's disease, arc-welder's nodulation) chronic inflammation of the lungs due to prolonged inhalation of dust containing iron salts; occurs in iron miners and arc welders. It is characterized by inflammatory tissue reaction mainly in the lymphatic tissues of the lungs and by diffuse, nodular shadows in the x-ray film. May also mean the discoloration of any part by an iron pigment or an excess of iron in the blood.

signature doctrine see DOCTRINE OF SIGNATURES.

sigmoid flexure (pelvic colon, colon sigmoideum) the loop formed by the lower end of the descending colon as it joins the rectum.

sign an objective symptom. A symptom or abnormality of the patient which is readily recognizable by the clinician and often by the patient. Hahnemann used 'sign' and 'symptom' interchangeably. See SYMPTOM.

silicosis (stone-mason's disease) sclerotic changes in the lungs due to irritation caused by inhalation of dust as a result of various occupations. The most prominent symptoms are pain in the chest, cough, little or no expectoration, dyspnea, fatigue after slight exertion, and sometimes cyanosis.

silphium the rhizome of Indian cup (*Silphium perfoliatum*), a plant employed as a tonic alterative.

similar disease see DISSIMILAR DISEASE.

simile (partial simillimum, L. 'similar') a remedy which is close to the simillimum but not exactly on target as the simillimum would be. Hahnemann recommended using a simile in cases with too few symptoms to accurately prescribe on. This was done in order to hopefully get more symptoms to surface, allowing a clearer picture of the simillimum to come forward. See SIMILLIMUM.

"Of course there can be only one *simillimum,* since only once remedy can be the 'most similar'. But God is merciful, and other remedies, while only 'similars' *(similes),* can still be of assistance."—C. Coulter, *Portrait of Indifference* (1989).

similia similibus curantur from the Latin, 'likes are cured by likes'. The homeopathic formula expressing the law of similars (the doctrine that any drug which is capable of producing morbid symptoms in the healthy will remove similar symptoms occurring as an expression of disease). Another version of the formula, the one employed by Hahnemann, is *similia similibus curentur,* 'let likes be cured by likes'; this is guide to practice, the former being a statement of fact. *'Curantur'* is the passive indicative of the Latin word meaning 'to cure', thus it simply means 'are cured' as a statement of fact, while *'curentur'* is the passive subjunctive or imperative, meaning 'let them be cured' or 'they should be cured.' The opposite is *contraria contrariis curentur* or allopathy.

simillimum (similimum) (L., the superlative of *simile:* 'the most similar') the remedy that most closely corresponds to the totality of symptoms. It is the most similar remedy corresponding to a case, the one best covering the true totality of symptoms, and when found, is always curative (or in incurable cases, it is the best possible palliative remedy).

Homeopathy essentially is the application of the law of similars. The practitioner only has to deal in two areas: the patient with his/her symptoms and the drug with its symptoms as produced in the healthy person or prover. When one can create the correspondence or bridge between the two a sure and speedy cure results. This is very simple, yet we all know this is very, very hard. This brief description is the tip of the iceberg. It takes you five minutes to read this, it will take you forty years to understand it. This is homeopathy. Hahnemannian similarity "exists between the patient's characteristic symptoms and the characteristic symptoms of the drug."—Wm. Boericke.

"Homoeopathists are too ready to prescribe for single, prominent symptoms, selecting sometimes a different drug for each symptom, when in reality, the patient's symptoms should all be taken as a unit and a single drug selected to cover the whole. . . . The hunting down of isolated symptoms may be said to be unsatisfactory, for by so doing one avoids the general review of the whole case as an entity."—*Primer of Materia Medica* (T.F. Allen).

In the Bible one may find Moses using the simillimum when he took the golden calf the Hebrews had made and melted it and crushed it into a powder and put it into water and gave it to the Israelites to drink.

Simmond's disease (hypopituitary cachexia, hypophyseal cachexia) a condition due to destruction of the anterior lobe of the pituitary by infection, trauma or tumors and characterized by emaciation, weakness, psychic changes, and lowered temperature, metabolism, and blood pressure. Weight loss is extreme, the body hair disappears, and there is a general atrophy of the organs. This disease is progressive and usually fatal. First described by M. Simmonds (1855-1925), a German physician.

sinapism a poultice made of mustard and vinegar. A cataplasm made with *Sinapi* (white or black mustard seed) which acts as a rubefacient.

sinciput (bregma) the upper half of the cranium; in the strictest sense, the anterior part of the head just above and including the forehead.

sine qua non a person or thing which is of absolute necessity (L. 'without which, nothing').

singultus hiccup.

sinistral relating to the left side. Left.

sinking fever pernicious fever. A deadly, destructive or serious fever.

sitology science or study of dietetics.

Sjogren's syndrome/disease (Sjogren-Mikulicz syndrome, Gougerot-Sjogren disease, sicca syndrome, keratoconjunctivitis sicca) dryness of the mucous membranes, purpura/spots on the face, and bilateral parotid enlargement, seen in menopausal women and often associated with rheumatoid arthritis, Raynaud's phenomenon and dental caries. Changes in the lacrimal and salivary glands occur as well. OSD (ocular surface disease, 'dry eyes') is a diagnostic sign.

SK Skinner potency. See POTENCY.

Skene's glands (paraurethral glands) mucus-secreting glands on the wall of the female urethra, first described by American gynecologist A.J.C. Skene (1838-1900)

Skinner potency see POTENCY.

slough to separate from the living tissue, as dead tissue would fall away from live tissue.

S.L.(s.l., sl) abbreviation for saccharum lactis. See SACCHARUM LACTIS. May also refer to sublingual. SQ refers to 'subcu' (subcutaneous).

small of the back the lower region of the back. The sacral/lumbar area on the dorsal side of the body.

small remedy a remedy with few symptoms. This does not mean the remedy is rarely used. On the contrary it may be used frequently. It just means the remedy is known to elicit few symptoms. Often a small remedy has well- documented symptoms (in bold type) and is frequently employed, e.g., *Calendula off., Symphytum, Crataegus.*

smallpox see VARIOLA.

smegma a white, cheesy, sebaceous secretion of Tyson's glands which collects under the prepuce (foreskin) of the penis.

smut any of the various plant diseases caused by fungi of the order *Ustilaginales* which results in the formation of black, powdery masses of spores on the affected parts.

smutty dirty, blackened, smudged; also, obscene.

snow headache headache as a result of conjunctival irritation caused by the reflection of bright sunlight from snow. Other symptoms include photophobia, blepharospasm, and burning pain in the eyes.

snuff to inhale forcibly through the nose; also, pulverized tobacco to be chewed or inhaled.

snuffles an obstructed condition of the nose. Obstructed nasal breathing, especially in the newborn infant, then often due to congenital syphilis.

sobriquet (soubriquet) an assumed name. A fanciful name or appellation. Nickname.

soft palate (velum pendulum palati) the soft part of the palate (the roof of the mouth) which forms two arches, affixed laterally to the tongue and pharynx. The rear portion of the top of the mouth.

solis ictus sunstroke (L., 'blow from the sun').

somnambulism (nyctobasis, noctambulism) sleepwalking. A sleep disorder in which a person walks, writes, or performs other complex acts automatically while somnolent (drowsy, semicomatose), having no recollection upon awaking of what he has done.

somnifacient causing sleep, hypnotic.

somnipathy any sleep disorder.

somnolence drowsiness, sleepiness.

sonorous having or producing a full, deep, or rich sound. Impressive; grandiloquent.

sopor stupor; an unnaturally deep sleep. A constant drowsiness.

soporic (soporific) sleep inducing.

sordes the dark brown or blackish crust-like collection on the lips, teeth, and gums of a person with severe typhoid or other low fever (L., 'filth, dirt').

soroche see MOUNTAIN SICKNESS.

sorrel a brownish orange to light brown color.

sotto voce uttering in a low voice or undertone (It., 'under the voice').

soubriquet see SOBRIQUET.

souffle a soft blowing sound heard during auscultation (auditory examination of the patient, as with a stethoscope).

spagyric/ism (Paracelsian) (Gr. *spao*, 'to tear open, divide'; *ageiro*, 'to collect, join, bind or gather together') a manufacturing process during which raw materials are broken down or separated. This 'tearing-down' process somehow cleanses or purifies the substance and when re-united it becomes a more dynamic or effectual substance. It means the application of alchemical methods to produce medicines. "Spagyric tinctures are prepared in a way that 'opens' the plant and through its own process liberates stronger curative powers. It is less interested in isolating and extracting only the pharmacologically active portion of the plant and therefore is more synergistic in principle, working with nature."—*Homeopathy in Pittsburgh* (3:1, p. 3, 1994). The homeopathic remedy is in reality a spagyric medication as in the preparation process it is broken down (diluted) and then joined again (succussed). The finished remedy is definitely far removed from the original starting substance.

Paracelsus believed in the essential importance of spagyrical/alchemical knowledge in the understanding and treatment of disease. Spagyrics and alchemy should not be considered precursors to modern chemistry, but rather as another way in which to view the powers of nature.

The Indian science of Ayurvedic medicine is very alchemical in nature. For example, the Ayurvedic metallic oxide remedies are calcined, or heated without melting, before immersing them into the juice from selected plants. This process may be repeated a number of times according to the recipe for that particular item. Loha-bhasma is such a remedy whose principle ingredient is iron. When administered it raises the hemoglobin count, without any of the side-effects associated with Western iron tonics. See ANTHROPOSOPHY, ALCHEMY.

spaniomenorrhea a scanty or scarce menstrual flow.

spasm an involuntary convulsive muscular contraction; convulsion or cramp.

spavin a disease of the hock-joint of the horse (corresponding to the ankle joint in man), marked by inflammation and swelling. There are two types, bog spavin (an infusion of lymph that enlarges the joint) and bone spavin (a bony deposit that stiffens the joint).

specific (specificum) a remedy which in virtually all cases and under all circumstances is curative of a certain condition, e.g. *Ledum* is a specific for violet-black bruises. Do not confuse this with the allopathic definition as used in the 1700s, which meant a drug whose effectiveness could not be explained.

specific gravity (SG) the weight of any volume of substance compared with that of an equal weight of water. The SG of water is set at 1.0.

specious sophistry an argument or logic having the ring of truth but which is actually implausible or deceptive.

spectres ghosts.

spermatic pertaining to sperm, as the spermatic ducts.

spermatorrhea an involuntary discharge of semen without orgasm.

sphacelus moist gangrene. A slough, a soft mass of necrotic matter.

sphenoid one of the cranial vault bones (Gr., 'wedge-like').

spica having a figure-eight appearance, especially used to describe a method of bandaging which the successive strips overlap slightly, giving the appearance of an ear of wheat or barley.

spina bifida (hydrorrhachis congenita) see BIFIDA.

spina ventosa swelling of a bone (giving the appearance of a bone filled with air) as a result of tuberculosis, bone decay, or cancer.

spinal meningitis (cerebrospinal fever) inflammation of the meninges of the brain and spinal cord. An acute, infectious epidemic meningitis that is often fatal, caused by *Neisseria meningitidis*.

spiritus nitri dulcis (spiritus aetheris nitrosi, sweet spirits of nitre) an alcoholic solution of ethyl nitrite containing 5% of the crude ether, formerly used in the mid to late 1800s as a diaphoretic, diuretic and antispasmodic.

spittle saliva.

splanchnic referring to the spleen.

splenalgia (splenodynia) pain or neuralgia in the spleen.

splenitis inflammation of the spleen.

spoiled case a homeopathic case which is supposedly considered incurable for example because the patient was prescribed too many remedies, either correct or incorrect. Whether such a phenomenon exists is still being debated.

spondylotherapy a system of spinal therapeutics and diagnostics developed by Albert Abrams. Here concussion made at spinal centers is used to affect the organs and parts of the body.

spoon meats soft or liquid food for taking with a spoon, especially by infants or invalids.

spoon nail (celonychia) a deformity of the nail marked by a concavity of the surface.

sporadic referring to an acute disease affecting only a few individuals here and there, in contrast to epidemic and endemic diseases.

spotted fever (cerebro-spinal meningitis, tick fever) a malignant epidemic fever, with lesions of the cerebral and spinal membranes. Any of the various and often fatal infectious diseases, such as typhus and Rocky Mountain spotted fever, caused by *Rickettsiae,* that are transmitted by ticks and mites and are characterized by skin eruptions. See TYPHUS.

sprue 1) aphthae or thrush. 2) a tropical diarrhea as described under PSILOSIS.

spurious false, not genuine.

sputum expectorated matter; saliva substances mixed with foreign material from the respiratory tract.

squamous having the shape of scales; scale-like.

squill a root or bulb of the sea onion often used as a diuretic or expectorant.

SR abbreviation for *Synthetic Repertory* (Barthels).

STDs sexually transmitted diseases.

St. Anthony's fire (malignant erysipelas) see ERYSIPELAS, ERGOTISM.

St. Vitus' dance (chorea, Sydenham's chorea) a disorder characterized by irregular, spasmodic, involuntary movements of the limbs or facial muscles. St. Vitus was a martyr under Diocletian: at one time the superstition prevailed that dancing before his image would ensure good health for the following year.

St. Yves' salve a salve formerly employed in ophthalmic disease/infections containing primarily red oxide of mercury.

staphylitis inflammation of the uvula.

staphylorrhaphy a surgical operation to unite a cleft palate, consisting of paring and bringing together the edges of the cleft.

staphyloma a bulging of the cornea or sclera due to an inflammatory softening.

stasis stagnation of the blood or other fluids.

status a severe condition; intractable. An abnormal state or condition.

status biliosus being in a bilious state caused by excessive bile secretions.

status epilepticus a condition in which epileptic attacks occur in rapid succession, the patient not regaining consciousness during the interval.

status gastricus (saburra, *embarras gastrique*) foul stomach as a result of imperfect digestion or morbid, decaying products of the gastric secretions.

status morbi the state or status of the disease or illness.

status praesens the state of the patient at the time of the examination.

statuvolence artificial somnambulism. The induction of sleep walking through the use of hypnosis/mesmerism.

stearoptene a tough, crystalline solid which separates out from a volatile oil which has been standing for some time or has been subjected to cold; sometimes called a camphor.

steatoma a fatty tumor, lipoma. A sebaceous cyst.

stellate star-shaped.

stenocardia angina pectoris.

stenosis a narrowing of any canal, a stricture; especially a narrowing of one of the cardiac valves.

stercoraceous relating to or containing excrement or fecal material.

sternal pertaining to the chest.

sternocleidomastoid pertaining to the sternum (breastbone), the clavicle, and the mastoid process (behind the ear), as the sternocleidomastoid muscle.

sternum the breast bone.

sternutation sneezing.

stertorous referring to loud snoring, a noisy inspiration occurring in coma or deep sleep.

Stevens-Johnson syndrome a condition in which the bullous lesions of erythema multiforme are accompanied by constitutional symptoms, with high fever, prostration and involvement of the conjunctiva or mucous membranes. See ERYTHEMA MULTIFORME.

sthenic strong, active. Having excessive force or vigor. For example, a sthenic fever is a fever with a strong bounding pulse, high temperature, and active delirium.

stibium antimony. *Stibium tart.* is *Antimonium tart.*

stitch sudden sharp tearing, pricking, sticking, or shooting pain usually of momentary duration.

stomacace (stomatocace) an ulcerative inflammation of the mouth; putrid sore mouth. Canker or scurvy of the mouth.

stomachic an agent which improves appetite and digestion.

strabismus a lack of parallelism of the eyes. One eye pointing in a different direction than the other. An involuntary turning of the eyeball out of the natural axis of sight, yet the eye can still be voluntarily turned in the opposite direction. The optical axis cannot be directed to the same point, thus an object appears fuzzy and the individual 'squints' in order to see clearly. Thus in some of the older literature 'strabismus' and 'squinting' are used synonymously.

strange, rare and peculiar see SYMPTOMS.

strangury a urinary disease characterized by a slow and meager excretion of urine; difficult urination, attended with pain and dripping.

strawberry mark a reddish birth-mark or naevus.

strawberry tongue a beefy-red tongue with inflamed papillae.

stria (pl. striae) a stripe, band or line and distinguished by color, texture, depression, or elevation from the surrounding tissue.

stricture a contraction, circumscribed narrowing or stenosis of a duct or tube. 'Urinary s.', constriction of some part of the urinary apparatus (urethra, neck of the bladder, or its opening) making urination impossible or restricted and accompanied by severe pain.

stridor a peculiar harsh, vibrating sound produced during expiration.

stridulous harsh, grating, or shrill (referring to sound).

stroma the framework or connective tissue of an organ, gland or other structure, as distinguished from the parenchyma (the specific tissue of a gland or organ which is responsibile for carrying out its function), e.g., the stroma of the kidney is that tissue which holds the kidney together, the parenchyma is that tissue which filters and excretes the fluids. Cf. PARENCHYMA.

stone 14 pounds. Part of a series of Anglo-Saxon weights which starts with the clove. Two cloves equal a stone, two stones make a quarter and four stones make a half hundredweight. Two half hundredweights make a hundredweight, and twenty hundredweights make a tone (2,240 pounds). Even today it is a common measurement in England, e.g. a person's weight might be given as '10 stone 5', meaning '145 pounds'.

strophulus (tooth rash, red gum, lichen infantum, miliaria rubra) a form of miliaria occurring in infants and often unilateral. Miliaria or sudamina is a disorder of the sweat glands with obstruction of their ducts.

strophulus pruriginosus (prurigo) an eruption characterized by disseminated, intensely itching papules. A chronic inflammatory disease of the skin characterized by small, pale papules and severe itching. The papules are deeply seated and are most prominent on the extensor surfaces of the limbs. The disease begins in early life.

struma scrofula, goiter or bronchocele. A scrofulous tumor. See STRUMOUS.

strumitis inflammation and swelling of the thyroid gland.

strumous (scrofulous, King's evil) goitrous. Also referring to tuberculosis of the cervical lymph nodes. A constitutional condition with glandular tumors and a tuberculous tendency.

strumous diathesis (scrofulous diathesis) a constitutional condition with glandular tumors and a tuberculous tendency.

strumous ophthalmia see SCROFULOUS OPHTHALMIA.

strumous phlyctenular keratitis the inflammation of the corneal conjunctiva with the formation of small red nodules of lymphoid tissue as a result of tuberculosis.

stupe a compress or cloth wrung out of hot water, usually impregnated with turpentine or other irritant, applied to the surface of the skin to produce counter-irritation.

stupefaction great astonishment or consternation. 'Stupefy', to dull the senses, put into a stupor.

stupor inactivity of the sense. Mental numbness, sluggishness or a deep drowsiness.

stymatosis a violent erection of the penis in combination with bleeding.

styloid peg-shaped. Shaped like an instrument for writing.

stype a tampon.

styptic having an alum, aluminum or tannic acid taste. An agent that checks hemorrhage by causing contraction of the blood vessels.

sub-maxillary of or situated below the lower jaw, or associated with the submaxillary gland.

subdelirium a slight or muttering delirium with lucid intervals.

subinvolution imperfect return to normal size after functional enlargement. An arrest in the normal involution of the uterus following childbirth, the organ remaining abnormally large.

subjective symptom see entry under SYMPTOMS.

subluxation a partial dislocation. A term often used to describe spinal vertebrae which have become dislocated from their normal position. Chiropractors correct subluxations by special manipulations which they feel increase nerve flow, while osteopaths feel that their manipulations work because they increased blood flow. Both are no doubt correct.

subsultus an abnormal jerking or twitching.

subsultus tendinum a twitching of the tendons, especially noticeable of the hands and feet, as seen in low fevers.

subtile subtle, elusive. Thin or penetrating.

subungual under the finger- or toenail.

succedanea relating to or acting as a substitute. Pertaining to that which follows.

succus a vegetable juice; an animal secretion. The fluid constituents of the body tissues. More specifically, a preparation obtained by expressing the juice of a plant and adding to it sufficient alcohol to preserve it (as opposed to an extract or tincture, in which the primary ingredient is alcohol/water).

succussion shaking; the process of potentization (vigorously shaking with impact the properly diluted homeopathic remedy). Hahnemann, according to his method (though he changed it several times), suggested that the vial be held in the hand and with an up-and-down motion of the forearm strike the vial against the opposite palm or a leather-bound book at least ten times. Today mechanical means are also employed to accomplish this potentizing process. See POTENCY.

sudamen (pl. sudamina) an eruption of translucent, whitish vesicles, due to a noninflammatory disturbance of the sweat glands, which consists of a collection of sweat in the ducts of the sweat glands. Very transitory, occurring after excessive sweating.

Sudeck's atrophy/syndrome (traumatic osteoporosis) acute bone wasting or septic necrosis following injury. An acute atrophy of a bone, more commonly one of the tarsal or carpal bones, following a slight injury such as a sprain or strain. After P.H.M. Sudeck (1866-1938), a German surgeon.

sudoresis (diaphoresis) perspiration or sweating.

sudorific that which causes perspiration.

sudoriparous producing sweat.

sudorrhea (dermatitis seborrheica, eczema seborrheicum, seborrhea sicca) an acute inflammation of the skin occurring usually on oily skin in areas having large sebaceous glands; may be due to a fungus. Characterized by dry, moist, or greasy scales and by crusted yellowish patches, remissions, exacerbations, and itching.

suffuse to spread through or over (as with liquids). To pour into.

sugar diabetes see DIABETES MELLITUS.

sugar of milk milk sugar or lactose. See SACCHARUM LACTIS.

suggillation (ecchymosis) bruise, black-and-blue mark.

suis pig, swine or hog (a term associated with sarcodes, i.e., a 'suis organ preparation' refers to a sarcode made from healthy pig tissue).

sulcus a groove, depression or furrow, especially in reference to the sutures of the brain.

sulphuretted combined with sulphur.

summer complaint see CHOLERA INFANTUM or CHOLERA MORBUS.

superannuated obsolete or antiquated. Set aside, discarded as old-fashioned.

supercilium the eyebrow.

superior in anatomy, higher; denoting the upper of two parts; toward the vertex.

supinate to turn the arm or hand so that the palm faces upward, or to roll the foot outwards so the instep is rolled up. To lie on the back.

supplication an earnest or humble appeal

suppression the act of driving a disease deeper inward, against Hering's Law. For example, a skin eruption is a manifestation of the conflict between the vital force and the disease and if suppressed (driven inward by any number of means) then the disease will appear later often in a more serious form. See HERING'S LAW.

"A forcible concealment or masking of perceptible manifestations of a disease condition without the cure of the disease."—S.C.F. Hahnemann, *Organon of the Medical Art* (O'Reilly trans., p. 354).

suppurate to produce pus.

supra- a prefix signifying upon or above.

supra-orbital above the eyeball.

suprarenal gland adrenal gland, the gland responsible for secretion of adrenalin (epinephrine), so called because it sits above the kidney ('renal').

suprasternal (episternal) above the sternum.

suprasternal fossa the throatpit; the depression in the midline of the base of the throat above the upper border of the sternum.

sural relating to the calf or the leg.

surdity (surditis, surditas) deafness.

surfeiting overeating. Overindulging in food or drink.

susceptibility the degree of sensitivity to outside influences. Homeopathy as well as other holistic therapies aim to decrease a person's susceptibility/sensitivity to disease-producing influences. 'Susceptibility' to a remedy means the patient either reacts well or perhaps over-reacts to it.

susurrus a soft murmur in an aneurysm.

Sutton's Law Willie Sutton, a famous bank robber, said, when asked why he robbed banks, "because that's where the money is." In medical terms, Dr. W.S. Dock, supposedly the greatest diagnostician, said, "Go to the patient because that's where the diagnosis is.... It is paramount to talk with the patient and observe the patient with focused, painstaking attention to detail because therein lies the key to the diagnosis."

swarthy having a dark or sunburned complexion.

swashing the sound of a splash of water or liquid.

sweating-sickness/fever (miliary fever, sudor anglicus) an infectious disease characterized by fever and profuse sweating with the formation of sudamina.

Swedenborgian member of a Protestant sect, founded in 1788 by Robert Hindmarsh, a London printer, based on the teachings of Emanuel Swedenborg (1688-1772, nee Swedberg), a Swedish scientist and mystic. Swedenborg's spiritual awakening occurred at the age of 57 when he claimed to have direct contact with the spiritual world. Up until then his life was devoted to earth science, metallurgy, and engineering. He invented a machine gun, a submarine, a new type of lock, a hydraulic engine, an air ship, a mechanical musical instrument and a mercury air-pump! From that late spiritual awakening until his death at the age of 84 he devoted himself to spiritual studies. He taught that Jesus was the one and only God, that there is a spiritual sense to the Scriptures and there are correspondences between nature and spirit. The Swedenborgian place of worship is called the Church of the New Jerusalem.

Many of the founding fathers of homeopathy in America were Swedenborgians, most notably Kent. Others were Gram, Hering, Holcombe, Farrington, Wesselhoeft, and C.G. Raue, who wrote *Psychology as a Natural Science Applied to the Solution of Occult Phenomena* (1889). Boericke & Tafel (Phila.) and Otis Clapp (Boston) were major distributors of Swedenborg's writings in America. Kent decided to arrange his repertory based on the Swedenborgian principle of 'from above downward'.

Richard DeCharms wrote an eight page paper, 'Hahnemann and Swedenborg: or the affinities between the fundamental principles of Homoeopathia and the doctrines of the New Church' (Anglo-American New Church Repository, Nov. 1850), and four years later he penned *A Defense of Homeopathy Against her New Church Assailants; or a full and fair view of the case of allopathy and chronothermalism vs. homoeopathy, as tried by the New Church judicative principles* (New Jerusalem Printer, 1854, 200pp.)

sweetbread the pancreas and thymus of calves or other young livestock prepared as a cooked edible dish.

sweetmeats any delicacy made with a sweetening agent; candy.

swimming of the head vertigo.

swoon (syncope) fainting. A temporary loss of consciousness due to lack of blood supply to the brain.

sx. abbreviation for 'symptom' or 'symptoms'.

sycosis (Gr., *sykon,* 'fig', 'fig-wart') 1) an inflammatory disease affecting the hair follicles, usually of the beard, characterized by papules, pustules and tubercles. 2) Hahnemann's term for the constitutional effects of the gonorrheal virus/miasm or the chronic miasmatic form of gonorrhea whose predominant symptoms are the overgrowth of tissue. See MIASM.

sycoma a pendulous fig-like growth; a large soft wart.

sycotic referring to the miasm, sycosis.

Sydenham's chorea see CHOREA. A condition first described by the English physician T. Sydenham (1624-1689). He described measles and differentiated it from scarlet fever. He also wrote a classic description of gout.

sympathetic powder (powder of sympathy) a special powder which, when applied to the bloody/torn clothing of a wounded person, assisted in the healing of the wound. The wound was also washed and cleansed. See WEAPON OINTMENT.

symphysis pubis the juncture of the pubic bones.

symphysis (pl. 'symphyses') a junction where two bones meet, e.g., sacroiliac, the skull sutures. 'Symphysis pubis', the line of union of the pubic bones.

symptoms (abbrev. 'sx.') the phenomena of disease which lead to complaints on the part of the ill person. Signs and symptoms are the only perceptible form of disease ('dysfunctional vital force'), and their full comprehension is necessary to intelligently understand the patient's loss of well-being. A sign is generally understood to be objective (red stripe down the middle of the tongue, fever, sweating, etc.), while a symptom is subjective and conveys how the patient feels, e.g., "my leg hurts" is a symptom, albeit not a very good one. Then the clinician needs to ask the patient, "Give me more of your subjective feelings [symptoms]." Encouraging the patient to open up, the practitioner will receive more information about the patient so as to help the practitioner perceive the nature of the illness and thus the curative remedy. Before going on to defining the myriad terms for symptoms which practitioners have coined over the years, it can be said that in the evolution of the disease picture, symptoms precede signs.

Suppose an individual comes with a complaint of dropsy in the feet (a sign). According to the theory of 'symptoms preceding signs', this patient would have had some unusual symptomatology prior to the development of the dropsy. And if the patient had been sufficiently aware of those symptoms a visit to the health practitioner might have occurred. During this visit the competent practitioner would have gathered an adequate amount of symptoms to *perceive* the patient and thus administer the curative remedy. Thus the dropsy would never have developed. This does not

symptoms *(cont.)*

mean signs are unimportant. They have their importance, especially in comatose patients, infants, the insane, patients with language barriers and uncooperative patients. "We always have to evaluate the place of the symptoms in the life of the patient."—R. Moskowitz

The complete description of a symptom includes its a) location, b) sensation, and c) modality (circumstances of occurrence and aggravation/amelioration, symbolized by < and >, respectively).

A symptom is basically an abnormal sensation experienced by a person as a whole or in a part of the body. The location includes the area and site, how the symptom extends, and the direction in which it spreads. The patient's description should give causative factors, the setting in which the sensation was first experienced, and conditions which increase or decrease the symptom and discomfort (modalities). Modalities are conditions which influence or modify the patient's symptom, and include time, temperature, weather, motion, emotion, menstruation, position, perspiration, and eating. There are two types of modalites: those which apply to the person as a whole and those which apply to the patient's complaint. Thus the patient may feel better in general with warmth, yet warmth may worsen his headache.

One last point before defining individual symptoms is this: The totality of symptoms is used to select the remedy; however, it is usually not the totality which directs our attention to a certain remedy. Usually what happens is that out of that totality comes a prominent/keynote/leading symptom which leads us to think of the remedy first. Then we compare the totalities. In Paragraph 104 of the *Organon* Hahnemann said, "When the totality of the particular symptoms characterizing the case at hand or, in other words, the picture of any given disease, is drawn exactly, the most difficult task has been accomplished." See ONE-SIDED CASE.

"Symptoms are but the language of nature, talking out as it were and showing as clearly as the daylight the internal nature of the sick man or woman. ... It is nonsense to say that prior to the localization of the disease, the patient was not sick."—*Lectures on Homoeopathic Philosophy* (J.T. Kent).

"Symptoms are the outward and visible signs of the inward disturbance of the vital force which will ultimately produce morbid states, and when these symptoms are removed the disease ceases to exist."—*Principles and Art of Cure by Homoeopathy* (H.A. Roberts).

absolute symptoms (basic sx.) symptoms which appear in most diseases and in most provings. They have little value in determining the specific homeopathic remedy needed, but do, when taken together, offer a beginning. Such symptoms include malaise, headache, weakness, dyspnea, cough,

symptoms, *cont.*

eructations, fever and pain.

accessory symptoms 1) see new symptoms. 2) "...when the imperfect medicine is used, some befallments will then emerge which were not to be found earlier in the disease. These are accessory symptoms of the not-completely-fitting medicine." - Organon (O'Reilly trans., P. 163, p. 174)

accidental symptom an occasional symptom which just doesn't seem to fit the pattern. It does not help in the diagnosis or in the selection of the remedy and actually lends confusion to the case. These symptoms should be, for the most part, ignored.

alternating symptoms symptoms felt when others disappear or subside, for example, asthma and the cutaneous eruptions of eczema, or constipation alternating with diarrhea. See *Organon*, Para. 232, 6th Ed.

associated symptom see CONCOMITANT SYMPTOM.

auxiliary symptom see CONCOMITANT SYMPTOM.

basic symptom see ABSOLUTE SYMPTOM.

characteristic symptom see PECULIAR SYMPTOM.

"But it must never be forgotten that *without* the *characteristics, ...* there can be no *individualisation,* and without *this* there can be no *accurate homoeopathic prescription."—Homoeopathy: The Science of Therapeutics* (C. Dunham).

The combination of a common symptom with a concomitant symptom may evolve to become a characteristic symptom.

chief complaint (main symptom, entering complaint) the illness, the reason why the patient has come to see the practitioner.

clinical symptom a symptom which does not appear in the proving of a remedy yet has been observed to be relieved by that remedy. (Since provings are stopped before pathology develops, some symptoms will only appear in clinical or toxological data. Others probably would appear if the proving were continued long enough.) "As an example, [material doses of] Granatum always produces dizziness when given for intestinal parasites. Thus inadvertently one of its main actions was discovered, and since then, in a case of dizziness, one always thinks of *Granatum*—a purely clinical application."—Garth Boericke.

common symptom (diagnostic symptom) a symptom all persons have who are suffering from the same disease.

"A symptom may be common to all cases of a certain disease, and therefore of no great use in picking out the individual remedy for a particular case of that disease; or it may be common to a very great number of drugs, and therefore indicate one of a large group of remedies only; and so of very little use in repertorising."—*Repertorising* (M. Tyler & Sir John Weir).

"The common symptoms, without the peculiar symptoms, may give a

symptoms, *cont.*

good understanding of a given case except for prescribing. Common symptoms alone will lead to failure of the prescription."—*New Remedies* (J.T. Kent).

"Common symptoms are such as are pathognomonic of diseases and of pathology, and such as are common to many remedies and are found in large rubrics in our repertories; e.g., constipation, nausea, irritability, etc."—*A.B.C. of Homoeopathy* (R.H. Langbridge).

The combination of a common symptom with a concomitant symptom may evolve to become a characteristic symptom.

complete symptom one which has its location, sensation, extensions, and modalities clearly indicated and defined. It is possible to select the remedy based on a single complete symptom. The symptom 'weakness' is common, yet becomes peculiar if 'it comes on only while eating' or 'after stool.'

"A complete symptom has four component parts: Sensation, Location, Modalities and Concomitants."—*Some Clinical Experiences* (E.E. Case).

concomitant symptom one occurring with or co-existing with the chief complaint, whether in the same general area or at a removed location. For example, a throbbing headache accompanying acute diarrhea, or right molar tooth pain accompanying blurred vision are considered concomitant symptoms to the chief complaints of acute diarrhea and blurred vision. Often the patient does not consider such symptoms to be very important because they are not a great source of bother to him. Yet they are important to the selection of the remedy. Concomitants usually occur at the same time as the chief complaint. There are at least 21 remedies having 'thirstlessness during fever', yet with the concomitant symptom of 'scanty urine' one remedy comes to mind, *Puls.* Eizayaga calls concomitant symptoms 'satellite' symptoms.

The combination of a common symptom with a concomitant symptom may evolve to become a characteristic symptom.

confirmatory symptom a symptom underlined three times in case taking. When taking a case, symptoms are underlined from one to three times depending on their severity or prominence.

contingent symptom see PECULIAR SYMPTOM.

contradictory symptom according to H.A. Roberts, one "which a patient may repeat in one breath and refute in the next . . . or [ones which] are contradicted in a review of the case."

determining symptom (secondary sx.) one related to the main symptom (chief complaint) and frequently found within the general symptoms. For example, the chief complaint is "long lasting diarrhea with fever and aversion to food" which indicates *Ant. c., Ars., Chin., Nux m., Phos.,* and symptoms, *cont.*

Puls. A secondary/determining symptom is necessary to choose one of the six. In this patient it is found that the "fever regularly lasts a certain amount of time," pointing to *Ant. c., Cina, Ign.,* and *Sabad.* This symptom helps to verify *Ant. c.* This symptom can also be called a characteristic symptom. If the symptom were even smaller, e.g., the time span being 4 to 8 PM, *Hell.* or *Lyc.* might alone determine the remedy. This is a peculiar/rare/strange symptom. This example also serves to show that some symptoms can be called by more than one name (a secondary symptom can be a characteristic or rare symptom. The peculiar or rare symptom can be called a keynote or leading symptom).

eliminative symptom one which the practitioner uses to repertorize the case. They are termed eliminative as they are used to gradually 'eliminate' remedies from the case, gradually narrowing the list down to a half-dozen or fewer. Then one does further comparative work in the materia medica to select the simillimum. One looks for eliminative symptoms in the mentals, modalities or a common symptom with an unusual flavor to it. One might consider this to be a keynote symptom which is used as the first symptom for repertorization. Since it indicates just a few remedies, it serves to eliminate a large number of remedies.

etiological symptom a symptom related by the patient to the onset or development of his/her disease (consequence of shock, fears, emotional upsets, etc.); also symptoms discovered by the practitioner to be related to the onset (germs, virus, high levels of physiological or metabolic substances).

first symptoms see OLDEST SYMPTOMS.

food symptoms desires, aversions, cravings, loathings, and adverse reactions are considered secondary symptoms and are very valuable for the remedy selection.

functional symptom one related to the functioning of the affected organ, usually preceding organic or pathological changes. These symptoms are of little importance (unless of course, they are accompanied by symptoms in another location). "Functional symptoms of an affected organ are of much less value than symptoms which occur in other parts during the excess of the function of that organ."—Wm. Boericke.

In gonorrhea, for example, if a burning pain is felt in the urethra during or after urination it is a symptom of little value. But if pain in the testes is felt during urination this symptom takes on greater importance and cannot be ignored. In indigestion, when the patient says he has stomach pains after eating, this is a functional symptom. It is not much help in choosing a remedy, yet if the accompanying symptom of headache or dizziness after eating is present this then becomes an important symptom. This example also serves to show how symptom definitions change. Here a functional symptom plus the concomitant symptom unite to become a peculiar symptom.

general symptom (absolute symptom) one which encompasses the whole person; the 'I' symptoms: "I feel better in the cold weather/while walking/ after a nap." These are symptoms which pertain to and characterize the patient and are not part of the disease. The 'I' symptoms refer to the whole person. Dreams come under this heading only if a dream is repeated over and over.

Sometimes just referred to as 'generals', this grouping can be divided into five areas: 1) *mentals*, the general psychological make-up of the person (emotional reactivity, depressive tendency, perfectionism, claustrophobia, fears, romantic tendencies, etc.) If mentals are well-defined, they may be of the highest significance in finding the simillimum. Mentals are not necessarily pathological. If a person is melancholic with perfectionistic tendencies, it doesn't mean *Arsenicum* needs to be prescribed, it is just the way the person is. If the mentioned symptoms were very pronounced and reaching a pathological state then the prescriber might consider *Arsenicum.* 2) *general modalities*, what makes the person feel better or worse (time of day/year, types of foods/drinks, environmental aspects). 3) *desires and aversions*, related to the general modalities in that we desire what makes us feel better and avoid things which disturb us. 4) *pathological predisposition*, whether the problem has existed in the past or still exists, for example, a susceptibility to recurring bronchitis or skin affections, etc. 5) *anatomical or physical structure* plays a role in helping to find the simillimum, as you would not give a lot of consideration to *Calc. carb.* if the patient is tall and thin.

A negative general is the absence of an expected symptom in a case. For example, if a patient's physical complaint is not aggravated by a change in weather, remedies like *Phos., Silicea, Tuberc.,* and *Rhod.* can usually be excluded. Yet one must be cautious as absence of a symptom should not allow one to assume it is not there. Perhaps the symptom was not elicited. The absence of this symptom should be noted in your case taking.

guiding symptom one which points clearly and unequivocally to a specific remedy, even when the symptom is a minor one.

incomplete symptom one lacking a description of a) location, b) sensation, and c) circumstances of its occurrence, concomitants, and modality (aggravation or amelioration). Thus a symptom lacking any of these three is termed an 'incomplete symptom'.

keynote symptom (leading symptom) one which is so apparent, so clear, that it suggests a small group of remedies or even a single remedy. For example, pain in the right shoulder blade points to *Chelidonium.*

Keynotes are actually peculiar symptoms which have taken on a highly characteristic flavor and tend to point almost directly to a remedy, yet if keynotes are taken as final and the generals do not confirm them, failures often result.

Many of the great homeopathic prescribers (Lippe, Allen, Boger) were very successful keynote prescribers, but you must realize that they had keen 'totality perceptions' and thus would not allow false-positives to sway them.

late symptom (recent sx.) the latest expression of a disease, usually valuable in determining the remedy, especially in acute diseases.

leading symptom (keynote sx.) see KEYNOTE SYMPTOM.

local symptom (particular sx.) one related to the site of pathology. Laterality (right or left sidedness) and anatomical appearance are considered. A local symptom in several different areas can be considered a general symptom (e.g., red orifices = *Sulphur* or *Acidum Nitricum*).

Locals are symptoms associated just with the chief complaint. For example, a patient is seen for hip pain. He describes his symptoms as better with motion, worse on wet, humid days, with lancinating pains upon lying on the right side and a warmth which seems to radiate from the painful area. These are symptoms directly associated with the hip and are termed local. Some may refer to local symptoms as particulars. Do not confuse local *symptoms* with localized *sensations.* Sensations or localized sensations, if pronounced enough, may act as keynotes/leaders steering you to the correct remedy. For example, the symptom 'lancinating pains in the sacrum on stooping, extending into the buttocks' is a localized sensation.

"The physician spoils his case when he prescribes for the local symptoms and neglects the patient."—*New Remedies* (J.T. Kent).

main symptom (chief complaint) see MAJOR SYMPTOM.

major symptom (chief complaint, main sx.) the one of greatest concern to the patient. To the adult with eczema it is the skin eruptions, in one with arthritis it is the pain in the joints. The major symptom is the symptom the patient considers to be his illness. Yet the major symptom may not be that important to the practitioner in the selection of the remedy.

minor symptom one obtained by deeper questioning of the patient, such as the patient's desires and aversions to foods or various sensitivities to weather. They may not have any connection to the major symptom. To the patient they may not seem relevant to his problem yet may be of great importance to the selection of the remedy.

new symptoms symptoms which emerge after the course of treatment has begun. They may be divided into three areas: 1) the re-occurrence of old symptoms in reverse chronological order, according to Hering's Law. If you are aware of this, there is no need to prescribe a remedy, just wait, and they should gradually dissipate. 2) proving symptoms. The patient, after taking the constitutional remedy, begins to prove the remedy with symptoms which he didn't have before. Usually these symptoms rapidly disappear. If the remedy is repeated, the symptoms will aggravate. 3) symptoms of a detoxification nature. As the cure progresses, cutaneous affections, mucosal discharges, etc. may occur. These are good, should not be suppressed, and with time will diminish.

"If a great number of new symptoms appear after the administration of a remedy, the prescription will generally prove an unfavourable one. The greater the array of new symptoms coming out after the administration of a remedy, the more doubt there is thrown upon the prescription."—*Lectures on Homoeopathic Philosophy* (J.T. Kent).

objective symptom one which is quantifiable and generally observable by the physician. For example, 'I have a fever' or 'my throat is red and pimply' are objective symptoms, as opposed to 'I feel better when I lie down', which is subjective. Physiological and laboratory findings are objective.

"Objective symptoms, those that are seen by the careful observer, have more importance in child life than in adult life, because through them we see the expression of the child's disposition and desires."—*Principles and Art of Cure by Homoeopathy* (H.A. Roberts).

"An objective symptom is one which not only the patient but others can determine by any of the five senses."—*Handy Book of Reference* (G. Royal).

oldest symptoms symptoms associated with the patient's first departure from good health. These are symptoms associated with chronic disease and are of the highest value, yet are useful in the treatment of acute disease, e.g., in cholera, the side on which it began may determine the choice of the remedy.

"The oldest symptom is of particular value before there was any treatment."—Wm. Boericke.

"Old symptoms reappearing are a step in the right direction, as we know; therefore a group of entirely new symptoms appearing after the administration of a remedy is evidence that we have made a decided step in the wrong direction."—*Principles and Art of Cure by Homoeopathy* (H.A. Roberts).

particular symptom (local sx.) a 'my' symptom (versus an 'I' symptom of the generals), referring to a part of the body or to the disease. These symptoms are generally less important than the generals unless they are peculiar. 'My head aches' is a useless particular symptom, but if the symptom is 'My head aches only between 10 AM and 2 PM', this is peculiar (even

symptoms, *cont.*

strange and rare) and indicates *Nat. mur.*

"And now, at last, you come to the *Particulars*—the symptoms that bulk so largely for the patient, and for which he is as a matter of fact, actually consulting you. You will have taken them down first . . . but you will consider them last: for these symptoms are really of minor importance from your point of view (certainly in chronic cases) because they are not general to the patient as a living whole, but only particulars to some part of him.

"Among the *Particulars*, your first-grade symptoms will always be anything *peculiar,* or *unusual* or *unexpected,* or *unaccountable.*

"Remember! *The more uncommon a symptom is, the more valuable; the less you can account for a symptom and the more intensely personal it is, the more important.*"—*Repertorising* (M. Tyler & Sir John Weir).

"What a patient fancies or fears, desires or dreads, is often of inestimable worth in fixing the value of a symptom."—*Handy Book of Reference* (G. Royal).

"But it must never be forgotten that *without* the *characteristics,* . . . there can be no *individualisation*, and without *this* there can be no *accurate homoeopathic prescription.*"—*Homoeopathy: The Science of Therapeutics* (C. Dunham).

pathogenetic symptom a symptom surrounding the onset or evolution of the disease.

pathognomonic symptom one fundamental and distinctive for the diagnosis, e.g., hyperglycemia in diabetes. If such symptoms are not present, the diagnosis of a particular disease cannot be made. "The modalities of a drug are the pathognomic symptoms of the materia medica."—Wm. Boericke.

pathological symptom an objective expression of the disease, such as hypertension, anemia, fibrillation, bleeding, fever, profuse watery diarrhea.

peculiar symptom (strange sx., rare sx., contingent sx., characteristic sx.) one often serving to point directly to the curative remedy. Alone these symptoms may be of no special value, but can take on great value by paying attention to their modalities. They are symptoms of an unusual nature and in turn give the case a pronounced flavor of individuality. For example, thirstlessness during fever, or a migraine, worse coughing and better by hot drinks. It may be a symptom which is not necessarily related to the chief complaint. "Those [symptoms] which vary with the individual and are not essentially pathognomic of the disease, but always of the individual patient."—Wm. Boericke.

253

symptoms, *cont.*

physical symptom one found upon examination by the practitioner, such as color of skin, shape of nails, appearance of the tongue, etc.

psychic symptom (nervous sx.) a mental symptom. See GENERAL SYMPTOM.

rare symptom one which very few patients and very few remedies have.

recent symptom see LATE SYMPTOM.

satellite symptom see CONCOMITANT SYMPTOM.

secondary symptom see DETERMINING SYMPTOM.

strange, rare, peculiar symptom (peculiar symptom) one that is striking, unique, or exceptional: a particular sensation, a striking modality or a concomitant symptom. For example, fever without thirst (*Bell.*), wasting with excessive eating (*Iodum*), or a chilliness yet aggravation from heat (*Puls.*) See PECULIAR SYMPTOM.

subjective symptom one described by the patient as his feelings or sensations. One must realize that patients vary in their ability to express and describe their sensations.

"A pure subjective symptom is one which the patient alone can feel and express, one which the doctor can neither see, hear, etc."—*Handy Book of Reference* (G. Royal).

symptom complex (syndrome) the aggregate of signs and symptoms which make up the morbid state and constitute the disease picture. For example, diabetes mellitus has a number of characteristic symptoms (frequent urination, extraordinary thirst, increased appetite, weakness and emaciation) which serve to describe the essence of diabetes.

symptomatic treatment the treatment of a single symptom rather than treatment based on the totality of symptoms.

synalgia reflex or referred pain (pain felt at a part remote from the seat of the causative lesion).

synchisis presence of bright shiny particles in the vitreous body of the eye.

synchronous occurring at the same time or simultaneously.

syncope fainting, a swoon; a sudden fall of blood-pressure or failure of the cardiac systole, resulting in cerebral anemia and more or less complete loss of consciousness.

syncope anginosa see ANGINA PECTORIS.

syndesmitis depending on the context it may mean inflammation of a ligament, or conjunctivitis.

syndesmos a ligament.

syndrome (disease) the aggregate of signs and symptoms which make up the morbid state and constitute the disease picture. See SYMPTOM COMPLEX.

synechia an adhesion, specifically of the iris to the cornea or to the capsule of the lens.

synocha (febris synocha) a continued fever.

synochal fever (synochus) a continued fever.

synovial crepitation the production of crepitant-like sounds (grating) in the joints. See CREPITANT.

synovitis inflammation of the synovial membrane (the lining which creates a sac encompassing a joint) which is usually painful on motion and prone to swellings.

syntaxis a joint or articulation.

syntexis an emaciation or wasting.

synthetic remedies a combination of two usually proven remedies to form a new entity which may nor not be proven in the homeopathic sense. *China ars.* is an example of a synthetic remedy which has been proven as such.

Knowing what the two proven remedies are, one may then synthesize or project what the action and use of the new remedy might be. For example, *Aurum arsenicum* and *Aurum iodatum* are combinations of *Aurum* and *Arsenicum* or *Iodatum*, respectively. As separate entities, they are in the homeopathic literature and their separate provings are available. But the two together, the synthetic remedy (*Aurum ars.* or *Aurum iod.*) may never have been proven. One looks at the two separate provings and attempts to deduce what effects the new combination would have. This is really not a reliable method for ascertaining the actions of combined substances.

syphilides (syphiloderma) skin eruptions due to syphilis. Nearly any type of skin lesion can be produced by *Treponema pallidum*, the bacteria which causes the disease syphilis.

syphilis (morbus gallicus, 'chancre') contagious venereal disease characterized by a variety of lesions of which the chancre, the mucous patch and the gumma are distinctive. It is caused by *Treponema pallidum* and is usually acquired during sexual intercourse.

From the protagonist of the most famous medical poem *Syphilis. Sive Morbus Gallicus* (Girolamo Fracastoro, 1530).

syphilitic refers to syphilis or the miasm arising from either suppressed or inherited syphilis. The destruction of tissue is the characteristic symptom of the syphilitic miasm. See MIASM.

syphiloderma the skin manifestations of syphilis.

syrygmus a ringing, buzzing, or tinkling sound in the ears.

syzygy unison, alignment in a straight line or alignment in purpose (Gr. *syn*, 'together', and *zygon,* 'yoke').

TT tablet triturate, trit. See TRITURATE.

tabacosis chronic tobacco poisoning, especially as seen in the tobacco industry as an occupational disease. Symptomatology would be similar to nicotinism.

tabes emaciation; gradual, progressive bodily wasting.

tabes dorsalis (locomotor ataxia, spinal atrophy) see TABES. A chronic progressive hardening of the posterior spinal roots, cord, and the peripheral nerves leading to ataxia (muscular incoordination), neuralgia, lancinating pains, muscular atrophy, disorders of the joints, and paralysis.

"Cannot walk backwards. Cannot walk in the dark or with eyes closed without staggering."—Stacy Jones, M.D., *Bee-Line Therapie and Repertory.*

tabes mesenterica tuberculosis of the abdominal glands (mesenteric and retro-peritoneal lymph nodes) most commonly seen in children and accompanied with a progressive wasting of the body.

tablet triturates (TTs, trits) see TRITURATE.

tachycardia a fast heart rate usually in excess of 100 beats per minute.

tachypnea rapid breathing.

taciturn reserved, habitually silent, disinclined to talk.

tactile relating to touch or to the sense of touch.

tactitation tossing of the body; restlessness.

taedium vitae weariness of life, disgust for life (L. 'irksomeness, tediousness, weariness of life').

taenia a band or band-like structure. A genus of tapeworm which are ribbon-like (bandlike), segmental flatworms. See TENIASIS, TENICIDE.

talalgia (tatalgia) pain in the heel (L. *talus,* 'heel, ankle').

talipes (club foot, cyllosis, kyllosis) a congenital malformation of one or both feet in which the forefoot is inverted and rotated, accompanied by shortening of the Achilles tendon and contracture of the plantar fascia. There are four main varieties: t. varus, t. valgus, t. equinus, and t. calcaneus. (L. *talus,* 'heel, ankle', and *pes,* 'foot').

tallow (suet, sevum) the solid fat of cattle and other ruminants.

tannin (tannic acid, gallotannic acid, tannicum) a light greenish yellow powder which is styptic and astringent and used primarily to relieve diarrhea.

tapeworm see TAENIA.

tapis an archaic term meaning 'under consideration'.

tar water mania tar water therapeutically used as a cure-all. A quart of tar was stirred into a gallon of water and allowed to sit for 48 hours then decanted. The liquid was then administered for a variety of ills and became somewhat of a panacea. It was promulgated by Bishop Berkley.

tarantismus desire for dancing and music, from the belief that the bite of the tarantula can cause this.

Tarantism/tarentisme was a sickness characterized by an uncontrollable urge to dance. It reached epidemic proportions in southern Italy in the 15th through 17th centuries.

"It afflicted girls of strict religious families; a hysterical insanity. They could only be cured if they danced for three days to inciting music in an abandoned church and cut themselves with knives or swords. The dance ended when they collapsed exhausted to the floor. Unfortunately, the hysterical attacks often reoccurred once a year and the whole ritual had to be repeated. The attacks have always been related to the bite of the Tarentula spider, but it is usually a spontaneous hysteria; the bite of the spider is not poisonous."—M. Pelt (*Homoeopathic Links,* 3/95, p. 46)

tarsal 1) the ankle area or that area between the leg and the metatarsus. 2) pertaining to the tarsus (outer edge) of the eyelid.

Tart. stibiatum Antimonium tartaricum.

tartar a white, brown, or yellow-brown deposit at or below the gum line of the teeth.

tartar emeticus (tartarized antimony) a mixture of antimony and potassium tartrate designed to induce vomiting when given by mouth. Sometimes refers to *Ant. tart.*

taxis the manual reduction (placing in its normal/natural position) of a hernia or prolapsed structure or organ.

taxonomy the science, laws, or principles of classification.

tautopathy a form of isotherapy, using a homeopathically-prepared allopathic medicine in order to counteract side-effects caused by that particular allopathic medication, e.g., giving homeopathic *DPT* to counter the ill-effects produced by the DPT vaccine or giving homeopathic *Valium* to counter the ill-effects produced by Valium. To carry this one step further, some practitioners feel it necessary to treat the allopathically-dosed patient in this manner before commencing homeopathic treatment.

teacher "The best teacher you'll ever meet will be your patient."—J. Imberechts. "Errors are (or contain) often the germ of truth where the mind without a teacher is obliged to teach itself."—von Grauvogl.

teat the nipple.

tectum (tectorium, tegmen) any covering or structure which acts as a roof.

tedium a feeling or a period of time characterized by dullness, boredom, weariness, or slowness; a sense of time passing too slowly with little of interest.

tegument an outer covering; integument, the skin. See INTEGUMENT.

telangiectasis (vascular naevus, mother's mark) a chronic dilation of groups of capillaries (small blood vessels) causing dark red blotches on the skin.

telangiosis any disease of the capillaries and terminal arterioles.

telluric earthly. Of or relating to the earth or soil.

temporal pertaining to time. Also, referring to the temple (the side of the forehead), as the temporal bone or artery.

tenacious holding or tending to hold firmly; persistent; stubborn. Clinging to another object or surface; adhesive.

tenesmus the straining at stool or while urinating which proves ineffective or only the passage of a small quantity of stool or urine occurs. Having the urge to go but with no result. An involuntary contraction, sometimes painful, of the anal or bladder sphincter. 'Vesical tenesmus' indicates bladder/urinary tenesmus.

tenesmus vesicae bladder straining. Straining to relieve the bladder but little or no evacuation results.

teniacide (tenicide) a remedy which destroys tapeworms.

teniasis the presence of a tapeworm in the intestine.

tenodynia (tenalgia) pain in a tendon.

tenositis (tendinitis, tendonitis) inflammation of a tendon.

terebinthine containing or resembling turpentine, which has diuretic properties.

teres round and long, referring to muscles and ligaments (L. *terere,* 'to rub').

terrain the patient's 'soil' or the 'earth'. In other words, the ubiquitous connective tissue which consists of mesenchymal cells, leukocytes, nerve endings, blood and vascular networks, and extracellular matrix *(vide).* Thus if the 'sea' in which one lives is toxic, the ability of the body to protect itself from infections or recover from trauma is impaired, as is the person's ability to thrive. This is where many methods of treatment, both homeopathic and nonhomeopathic, focus in order to raise the patient's overall level of health. For instance, the homotoxological approach, with its plethora of complex remedies, attempts to improve the functioning of the bodily metabolic processes and increase or support the eliminative activities.

tertian recurring every third day, counting the day of the paroxysm as the first; every other day, e.g. Monday, Wednesday, Friday, Sunday.

tertiary third in order; the third and usually most serious stage in the progression of a disease.

tertiary syphilis the third stage of syphilis, characterized by severe skin lesions and the formation of gummae (masses of sticky, fibrous matter) throughout the body. Aortic aneurysm may occur as well as involvement of the central nervous system, causing meningitis, tabes dorsalis, and paresis.

testalgia testicle pain.

tetanic relating to tetanus. Tonic muscular contractions (continuous and steady).

tetanus (lockjaw) an acute infectious disease characterized by intermittent painful tonic spasms of voluntary muscles and convulsions caused by the toxin of *Clostridium tetani* acting upon the central nervous system.

tetanus narcolepsy a condition involving both narcolepsy and tetanic convulsions or spasms.

tetanus nascentium (tetanus neonatorum) a form of tetanus affecting newborn infants, especially in the West Indies, possibly due to infection through the open end of the severed umbilical cord.

tetter a broad, common term for various skin eruptions, particularly herpes, eczema, pemphigus, and psoriasis. Eating tetter (lupus), honeycomb tetter (favus), moist tetter (eczema), scaly or washerwomen's tetter (psoriasis or scaly eczema), milky tetter (milkblotch or milk scall), running tetter (impetigo), tarsal tetter (blear-eye, eruptive disease of the eyelids).

tettery eczematous.

thalassaemia (thalassanemia, hereditary leptocytosis, Coolie's anemia) an inherited disease primarily occurring in the Mediterranean region characterized by an enlarged spleen, bone changes and alterations in the pigmentation of the skin.

thalassotherapy treatment of disease by residing at the seashore, by sea bathing, or by going on a sea voyage.

the plague see BUBONIC PLAGUE.

theism ('tea-drinkers' disease') the toxic condition produced by the excessive use of tea, i.e., nervousness, cerebral excitement, then later mental and bodily depression. With continued use the patient develops heart irregularities and digestive disturbances, nightmares and nervous trembling. The best treatment is exercise and an open-air life.

thelalgia pain in the nipple.

thelitis inflammation of the nipple.

thenar the fleshy part of the palm of the hand.

theomania a religious insanity or melancholy. Insanity in which the individual believes that he is God.

thermic relating to heat.

Thomsen's disease (ataxia muscularis, myotonia congenita) a hereditary disease characterized by tonic spasms in the voluntary muscles with an abnormally slow relaxation after contraction, resulting in muscular stiffness. First described by Danish physician A.J.T. Thomsen (1815-1896).

Thomsonianism (steam system) a system of medical therapeutics, popularized by Samuel Thomson (1769-1843) in the 1800s, using herbal formulations.

Using herbs does not sound unusual to us, but back then it was, as doctors primarily used drastic measures (bloodletting, strong or toxic chemicals and medicines) to treat the ill. Thomson, who wrote *New Guide to Health, or Botanic Family Physician* (1822) and whose main slogan was "Every man his own physician", described his method as relying upon two approaches, botanical medications and external steaming. He believed that "heat is the substance of life and that this primordial principle of life may also be its renovator and restorer of health . . . to increase the internal heat, remove all obstructions of the system, restore the digestive powers of the stomach, and produce a natural perspiration." The Botanico-Medical College of Ohio (Cincinnati) was founded in 1838 and in 1839 the Southern Botanico-Medical College was organized.

Thomson developed his thoughts into a method, patented it (in 1813 and 1823), and sold rights to practice it. Later his followers, some three million strong, joined together with herbalists to form the Eclectic Medical Institute; however, a schism occurred within the membership. Thomson split off to head the U.S. Thomsonian Society, while Alva Curtis (1797-1881) organized the Independent Thomsonian Botanic Society. Later Curtis and Wooster Beach (1794-1859) joined to form the Reformed School. In 1830, they formed the reformed Medical College of Worthington. See ECLECTIC, PHYSIOMEDICALISM.

A good resource for herbal information is the American Botanical Council, PO Box 201660, Austin, TX 78720.

thoracic referring to the chest.

three parallels of Hahnemann (three parallels of force) a) plane of vital force of the organism, b) plane of disease cause, c) plane of medicinal substance.

thromboangitis obliterans (Winiwater's disease, Buerger's disease) inflammation of the walls of medium-sized veins and arteries and the surrounding connective tissue, especially of the legs of middle-aged and sometimes young men. Occlusion may occur and gangrene is common.

Described by two physicians, Alexander von Winiwater (1848-1916), a German surgeon, and Leo Buerger (1879-1943), a New York doctor.

thrombocytopenia purpura see PURPURA HEMORRHAGICA.

thrombosis the formation, development, or presence of a clot.

thrush an oral fungal infection characterized by white eruptions in the mouth.

thymion a wart.

thymol (thymic acid) an aromatic liquid principally used both internally and externally as an antiseptic. Used specifically in uncinariasis (see ANKYLOSTOMIASIS).

tibia the shin bone.

tic a nervous problem with involuntary movements of any part of the body. Tics around the eyes (lower eyelid) are common in most people at one time or another. They are usually caused by a build-up of tension and fatigue and an inability to relax. Hereditary factors may also play a role.

tic douloureux (prosopalgia, facial neuralgia) a habit spasm. A twitching neuralgia of the trigeminal nerve (Fr., 'painful tic'). See FACEACHE.

Tiegel's contracture the definition for this term could not be found. However, it is probably similar to Thomsen's disease. 'Contracture' means a state of permanent muscular contraction. See THOMSEN'S DISEASE.

time "Time does not respect what you do without taking time into account."— J. Imberechts. In homeopathy, 'time' can refer to 'times of the remedies', the concept that remedies may work more effectively when given at certain times, e.g., some clinicians have found that if *Sulphur* is the simillimum or indicated remedy it would best be administered late in the morning (11 AM), or if *Nux v.* is indicated it is best given in the evening. In a related area, some remedies are known to relieve symptoms if they appear during certain hours of the day, e.g., *Arsenicum* has a modality of < midnight, or *Lycopodium* is < 4 to 7 PM. Some common terms for times of day, and their exact meaning:

Morning (5 AM to 10 AM)	Forenoon (10 AM to noon)
Noon (noon to 1 PM)	Afternoon (1 PM to 6 PM)
Evening (6 PM to 9 PM)	Night (after 9 PM to 5 or 6 AM)

tincture an alcoholic or hydroalcoholic solution prepared from a medicinal substance usually of plant origin. 'Mother tincture' is a term particular to homeopathy and means a water-alcohol solution of any substance from which homeopathic potencies are made from. The strengths of tinctures are not uniform, because the percentage of alcohol depends on whether the active ingredients in the plant are alcohol- or water-soluble.

tinctura nervina Bestuschefii (spiritus ferri chlorati aethereus, Lamotte's Golden Drops) a mixture of ether, alcohol, and perchloride of iron used as an iron tonic and astringent "adapted to weak and relaxed conditions of the stomach and bowels and to anemic symptoms generally."—*A Treatise on Pharmacy* (E. Parrish).

tinder readily combustible material, such as dry twigs, used to kindle fires.

tinea (porrigo decalvans) fungal skin disease; ringworm. Today there are eight forms of *Tinea* (dermatophytic) infections: *Tinea corporis* (ringworm of the body), *Tinea cruris* (ringworm of the groin, jock itch), *Tinea pedis* (ringworm of the foot, athlete's foot), *Tinea barbae* (ringworm of the beard, barber's itch), *Tinea capitus* (ringworm of the scalp), *Tinea manuum* (ringworm of the hand), *Tinea unguium* (ringworm of the nail), *Tinea versicolor* (pityriasis versicolor).

tinea annularis (tinea capiti/us, scald head) ringworm of the scalp.

tinea ciliaris a fungus infection/ringworm of the eyelashes.

tinea circinata (herpes tonsurans) ringworm of the body, an eruption, usually annular (ring-shaped, circular) in form, occurring on the non-hairy parts of the body.

tinea cruris a pruritic affection clinically resembling eczema, involving the skin of the perineal region and inner side of the thighs, sometimes the axillae, and beneath the breasts in women. It is due to the presence of a fungus, *Trichophyton cruris.*

tinea decalvans see ALOPECIA AREATA.

tinea faciei (milk crust, milk scab) see PORRIGO CAPITIS.

tinea favosa (favus) ringworm of the scalp.

tinea tonsurans ringworm of the scalp.

tinea tarsi see BLEPHARITIS.

tinea versicolor (chromophytosis, pityriasis versicolor) an eruption of brownish yellow, branny patches on the skin of the trunk, due to the presence of a fungus, *Malassezia furfur.*

tinnitus (tinnitus aurium) noises or ringing in the ears.

tipsy drunk.

tissue salts/remedies see SCHUESSLER.

titaniform having enormous strength or power, as in 'titaniform [violent] convulsions'.

titillation 1) the act or sensation of tickling 2) pleasurable excitement or stimulation, often in the context of sexual stimulation.

titration the process of determining the strength of something, usually using a standardized solution as a reference.

tocology obstetrics, the branch of medical science dealing with childbirth.

Tokay wine a very sweet and highly alcoholic (12%) white wine from Hungary. Still available today, it was used therapeutically in the second half of the 19th century.

token a livid spot on the body which (supposedly) indicates the approach of death.

tolerization 'a form of vaccination via the gut'. Patients are orally dosed with small amounts of a protein which is either directly or indirectly involved in the sufferer's particular autoimmune disease.

This treatment for autoimmune disease emerged in the late 1990s and holds promise for the transplantation of mismatched tissues or body parts. Here patients can be pre-tolerized. Instead of having to wait for a good match they could be pretreated so they could accept a larger degree of incompatibility and still have a successful transplant. For example, patients with diabetes would be given insulin; those with multiple sclerosis would be given a protein from the myelin sheath (nerve tissue); and patients suffering from uveitis would receive a protein called S-antigen.

This method stimulates the immune system, helping the host to suppress autoimmune disease. It is another example of the allopathic community using the 'like cures likes' principle. The Chinese have known of this principle for several thousand years.

tolle causam 'remove the cause' (Latin). One of the three methods of cure outlined by Hahnemann, and the one he called 'the most sublime'. The other two were based on the Law of Contraries (allopathy) and the Law of Similars (homeopathy) .

tonic 1) characterized by continuous or steady tension, as a 'tonic muscle spasm'. 2) a remedy which restores weakened function and promotes vigor and a sense of well-being. Tonics are qualified by their affinity to a particular area of the body or organ, e.g., cardiac, digestive, general, nervine, or uterine. A bitter tonic is a tonic of bitter taste which acts chiefly by stimulating the appetite and improving digestion.

tonsillitis an inflammation of the tonsil(s) with pain, increased temperature, swelling, exhaustion and painful swallowing.

Many young adults with chronic, recurring tonsillitis had their tonsils (and sometimes adenoids) removed. This practice started in the 1880s when doctors proposed tonsil removal to 'cure' the problem. Soon this operation became the most popular surgical operation during that period (actually right through to the 1950s). In the 1930s medical historian R.F. Packard complained about the procedure as 'the slaughter of tonsils', and in 1947 the distinguished medical historian A. Castiglioni commented about the popularity of tonsillectomies: "lessened, the operation still constitutes a mainstay of the specialist budget."

took as in 'the vaccination took'. This means that vaccination was successful or the individual was successfully immunized.

toper a chronic drinker; drunkard.

tophus (pl. tophi) a urate deposit found in tissue, such as cartilage around the joints. May also refer to plaque on the teeth.

tormen see TORMINA.

tormina (sing. tormen) griping pains in the bowels. Gripe.

torpent torpid; or an agent which numbs.

torpid sluggish, inactive.

torpor sluggishness, numbness, insensibility, stupor. A condition of mental or physical inactivity or insensibility.

torrefy to parch or dry by heat.

torticollis (obstipitas lateralis, wry-neck, stiff-neck, caput obstipum) a spasmodic, painful contraction of the muscles of the neck, whereby the head is drawn to one side and usually rotated so that the chin points to the other side.

torus a smooth, rounded bulging seen at the base of a pillar or pillar-like structure; a doughnut shape in general.

toss to and fro to toss backward/forwards, side to side, very restlessly.

totality of symptoms all the symptoms and signs of a disease.

As suggested by P.P. Wells, it means not only the sum of the agggregate of the symptoms, but also this other and most important fact of all, in true homoeopathic prescribing, the totality of each individual symptom of the aggregate group. In other words, a single symptom is more than a simple fact; it is a compound, made up of a fact, with its history, its origin, progress, and conditions attached. If it is a cause of suffering to the patient, then in it are included all the circumstances of its aggravation or amelioration; as to the time of its greatest intensity, position, motion, rest; how affected by eating, drinking, or the performance of any bodily function; how affected, if at all, by different mental emotions; or by any other cause of increase or relief of suffering. All this is included in the 'totality' of each single symptom, and without all this the prescriber is ignorant of the intimate nature of the symptom for which he is to find a simillimum.

As an example, Stuart Close quotes Dudgeon: "Sensation as if the whole abdomen were hollow, and at the same time a perpetual movement in the bowels (with blue rings around the eyes), and when the attack comes on in the evening, it is for a short time combined with anxiety. We have here the statement of a fact, with its elements and concomitants of time, place, and circumstances, and all these together make up one, and only one, symptom, which is classified, for convenience of reference, under the general heading of Abdomen."

Tourette's disease/syndrome (Gilles de la Tourette's disease) a form of tic; motor incoordination with echolalia (involuntary repetition of a word or sentence just spoken by another person) and coprolalia (the involuntary utterance of vulgar or obscene words).

Named after the Parisian physician, Georges Gilles de la Tourette (1857-1904), who first described the phenomenon, "Maladie des tics convulsifs."

toxalbumin toxin, a toxic albumin.

toxemia blood poisoning; the presence in the blood of the poisonous products of any disease-causing bacteria.

toxicatio the state of being poisoned.

toxicology the study of the nature, effects, and detection of poisons and the treatment of poisoning.

toxoplasmosis an infection caused by the protozoan *Toxoplasma gondii*, having a symptom complex similar to Rocky Mountain Spotted Fever, including fever, rashes, lymphatic swellings, malaise and headaches. Encephalomyelitis, joint and muscular pains, lung and heart involvements and impaired vision (inflammation of the iris, ciliary body and choroid). Chronic infections may lead to the formation of large intracellular cysts and nodules.

trachea the windpipe. A thin-walled tube of cartilaginous and membranous tissue descending from the larynx (voice box) to the bronchi and carrying air to the lungs.

tracheitis inflammation of the lining membrane of the trachea.

trachelagra a gouty or rheumatic affection of the muscles of the neck, producing torticollis.

trachoma ('granular lids', granular conjunctivitis) a chronic contagious viral inflammation which causes excessive growth of the conjunctiva (the mucus membrane covering the eyeball and lining the eyelids). If a patch of greyish vascularized membrane covers the upper half (sometimes the whole) of the cornea this is called 'pannus' and is occasionally a complication of trachoma.

tract a distributed paper, pamphlet, or brochure which contains a declaration, appeal, or material which tries to persuade and educate the reader.

William Sharp's (1805-1896) *Tracts on Homoeopathy* contained twelve chapters/tracts designed to educate and defend homeopathy: 1) What is Homoeopathy?, 2) The Defense of Homoeopathy, 3) The Truth of Homoeopathy, 4) The Small Dose of Homoeopathy, 5) The Difficulties of Homoeopathy, 6) The Advantages of Homoeopathy, 7) The Principle of Homoeopathy, 8) The Controversy of Homoeopathy, 9) The Remedies of Homoeopathy, 10) The Provings of Homoeopathy, 11) The Single Medicine of Homoeopathy, and 12) The Common Sense of Homoeopathy.

traduce to slander or defame. To speak maliciously and falsely of.

tragus the small prominence of cartilage projecting over the meatus of the external ear.

transcendentalists see HIGH FLYERS.

transient temporary.

transudation the process of passing through, as sweat passes through the skin during perspiration.

tremulous shaky.

trench mouth see VINCENT'S ANGINA.

tribadism intercourse between women.

trichiasis inversion of one or more of the eyelashes causing irritation of the corneal conjunctiva.

trichinae referring to the genus of nematode worms, *Trichinella spiralis,* often found in inadequately cooked pork. The intestinal symptoms are due to the development of the worms' adult stage and the other symptoms due to the larval migration and subsequent tissue infiltration.

trichinosis a disease caused by eating inadequately cooked pork containing trichinae, a parasitic nematode worm infesting the intestines of various mammals, and having larvae that move through the blood vessels and become encysted in the muscles. It is characterized by intestinal disorders, fever, painful muscular swelling, pain, insomnia, prostration, stiffness, vertigo, and edema of the face.

trichomonas a genus of flagellate protozoa which are often responsible for recurrent vaginal infections *(Trichomonas vaginalis).*

trichophytosis (ringworm) a superficial fungus infection caused by species of *Trichophyton.*

tricuspid having three points or cusps, as in the tricuspid valve of the heart.

tridosha the Ayurvedic concept that matter is energetically composed of three aspects: Vata (air), Pitta (fire), and Kapha (water). Just as in Chinese medicine (which has five elements), these three can be ascribed to everything. In homeopathy the remedies have their tridosha characteristics, e.g., *Nat. phos.* is Vata, *Kali mur.* is Pitta, and *Ferr. phos.* nourishes all of three doshas. See *Tridosha and Homeopathy* (Bhattacharya).

trigeminal neuralgia (prosopalgia, tic douloureux, faceache, face ague) severe, paroxysmal bursts of pain in one or more branches of the trigeminal nerve; often induced by touching trigger areas in or about the mouth.

triplopia triple vision. Seeing three images in the visual field. Objects seem multiplied.

trismus lockjaw; a firm closing of the jaw due to tonic spasm of the muscles of mastication (chewing) from the disease of the motor branch of the trigeminal nerve. An early sign of tetanus. 'Trismus neonatorum' is tetanus of the newborn infant.

trit/s see TRITURATE.

triturate 1) to perform the process of trituration. 2) a homeopathic dosage form, as in 'tablet triturate' (TT, trits). This dosage form looks like a very small round flat button about 2mm high and 3mm in diameter and weighing approximately 60-65mg. It generally dissolves faster than the globule. Tablet triturates (trits) can be manufactured as placebos then sprayed with the appropriate homeopathic dilution or can be made up with the appropriate homeopathic medication already incorporated (see TRITURATION).

trituration the reduction of a substance to a minute state or division by means of long, continued rubbing or grinding. A method of remedy preparation by which the finely powdered, medicinal substance (usually insoluble in water or alcohol) is ground for a certain time with a pestle in a mortar with a certain proportion of lactose. In this process there is a progressive division and diminution of the medicinal substance. All potencies can be made this way, but it is only necessary to do it in this manner to the third centesimal trituration before 'insoluble' substances become soluble and further dilutions can be made via the standard method (using water and alcohol).

Some texts, in regard to a particular remedy, may say "give the 12th trituration." While this may refer to the remedy in powder or solid form, this does not necessarily mean to give the remedy in powder form, but just give it in the 12th potency, whether it be powder, globules/pellets, or liquid. See POTENCY.

"By the trituration of a medicinal substance and the succussion of its solution (potentization) the medicinal forces lying hidden in it are developed and uncovered more and more and the material is itself spiritualized, if one may use that expression."—*Organon*, Para. 269, 6th Ed.

trophic referring to growth, e.g., 'trophic changes of the nails' would mean the nails are showing abnormal growth patterns or changes.

trophoedema (hereditary lymphedema) a permanent pitting edema usually affecting the lower extremities. It is the swelling of subcutaneous tissues as a result of the blockage of lymphatic vessels or nodes, causing large amounts of lymph fluid to collect in the affected region.

tropical splenomegaly see KALA-AZAR.

troublous causing trouble, turbulent, troubled.

trypsin an enzyme found in pancreatic juice which breaks down protein.

tubercle the small, rounded nodules produced by tuberculosis.

tuberculosis (phthisis, consumption, TB) an infectious disease caused by the *Mycobacterium tuberculosis* (tubercle bacillus). It can affect any area of the body but most commonly affects the lungs. In 1944 it was the seventh leading cause of death in the USA. It causes acute inflammation and may or may not be productive or proliferative. If it is, tubercular lesions are formed in response to the irritant bacteria. Symptoms include cough, fever, a general malaise, weight loss, sputum formation, hemoptysis, pain, and dyspnea. However, these symptoms come on so gradually and insidiously that the disease may proceed onto an advanced stage.

It is postulated that TB first occurred 8000 years ago in the Middle East. It originated in animals as cowpox and crossed over to humans when cattle were domesticated. However, this does not explain why TB was found in Pre-Columbian America.

tuberculous peritonitis inflammation of the lining of the abdominal cavity caused by tuberculosis.

tubera ischiadica (ischial tuberosity) the bony prominence commonly called the hip bone.

tuberous covered with small, rounded projections; knobby.

tularemia see DEERFLY FEVER.

tumefaction the condition of becoming or of being swollen.

tumefied swollen.

tumescent swelling, becoming swollen, distended, or bulging. Usually describing a body part or organ.

tumid swollen or distended.

tumor a solid mass greater than 1 cm in diameter.

tumult a commotion, agitation, overaction, disturbed action.

tumultuous in a stuttering, disorganized, confused manner.

tunica vaginalis a layer of tissue (fascia) enveloping the testicle and spermatic cord in the scrotum.

turbid corpus vitreum cloudiness of the vitreous fluid of the eye.

turbid cloudy, muddy.

turbinate relating to the nasal bones, or concha. Any one of the three nasal conchae; a medial projection of thin bone from the lateral wall of the nasal cavity, covered by mucous membrane and designated by position as superior, middle, or inferior.

turgid rigid, erect, or stiff.

tussal (tussive, tussicular) relating to a cough. (L. *tussis*, 'cough').

tussiculation hacking cough.

tussis convulsiva see WHOOPING COUGH.

twinge a sudden momentary sharp pain. A darting sensation or pain.

twitter to utter a succession of light chirping or tremulous sounds, as a bird. To tremble with nervous agitation or excitement. Light, tremulous speech or laughter.

tyloma any callosity or callus.

tylosis a callosity or hardening of the edges of the eyelids.

tympanic like a drum.

tympanitic resonant or drum-like in tone. A term applied to an elastic, distended state of the abdomen, sounding like a drum when struck and usually caused by an accumulation of air.

tympanites (drum-belly, tympany) a bloating of the belly, caused by excess of air or gas. May refer to a drum-like sound.

tympanitis otitis media (commonly known as an ear infection).

tympanum ear drum.

type effect hypothesis see KOETSCHAU HYPOTHESIS/LAW.

typhlitis (cecitis) appendicitis. Inflammation of the cecum.

typhoid fever (ship fever, enteric fever, putrid fever) a systemic infectious disease carried by *Salmonella typhi,* which enters the body via food and water and lodges in the intestine and spleen. The principle lesions are an enlarged spleen and mesenteric lymph nodes. The intestinal mucous membrane is also affected by a catarrhal inflammation.

After an incubation period of 1-2 weeks the disease sets in with weakness, headache, pains and a tendency towards diarrhea and nosebleeds. The temperature gradually rises, becoming higher each successive evening, reaching a maximum of 104^0-105^0F in about 2 weeks. Then it begins to fall, reaching normal levels by the 4th week. After the first week a peculiar eruption appears which consists of rose-colored spots on the chest and abdomen. These disappear in another week. Nervous symptoms are prominent, consisting of headache, slight deafness, stupor, and a muttering delirium. Complications may occur, these being intestinal bleeding, perforation of the bowel, peritonitis, pneumonia and inflammation of the kidneys. The disease usually resolves itself in about four weeks, and prior to the introduction of antibiotics had a mortality rate of 12%.

typhoid a generic term for a species of low fever, characterized by debility.

typhus (jail fever, gaol fever, continued fever, classic typhus, ship fever, hospital fever, camp fever, dungeon fever, fleck typhus) a rickettsial disease *(Rickettsia prowazekii)* transmitted by lice *(Pediculus humanus)*. Symptoms produced after a 7-14 day incubation period include head, back and limb pains and fever rapidly rising to 104-105⁰ F. An eruption occurs on the 4th or 5th day as rose-colored spots scattered all over the body become hemorrhagic. Chief complications are a high fever, pneumonia and inflammation of the kidneys. Other symptoms may include dry tongue, stupor, delirium, and great prostration.

typology the study of types, as in a systematic classification of human beings according to their physical and psychological characteristics, e.g., persons who have similar bodily shapes and character particularities and similar pathological tendencies. That information is used to gauge or assess a person's weaknesses and strengths so that advice can be provided to restore or improve health and prevent disease. The ultimate purpose is to allow the person to realize his true self or potential.

The *Pulsatilla* 'typology' would mean persons who are especially sensitive to *Pulsatilla* and its therapeutic effects. Generally (but not always) they are women with blonde or light brown hair and blue eyes, mild-mannered and sensitive.

Typology may be used in assessing patients and finding remedies. You may wish to consult Leon Vannier's interesting *Typology in Homoeopathy*. He classified people into three constitutions according to their skeletal configuration. Carbonic *(Calc c.)*: "This man is literally a square. He is of medium build, with a square head, square white teeth, regularly set in his jaws. When his arms hang down the forearm forms a slight angle with the humerus. Phosphoric *(Calc. p.):* is tall, slender, graceful, with long, yellowish, but regularly shaped teeth. When his arms hang down, the forearm forms a straight line with the humerus. Fluoric *(Calc. f.)*: is the irregular type. He may be tall or short, but is likely to be malproportioned. His teeth are irregular in shape and do not fit well in his jaws. When his arms hang down, the forearm forms an obtuse angle with the humerus." - *The Layman Speaks,* 19:8, p. 266-7.

Typology is a vast subject explored by many persons, religions and cultures. For example, Hinduism has its typology in Ayurveda (Vata, Pitta, Kapha), Sufism is a prime influencer of the Enneagram, which has nine distinct personalities (consult Riso's *Understand the Enneagram: The*

Practical Guide to Personality Types. Also consult Eli Jaxon-Bear, Almaas, Naranjo, Palmer, H.F. Keyes, etc.).

Perhaps familiar to all is the Sheldon's typology which stratifies human beings into mesomorphs, endomorphs, and ectomorphs. Typing or classifying the 'human animal' is something which has been with us for thousands of years. It is in our nature to group and dissect, to categorize and deconstruct. It is part of human nature to constantly strive to understand the world and our fellow man. It is no wonder that 'typing' is so ubiquitous in the makeup of world cultures. There are astrological types, personality types in Eastern traditions, psychological typologies, Jungian types, mental typologies, business/leadership typologies, Native American typologies, etc. Consult *Who Am I?* (edited by Robert Frager, PhD.). See CONSTITUTION.

typus periodicity; periodical attacks.

tyriasis see ELEPHANTIASIS.

tyrranism sadism or a lust for cruelty.

ᴜ ᵁ U U U ᵁ ᴜ

ubi morbus ibi remedium 'where the sickness is, there is the cure' (L.).

ulcerative relating to or causing an ulcer or ulcers.

ulcus an ulcer.

ulcus cruris an ulcer located on the thigh or leg.

ulcus exedens see NOLI ME TANGERE.

uletic depending upon the context, relating to the gums or relating to a scar.

ulitis (gingivitis) inflammation of the gums.

ulnar pertaining to the inside (medial) aspect of the arm. Contrasted with 'radial' (the outside aspect of the arm).

umbilicus the navel.

undulant fever referring to the wavy appearance of the long temperature curve, marked clinically by repeated febrile paroxysms a week or more in duration, attended with enlargement of the spleen, profuse sweating, and painful swelling of the joints, separated by intervals of normal or nearly normal temperature.

unicist 1) one who prescribes homeopathic remedies in the classical way (one remedy at a time, usually in high potency). 2) The belief that there is but one venereal virus [*archaic*].

union by the first intention healing of wounds or cuts by adhesion (the growing together of the opposite surfaces of the wound) without suppuration or granulation. Healing by second intention occurs when suppuration and/or granulation is present (incarnation).

unguentum (pl. unguenta) ointment.

unrequited unreturned, as in 'unrequited love' (when one person loves another who does not return the sentiment).

uranist (urnist) a sexual pervert; archaic word for homosexual.

uremia a toxic condition of the blood from accumulation of urea and other urinary constituents, usually due to some form of kidney disease. Symptoms chiefly include headache, vomiting, dyspnea, insomnia, delirium, convulsion, and coma.

uresis urination.

urethra the canal through which urine is discharged, extending from the neck of the bladder to the point of emptying. In the male it is 8–9 inches long, in the female approximately 1.5 inches.

uretic relating to the urine. Increasing the excretion of urine, diuretic.

urethritis inflammation of the urethra.

uridrosis (urhidrosis) a condition in which some of the constituents of the urine, generally urea, are excreted in excessive amounts in the sweat.

urocele the leakage (extravasation) of urine into the scrotum.

urticaria a generic term for edematous hives or rashes. From the nettle, *Urtica dioica,* a weed which causes a stinging sensation and produces a rash which usually fills with fluid.

urticaria tuberosa (urticaria gigans, angioneurotic edema) urticaria occurring when the subcutaneous tissue is lax, being marked by the occurrence of large edematous, tumor-like swellings.

uveal pertaining to the middle coat of the eye, or uvea.

uvula the small fleshy finger-like appendage which hangs down from the roof of the mouth at the rear of the throat.

v v V V V v v

V.S. (venesectio, bleeding) an abbreviation for venesection. V.S.B., 'bleed in the arm' (venesectio brachii).

vaccinia (vaccina) see COWPOX.

vacillate to waver, be indecisive.

vaccination inoculation with a vaccine (a suspension of attenuated or killed microorganisms) in order to afford protection against that like disease, e.g., smallpox vaccine is administered to healthy persons to stimulate the immune system to recognize smallpox and eradicate it if the person becomes infected.

Edward Jenner (1749-1823) is considered the founder of immunology and coined the term 'virus', though he did not coin the term 'vaccination'. He also described anaphylaxis and is the first pioneer in the field of virology. His theories were collected into his 1798 book, *An Inquiry into the Causes and Effects of the Variolae Vaccinae, a disease discovered in some of the western counties of England, particularly Gloucestershire, and known by the name of the Cow Pox.*

This vaccination process spread around the world quite rapidly, i.e., India and America, where President Jefferson vaccinated his family and neighbors. Jenner discovered that persons who had had cowpox were immune from contracting smallpox. After experimentation he made his vaccine from the matter from the arm of a milkmaid who had been infected with cowpox and who had been known to be resistant to smallpox. This matter was, on May 14, 1796, inserted into James Phipps, a country boy. When exposed to smallpox he did not become infected.

vaccinosis the malaise or effects/sequelae caused by the administration of vaccines to healthy individuals, including fever, muscular aches, bone pain, and prostration. For interesting theories about the chronic effects, consult H. Coulter's *DPT: A Shot in the Dark.*

Boenninghausen first spoke of the similarity between smallpox disease and *Thuja* ('Uber die Heilkraft der Thuja gegen Menschenblattern' in *Allgemeine Homoopathische Zeitung*, 37/1849). The term 'vaccinosis' was coined by Dr. Goullon of Weimar in a paper he published on the subject in 1877. He related it to the sycosis as described by Hahnemann and related the symptoms occuring after smallpox vaccination to the symptoms of sycotic gonorrhea. Later, J.C. Burnett described the phenomenon

272

in *Vaccinosis and Its Cure by Thuja* (1884) where he reported his experiences curing the diseases following vaccination with *Thuja*. It is postulated that many of the ill-effects of today's vaccinations can be treated with *Thuja*.

vade mecum a useful item which a person constantly consults or uses (L., 'go with me').

vaginismus (vaginism) painful spasms of the vagina during sexual activity and/or preventing sexual intercourse.

vagitus the crying of an infant.

vagotonia an abnormal increase in vagus nerve activity. An abnormal slowness of the heart, faintness and a sudden loss of strength are the typical characteristics. Constipation, sweating, blood pressure instability, and involuntary motor spasms may also be present. "Let us also think of the trio of vagotonia: *Ipecac, Hydrocyanic acid, Lobelia inflata.*"—Rousseau & Fortier-Bernoville, *Diseases of the Respiratory and Digestive System of Children*, p. 63.

vagus/vagi the vagus nerve. See PNEUMOGASTRIC NERVE.

Valleix's point douloureux a tender point found in the course of certain nerves in peripheral neuralgias where they pass through openings in fascia or issue from bony canals. First described by F.L.I. Valleix (1807-1855), a French physician. (Fr. *douloureux*, 'painful').

valvulitis (dicliditis) inflammation of a valve, especially a heart valve.

varicella (chickenpox, waterpox) an acute infectious disease marked by an eruption of (usually) non-scarring vesicles. There is usually a slight fever which lasts from a few days to a week.

varicella coniformis a form of chickenpox where the characteristic vesicle eruptions resemble cones.

varices (cirsoid) enlarged and tortuous veins, arteries or lymphatic vessels.

varicocele (cirsocele) varicose veins of the testes; varicosities of the scrotal veins forming a soft, elastic swelling which feels like a collection of worms. It causes pain and a dragging, weighty sensation.

varicose swollen, knotted and tortuous, referring to blood vessels. A varicose ulcer is due to varicose veins. Adjective form of VARIX.

variegated marked by a diversity of coloration.

variola smallpox. An acute eruptive contagious disease marked at the onset by chills, high fever, backache, and headache; in from 2-5 days the constitutional symptoms subside (those symptoms just mentioned) and then the skin eruptions appear. These are at first papular, then in turn become vesicles and then pustules, which dry, form scabs and fall off leaving permanent scars (pock-marks).

varioloid resembling smallpox. A mild form of smallpox occurring in those who are relatively immune either naturally or as a result of a previous vaccination. The course of the disease is shortened and the different stages of the eruption follow each other rapidly, or the lesions may abort at any stage.

varix an enlarged and tortuous vein, artery, or lymphatic vessel.

vas vessel.

vascular deafness of Cooper deafness due to obstruction of the auditory tube. A.P. Cooper (1768-1841), an English surgeon, not only described this syndrome (1801) but also made a number of contributions in understanding the nature of hernias.

vasoconstriction a constriction or narrowing of blood vessels.

vault the rear portion of the throat, as in the pharyngeal 'vault'.

vaulted places cellars, basements, and other underground locations.

Vegatest a method of testing and diagnosing the health of an individual developed by H.W. Schimmel of Germany. Instrumentation is used to access the energy fields of the body, i.e., acupuncture sites, in order to diagnose and treat disease. Vegatest is an acronym for Vegetative Reflex Test (VRT). See FUNCTIONAL MEDICINE, ACUPUNCTURE, EAV.

Vega Rozenberg's boxes sixty or so categories of remedies which Vega Rozenberg has developed in his homeopathic prescribing approach.

vegetative dystonia autonomic nervous system dysfunction. 'Vegetative' refers to the fact that many of our bodily functions are plant-like or automatic (in other words, we don't think about them and these are under the control of the autonomic nervous system). 'Dystonia' refers to a disturbance in these 'automatic' functions, such as heart irregularities, sleep dysfunctions, and gastrointestinal distresses.

vegetative reflexes/nervous system the autonomic nervous system as it relates to the digestive system (reflexes which need not be given any thought as they are done automatically or reflexively).

velum any structure resembling a veil or curtain. That part of the back of the hard palate that extends back and downward, separating the mouth cavity from the pharynx.

velum palati the soft palate. See SOFT PALATE.

veneration a profound respect or reverence.

venereal disease a disease acquired primarily through sexual intercourse. This term was used by Hahnemann primarily in reference to syphilis and gonorrhea.

venery sexual intercourse (L. *veneris,* 'belonging to Venus', goddess of love).

venesection (V.S.) opening a vein to allow blood out. Bloodletting.

ventriculus (pl. ventriculi) a cavity, commonly referring to the stomach; i.e., 'cancer ventriculi' means 'cancer of the stomach'.

verdigris the greenish deposit upon copper vessels of copper salts (acetates) caused by oxidation.

vermiform wormlike.

vermifuge any agent that kills or expels intestinal worms.

vermin parasitic insects, such as lice and bedbugs.

verminosis infestation with worms.

vernacular pertaining to or existing in a particular locality; endemic.

verruca a wart. 'Verruca vulgaris' is another name for the common wart, which is usually seen over the hands, about the nails or on the arms or legs, and is more common in children. Lesions are horny projections of normal skin color but soon become dark with papillary projections. They are of various sizes but usually are round and from 1/3 to 2cm. in diameter.

In the 1800s, 'wart' was a very imprecise term/rubric as it could mean any growth on the skin, e.g., sebaceous cyst, wen, etc.

vertex the top or crown of the head.

vertigo dizziness, giddiness, a sensation of irregular or whirling motion, either of oneself or of external objects.

vertigo caduca the dizziness or giddiness attending the discharge of the caduca during childbirth. See CADUCA.

verum true, real, or genuine.

VES an acronym for a homeopathic computer software program, Vithoulkas Expert System.

vesical pertaining to the bladder.

vesical calculus bladder or kidney stone.

vesical spasm a spasm of the bladder.

vesical paresis a partial paralysis of the bladder.

vesicant an agent producing a bleb or blister.

vesication the formation of vesicles.

vesicle a small sac containing liquid or gas. A small blister no larger than 1cm in diameter caused by the accumulation of fluid between the upper layers of the skin, e.g., contact dermatitis, early chickenpox and herpes zoster.

vesicocele see CYSTOCELE.

vesicular erysipelas an acute, infectious disease due to the *Streptococcus* bacterium, characterized by a spreading inflammation of the subcutaneous tissues with formation of vesicles.

veta see MOUNTAIN SICKNESS.

vexation the state or condition of being annoyed, irritated, or harassed.

vibices the large purple spots which appear under the skin in certain virulent or fatal fevers.

vibriones an archaic term referring to *Vibrio,* the motile, comma-shaped bacillus which is the cause of cholera.

vicarial phenomenon see VICARIATION.

vicariation the transition of the disease from one phase to another. The supersession of one manifestation by another. Progressive and regressive vicariation is one of the principles of homotoxicology. 'Progressive v.' means the disease is worsening, 'regressive v.' means the disease is proceeding in a direction of cure, for example, the eczema-asthma syndrome (when the patient's asthma worsens the eczema seems to get better and vice versa).

"The supersession of one manifestation by another."—Werner Frase, M.D. See HOMOTOXICOLOGY.

vicarious acting for another. Acting as or being a substitute. Taking place in one part instead of another, e.g., 'v. menstruation' is a periodic loss of blood from the stomach (or other part) in cases in which normal menstruation is absent or suppressed.

vide (vid.) 'look to', 'see', 'refer to' the text or reference (L., imperative of *videre,* 'to look or see').

Vienna paste/caustic an ointment of *potassa cum calce.* A caustic ointment made up of equal parts of caustic potash and quicklime (CaO, burnt lime, unslaked lime, calcium oxide, unslacked lime).

Vincent's angina (trench mouth, diphtheroid angina, ulceromembranous angina) an ulceromembranous sore throat and stomatitis of the mucous membranes of the throat and mouth. Simply, an inflammatory condition with death of gum tissue. Pain is the characteristic feature; symptoms such as bad breath, salivation, a slight fever and malaise are common.

vinous wine-like. Having the nature of wine.

violaceous having a violet-blackish color.

viridis greenish, or having a green hue.

virilism the development of male secondary sexual characteristics in a woman; particularly the growth of hair.

virus 1) contagion or poison. The contagious or poisonous matter (from ulcers, snake bites, etc.) as applied to organic poisons. 2) One of a group of microbes smaller than bacteria consisting of a core of a single nucleic acid surrounded by a protein coat, having the ability to multiply only within a living cell). Unknown to 19th and early 20th century medicin, it was archaically defined as a special contagion, imperceptible to our senses, which acts in exceedingly minute quantities to cause disease in the body.

vis medicatrix naturae the natural curative power, the power inherent in the organism of overcoming disease without the aid of any therapeutic agencies. (L. 'the healing power of nature').

viscera the contents of the body cavities. Internal organs, especially those contained within the abdominal and chest cavities.

viscid thick and adhesive; sticky.

vital force that energy which maintains life in the individual. It is unique from person to person, each being endowed with his or her own quality of it. The vital force is a unique principle distinct from chemical or physical phenomenon. See VITALISM.

"Vital Force and Soul are in the cell as well as in the body. The same thing rules the remedy and, stripped of its grossness and placed upon the tongue, it will be taken into the economy instantly. I went a thousand miles once to place a dose of *Zincum* on the tongue of a paralyzed woman who felt its effects in less than thirty seconds and in six weeks her paralysis left her." - J.T. Kent.

"In the healthy condition of man the Spirit-like Vital Force, the Dynamis that animates the material body, rules with unbounded sway and retains all the parts of the organism in admirable, harmonious, vital operation, as regards both sensations and functions, so that our indwelling, reason gifted mind can freely employ this living healthy instrument for the higher powers of our existence." - Hahnemann (*Organon*, P. 43)

vitalism the theory that all animal functions are dependent upon a special form of energy or force, the vital force, distinct from any other of the physical forces.

Vithoulkian homeopathy the practice of homeopathy based upon the philosophy and work of George Vithoulkas. Like Kentian and Hahnemannian homeopathy, it is classical homeopathy. Vithoulkian homeopathy differs from the others primarily in its approach to case analysis and in its reliance on remedy essences, keynotes, and case totality.

The essence consists of three elements: the causative factor of the patient's complaint, the timeliness or tempo of the complaint, and the center of the pathology. This essence approach also includes the personality and physical appearance of the patient. The keynote is a particular symptom which suggests a specific remedy. Totality of course includes repertorization. Vithoulkian homeopathy also places importance on understanding the concepts of 'layering', vital force and the three planes (mental, emotional, and physical) as they relate to disease and the individual. The model thus created allows the practitioner to determine the level of health and the effectiveness of treatment.

vitiate to impair the value or quality of. To make impure. To corrupt or render useless. To spoil.

vitiligo see LEUCODERMA.

vitreous glassy, resembling glass. The translucent fluid between the lens and retina. The fluid in the eyeball itself. See VITREOUS BODY.

vitreous body (corpus vitreum) a transparent jelly-like substance filling the interior of the eyeball behind the lens.

vitriol sulphuric acid.

vives enlarged glands, sometimes suppurating, on the side of the head below the ear. Young horses are particularly prone to developing such an affliction.

vivisection experimental research on living animals including operations, injections, blood tests, and feeding experiments. The dissection of living animals for purposes of study and investigation. An anti-vivisectionist is one opposed to these sorts of procedures and is opposed to cruelty to animals in general.

viz. (L. *videlicet*, 'see, it is permitted') that is to say; namely.

vola the palm of the hand or the sole of the foot.

Voll the surname of the scientist responsible for developing EAV.

Reinhold Voll (1909-1989) developed the first biofeedback unit for investigating homeopathy and acupuncture in 1954. He used this technology to cure his bladder cancer when medical colleagues had given him little hope. There are over 900 Voll-points on the body. Dr. Voll also did seminal work on the relationship between energetic disturbances in the body and tonsils, teeth cavitations, and ear and sinus infections: *Interrelations of Odontons and Tonsils to Organs, Fields of Disturbance, and Tissue Systems* (1978). See EAV.

volo-therapy this method of treatment is related to autosuggestion, telepathy and psychic cures, as it was developed by homeopath Sheldon Leavitt (1848-1933) who was interested in those phenomena. He wrote a large treatise, *The Science and Art of Obstetrics* (Gross-Delbridge, 2nd ed., 1892, 769pp). Towards the end of his life he became quite interested in the above-mentioned methods of healing and wrote *Psycho-Therapy in the Practice of Medicine and Surgery* (2nd ed., 1907, 247pp) and his last, *Volo-therapy: A new method of treatment for every form of disease and for the self-preservation of health* (1917, 119pp).

voluptuous devoted to or frequently indulging in sensual gratifications. A full and appealing form. 'Voluptuous itching', a combination of itching and sexual arousal.

volvulus a twisting of the intestine upon itself which occludes the lumen. It occurs most frequently in the sigmoid flexure.

vomer a slender thin bone of the nose forming the partition between the nostrils.

vomica an abscess of the lungs.

vomitus matutinus vomiting in the morning.

vorax voracious, ravenous. See LUPUS VORAX.

votary a person who is devoted (or even addicted) to some subject or pursuit.

vox the voice.

VRT vegetative reflex test. See VEGATEST, EAV, FUNCTIONAL MEDICINE.

vulnerary having curative qualities; useful in healing wounds.

vulnus a wound.

vulva (pudendum muliebre) the labia majora and the cleft between them. The external female genitalia including the labia majora, labia minora, clitoris, and vestibule of the vagina.

W W W W W W W

Waldeyer's tonsillar ring (Waldeyer's ring, Waldeyer's throat-ring) the incomplete ring of lymphoid tissue formed by the faucial, lingual, and pharyngeal tonsils. From the German anatomist H.W.G. von Waldeyer-Hartz (1836-1921).

Wartenberg's disease (chiralgia paresthetica) a weakening of the muscular control of the upper eyelid in facial paralysis, first described by American neurologist Robert Wartenberg.

wash-leather skin a trophic change in the skin, occurring in certain cases of chronic constitutional disease, in which the texture is altered and a silver coin drawn across the skin will leave a dark line.

Wassermann's reaction/test a diagnostic test for syphilis.

wasting disease a disease which lingers and weakens the body.

water canker (noma, canker) see NOMA.

water pox see VARICELLA.

waterbrash (heartburn, pyrosis) from the German terms *Wasseraufschwulken* and *Wurmerbeseigen* which both mean 'rising of water from the stomach into the mouth', as per *Guide to Kent's Repertory* (A.N. Currim, p. 129). It does not necessarily mean a watery, acid fluid regurgitated from the stomach, sometimes accompanied by nausea. Thus there could be a subtle difference between pyrosis and waterbrash.

waxen pale, smooth and lustrous. Covered with wax.

waxing kernels enlarged inguinal and submaxillary lymph glands in children.

weal see WHEAL.

weapon ointment/salve a complicated, compounded ointment applied to the weapon responsible for creating the wound, as well as to the wound itself. Supposedly this helped the wound to heal.

This form of treatment was popularly employed in the 19th century. This ointment, also called 'powder of sympathy' or 'sympathetic powder', was invented by Kenelm Digby, as described in his book, *Theatrum Sympatheticum . . .* (1661). The supposedly 'active' ingredient was powdered vitriol. A bandage was to be taken from the wound, immersed in the powder, and kept there till the wound healed. His book was widely translated and distributed.

Webb's remedy used specifically for the prevention of rabies: 2 oz. box-

279

wood, 2 oz. fresh rue leaves, and 1/2 oz. sage, mixed and used as a poultice which would absorb the poisons. It is listed in Hale's *New Remedies*.

Weil's disease (spirochetal jaundice) a disease caused by the spirochete *Leptospira icterohaemorrhagiae*, characterized by fever, nausea, headache, muscular pain and jaundice. Named after the German physician Adolph Weil (1848-1916), who first described it and differentiated it from other forms of acute jaundice.

wen a sebaceous cyst, especially one occurring on the scalp. A cyst containing oily matter.

Werlhoff's disease see PURPURA HEMORRHAGICA.

Werlhoffi morbus maculosus see PURPURA HEMORRHAGICA.

wesen a German word employed by Hahnemann to describe the essence of something. A person, animal, or plant has a *wesen*, as do diseases and medicines.

wheal the raised ridge or bump on the skin, often accompanied by itching and burning, characteristic of hives or urticaria.

whelk a wheal; a pustule; a tubercle or nodule on the face, ionthus. See CARBUNCLE.

whey-like resembling whey (the liquid part of milk separating from the curd in coagulation).

white flux diarrhea; mainly referring to diarrhea occuring in Native Americans during the 1800s.

white swelling tuberculosis of the joints (tubercular arthritis), as the affected joint takes on a glossy, bright appearance. The joints become rigid while the muscles around the joints waste away. There is swelling with an exudation of fluid and a dull pain which is < motion, pressure and jarring.

whites see LEUCORRHEA or FLUOR ALBUS.

whitlow (panaris, felon, panaritium, paronychia) a festering inflammation usually around the nail. It is usually superficial but may be deep-seated, affecting bone. See PANARITIUM.

wholistic see HOLISM.

whooping cough (pertussis, morbus cucullaris, tussis convulsiva) an acute infectious disease marked by recurrent attacks of spasmodic coughing continued until the breath is exhausted, then ending with a deep, noisy inspiration.

Wilder's Law a law which follows Koetschau's hypothesis and the Arndt-Schulz law but takes into consideration patients' varying sensitivities to given doses. From Joseph Wilder, who proposed thse theories in the1930s. He realized that what is small for one will be medium or large for another:

"The reaction to administration of a medicinal substance depends on the 'excitement' of the vegetative nerves. If 'excitement' is high, a stimulant will have little effect and may be 'paradoxically' depressant. By the same token, 'depressants' have less impact when the individual or system is already depressed."—H. Coulter, *Divided Legacy, Vol. 4*, p. 461, 1994. See KOETSCHAU'S HYPOTHESIS, ARNDT-SCHULZ LAW.

Willan's leprosy see PSORIASIS LEPRA.

willfulness obstinacy, stubbornness; unyielding determination.

Wilson's syndrome (hepatolenticular degeneration) a condition marked by muscular tremors, weakness, loss of weight, cirrhosis of the liver, mental deterioration and the Kayser-Fleischer ring (a golden brown or brownish green pigment behind the limbic border of the cornea).

Wilson's disease extensive dermatitis exfoliation, an acute or chronic inflammation of the skin, in which the epidermis is shed more or less freely in large or small scales. First described by English dermatologist Sir W.J.E. Wilson (1809-1884).

Winckel's disease a rapidly fatal disease of the newborn, marked by cyanosis, jaundice, hemoglobinuria, various hemorrhages, and fatty degeneration of the heart and liver. First described by the German obstetrician Franz von Winckel (1837-1911).

windgall a soft and puffy tumor.

Winiwater's disease (Winiwater-Buerger disease, thromboangitis obliterans) see THROMBOANGITIS OBLITERANS.

wiseacre a simpleton or one who affects wisdom. Can also mean the opposite, a wise man or sage.

womb the uterus.

wooden tongue see ACTINOMYCOSIS.

woolsorter's disease (anthrax, malignant pustule) the pulmonary form of anthrax caused by inhalation of dust laden with *Bacillus anthracis*; the symptoms are often obscure, pointing only to some mild pulmonary infection, but death is common and frequently sudden. See ANTHRAX.

worm colic colic induced by the presence of worms in the body.

wound, wall, mask the main concepts behind Ananda Zaren's philosophy of homeotherapeutics.

The *wound* is a sudden and unexpected event (or series of events) which forms a protective layer around the core. It is a negative impulse and has to be protected. The wound helps the practitioner to understand the patient and where symptoms have come from. Wounds can be large (betrayal, abandonment, war, fire, bone fractures, burns, abuse, head injuries, neglect) or small as when a child gets all As and one B on his report card and the father says: 'Why didn't you get all As?' or a child makes his bed and does a good job but the mother finds fault saying, perhaps in a negative tone, 'You didn't tuck that corner in!' These can be small woundings. The wound is never prescribed upon.

The *wall*, the second layer of defense or protection, is the adaptation which the individual makes to that trauma or wounding. It is the character structure. According to Zaren it does not shift over time-it is always there. It is where the energy is constricted; where the patient is suffering. The symptoms of this wall determine the remedy but only the most prominent or strongest symptoms (i.e., asthma, eczema, suicidal thoughts, panic attacks, PMS, chronic fatigue syndrome) are used in determining the remedy.

The *mask* is just that: an instrument which the patient uses, more often than not unconsciously, to deny real emotions. Thus an individual will feel more himself when acting superior, aggressive, haughty, etc. than when warm, admiring or compassionate. It is a role game, facade, or veneer which tries to keep others from seeing inside to the inner reality. Zaren says that this mask becomes part of the persons being. This mask can turn on and off whereas the wall is intact and present all the time. Examples include childishness, smiling, attitudes of 'everything is fine', or 'I can do it all' (inner strength), etc. The mask is not prescribed upon.

"In summary, the wound, wall, mask is a model that can provide a method for discerning and interpreting the symptoms of a case, such that the rubrics used and the remedy selected will address the central disturbance or core pathology." - Zaren, *Materia Medica: Core Elements of the Materia Medica of the Mind, Vol. I* (1993, p. 42).

writer's cramp/palsy/spasm (scrivener palsy, mogigraphia, graphospasm) an occupational neurosis affecting chiefly the muscles of the thumb and two adjoining fingers of the indicated hand, induced by excessive writing, violin playing, telegraphing, etc. It may occur in one of four main forms: spastic, paralytic, neuralgic, and tremulous. A scrivener was a professional writer, generally drawing up contracts or other prepared writings for a fee.

writhing twisting, squirming, or moving with a contorted motion, as if in pain.

wry neck (obstipitas lateralis, torticollis) a painful, stiff neck, a contraction, often spasmodic, of the neck muscles whereby the head is drawn to one side and usually rotated so that the chin points to the other side.

x x X X X x x

X⁰R an archaic acronym for the 30th centesimal potency.

XM another way of referring to the 10M potency. XMK is the 10M potency made according to the Korsakovian method. See POTENCY.

xanthodontous having yellow teeth.

xanthopia see XANTHOPSIA.

xanthopsia yellow vision. The condition in which objects look yellow, sometimes accompanying jaundice.

xanthelasma see XANTHOMA.

xanthoma (xanthelasma) a skin disease characterized by the presence of yellowish orange colored nodules or slightly raised plates in the skin, especially of the eyelids.

xenocritic one who criticizes other persons or concepts which one does not fully understand or know.

xenomenia (menoplania) vicarious menstruation. The discharge of blood at the time of menstruation from some place other than the vagina. it is thought to result from an increased capillary permeability related to the woman's menstrual cycle.

xenophobia a fear of strangers or foreigners.

xerasia a disease of the hair whereby it is very dry, brittle, and does not grow.

xeroderma (mild ichthyosis) a condition of roughened skin due to a slight increase of the horny layer and diminished cutaneous secretions. See ICHTHYOSIS.

xerophthalmia (xeroma) abnormal dryness of the eyeball.

xerosis dryness. The normal evolutionary sclerosis of the tissues with aging.

xerostomia dry mouth.

xiphoid (metasternum, processus xiphoideus, ensiform) sword-shaped, referring to the cartilaginous process, shaped like a sword-tip, which forms the lower extremity of the sternum (breastbone).

Y Y Y Y Y Y Y

yaws (zymotic papilloma) see FRAMBOESIA.

yclept 'known as', 'called', or 'named' (archaic).

yellow fever an acute infectious disease of tropical or subtropical regions of America caused by a virus harbored by the *Aedes aegypti* mosquito. After the bite and a period of incubation varying from a few hours to several days, the disease begins with a chill and pain in the head, back and limbs. The temperature rises rapidly to $103^0 - 105^0$ F, vomiting occurs, bowels become constipated, the urine is scanty and albuminous. A remission follows, after which, in severe cases, the temperature rises to its original height, jaundice develops and vomitus becomes black due to the presence of blood. Intestinal hemorrhages may occur. The disease is often fatal. A vaccine is available for this disease as are homeopathics, of course.

yellow saddle a yellowish discoloration of the skin across the bridge of the nose resembling a saddle. Often found on the faces of persons fitting the *Sepia* picture.

yerba herb (Spanish).

zZ**Z**Zzz

zeismus (zeism) the belief that pellagra is due to the ingestion of Indian corn/ maize. See PELLAGRA.

zephyr any gentle breeze. The west wind, named for the Grecian god Zephyrus.

Zinn's artery the central artery of the retina, first described by J.G. Zinn (1727-1759), a German anatomist.

zona see HERPES ZOSTER. 'Zona' means 'a belt or sash', and the most common form of herpes zoster or shingles is the lesional outbreak which wraps around the abdomen. Lesions may also appear on the face and neck.

zonesthesia (girdle-sensation, strangalesthesia) a sensation as if a rope were drawn about the body.

zoonosis any disease in man acquired from an animal, such as rabies.

zoster see HERPES ZOSTER.

zygoma the cheek bone. The arch formed by the union of the zygomatic process of the temporal bone and the malar bone.

zygomatic referring to the cheek bone.

zymosis fermentation. An infectious disease due to a fungus. The process of infection. Breakdown or decomposition; an archaic term for prostration and septicemia.

zymotic relating to fermentation. The zymotic doctrine/theory was in vogue during the mid to late 1800s and described infectious diseases as essentially a fermentative process. This term was used to describe a vast number of 'epidemic, endemic and contagious' diseases which acted in a similar way to the fermentative process. After a while the term became restricted to the chief fevers and contagious diseases, e.g., cholera, measles, scarlet fever, whooping cough, diphtheria, typhus, and typhoid fever. Compare to 'septic' in the 'fever' section of the repertory.

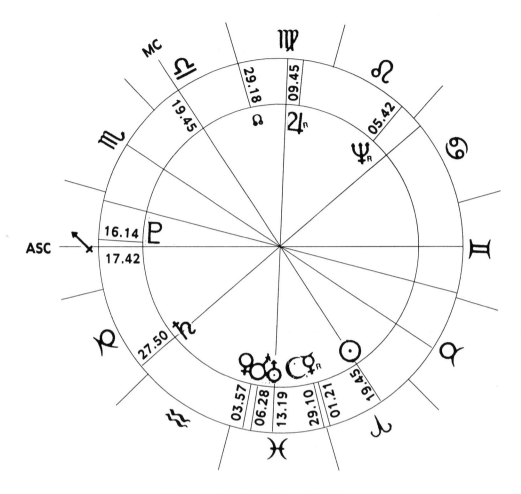

Christian Friedrich Samuel Hahnemann
geboren 10./11. April 1755 Mitternacht in Meißen

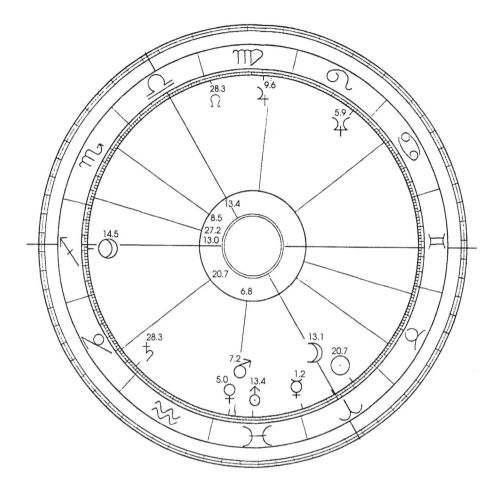

S.C.F. Hahnemann
April 10, 1755
23:40:12 MEZ
Meissen
13:28:00 O
51:10:00 N

Rising Sign is Sagittarius
Sun, Moon, and Mercury in Aires
Mars, Venus, and Uranus in Pisces
Saturn in Capricorn
Pluto in Sagittarius
Jupiter in Virgo
Neptune in Leo

Courtesy of Wolfgang Dobereiner, The Munich Rhythm Theory Press
Munich, West Germany

Abdominal Regions

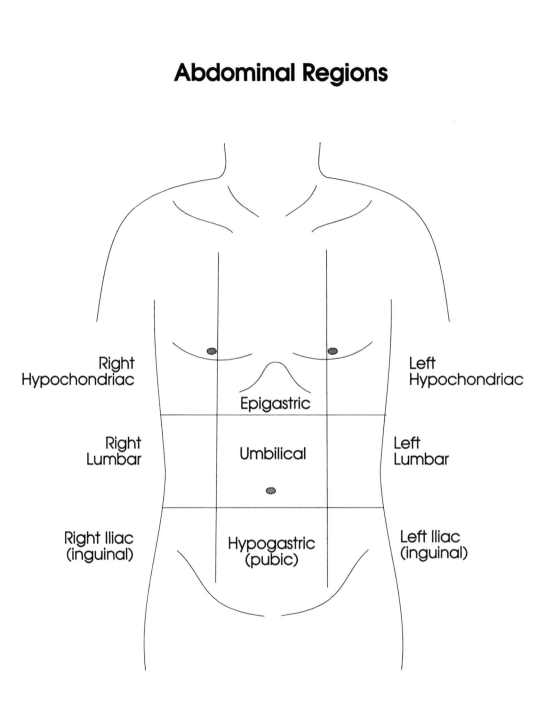

Right
Hypochondriac

Epigastric

Left
Hypochondriac

Right
Lumbar

Umbilical

Left
Lumbar

Right Iliac
(inguinal)

Hypogastric
(pubic)

Left Iliac
(inguinal)

Superior (cephalic)

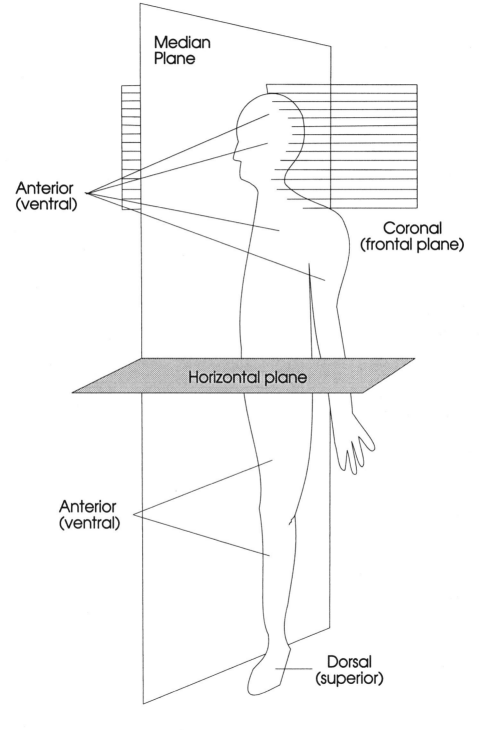

Median Plane

Anterior (ventral)

Coronal (frontal plane)

Horizontal plane

Anterior (ventral)

Dorsal (superior)

Inferior (caudal)

PRONUNCIATION KEY

a	short ă, a — mat, ask
ā	long — mate
ä	father, brother
e	short ĕ — bet, peck
ē	long — beat, easy
i	short ĭ — ill, tip
ī	long — ice, side
o	short ŏ — off, aw
ō	long — over
u	short ü ŭ u — pull, push
ū	long o͞o — union, youth, rule, shoot

LIST OF MEDICINES AND PRONUNCIATION.

Abelmoschus	ā´bel-mos´kus
Abies canadensis	ā'bi-ēz kăn-a-děn'sĭs
Abies nigra	ā'bĭ-ēz nī'gra
Absinthium	ăb-sĭn'thĭ-ŭm
Acalypha indica	a-kăl'ĭ-fa in'di-ka
Achyranthes calea	ak´i-ran´thēz kal´ē-ä
Acidum aceticum	ăs'ĭd-ŭm a-sē'ti-kŭm
Acidum benzoicum	ăs'ĭd-ŭm běn-zō'ĭ-kŭm
Acidum boracicum	ăs'ĭd-ŭm bō-răs'ĭ-kŭm
Acidum butyricum	as´id-um bū-ter´ĭ-kum
Acidum carbolicum	ăs'ĭd-ŭm kär-bŏl'ĭ-kŭm
Acidum chromicum	ăs'ĭd-ŭm krō'mĭ-kŭm
Acidum citricum	ăs'ĭd-ŭm sĭt-rĭ-kŭm
Acidum formicum	ăs'ĭd-ŭm fŏr'mĭ-kŭm
Acidum gallicum	ăs'ĭd-ŭm găl'lĭ-kŭm
Acidum hydrocyanicum	ăs'ĭd-ŭm hī-drō-sī-ăn'ĭ-kŭm
Acidum hydrofluoricum	ăs'ĭd-ŭm hī-drō-flū-ŏr'ĭ-kŭm
Acidum lacticum	ăs-ĭd-ŭm lăk'tĭ-kŭm
Acidum muriaticum	ăs-ĭd-ŭm mū-rĭ-ăt'ĭ-kŭm
Acidum nitricum	ăs-ĭd-ŭm nī'trĭ-kŭm
Acidum nitro-muriaticum	ăs'ĭd-ŭm nī-trō-mū-rĭ-ăt'ĭ-kŭm
Acidum oxalicum	ăs'ĭd-ŭm ŏx-ăl'ĭ-kŭm
Acidum phosphoricum	ăs'ĭd-ŭm fŏs-fŏr'ĭ-kŭm
Acidum picricum	ăs'ĭd-ŭm pĭk'rĭ-kŭm
Acidum salicylicum	ăs'ĭd-ŭm săl-ĭ-sĭl'ĭ-kŭm
Acidum sulphuricum	ăs'ĭd-ŭm sŭl-fū'rĭ-kŭm
Acidum tannicum	ăs'ĭd-ŭm tăn'nĭ-kŭm
Acidum tartaricum	ăs'ĭd-ŭm tar-tar'ĭ-kŭm
Aconitum Napellus	ăk-o-ni'tŭm nā-pel'lŭs
Aconitum e radice	ăk-o-ni'tŭm ē ra-dī'sē
Actæa racemosa	[See Cimicifuga racemosa]
Actæa spicata	ăk-tē'a spi-kā'ta
Adonis vernalis	ă-dō'nĭs ver-nā'lĭs
Adrenocorticotrophin	ā-drē´nō-kord-ē-kō´trō-fin
Æsculus glabra	ĕs'kū-lŭs glā'bra
Æsculus Hippocastanum	ĕs'kū-lŭs hip-pō-kăs'ta-nŭm
Æthusa cynapium	ē-thū'sa sī-nā'pĭ-ŭm
Agaricus muscarius	ā-găr'ĭ-kŭs mŭs-kā'rĭ-ŭs
Agaricus emeticus	ā-găr'ĭ-kŭs ē-mĕt'ĭ-kŭs
Agave americana	ā-gā'vē a-mĕr-ĭ-kā'na
Agave tequilana	ä-gä´ve tā-kē´lä-nä

Agnus castus	ăg′nŭs kăs′tŭs
Agrostemma Githago	ăg-rō-stĕm′ma jĭ-thā′gō
Ailanthus glandulosus	ā-lăn′thŭs glăn-dū-lō′sŭs
Aletris farinosa	ăl′e-trĭs far-ĭ-nō′sa
Allium Cepa	ăl′lĭ-ŭm sē′pa
Allium sativum	ăl′lĭ-ŭm sa′tĭ′vŭm
Alnus serrulata	ăl′nŭs ser-rū-lā′ta
Aloe socotrina	ăl′o-ē sō-kō-trī′na
Alstonia scholaris	ăl-stō′nĭ-a skō-lā′rĭs
Althæa officinalis	ăl-thē′a of-fĭs-ĭ-nā′lĭs
Alumen	a-lū′mĕn
Alumina	a-lū′mĭ-na
Aluminium metallicum	a-lū-mĭn′ĭ-ŭm me-tăl′lĭ-kŭm
Ambra grisea	ăm′bra grĭzh′e-a
Ambrosia artemisiæfolia	ăm-brō′zhe-a ar-te-mĭzh′e-ē-fō′lĭ-a
Ammoniacum gummi	ăm-mō-nī′a-kŭm gŭm′mī
Ammonium aceticum	ăm-mō′nĭ-ŭm a-sē′tĭ-kŭm
Ammonium benzoicum	ăm-mō′nĭ-ŭm bĕn-zō′ĭ-kŭm
Ammonium bromatum	ăm-mō′nĭ-ŭm brō-mā′tŭm
Ammonium carbonicum	ăm-mō′nĭ-ŭm kär-bŏn′ĭ-kŭm
Ammonium causticum	ăm-mō′nĭ-ŭm kaw′stĭ-kŭm
Ammonium iodatum	ăm-mō′nĭ-ŭm ī-o-dā′tŭm
Ammonium muriaticum	ăm-mō′nĭ-ŭm mū-rĭ-ăt′ĭ-kŭm
Ammonium nitricum	ăm-mō′nĭ-ŭm nĭ′trĭ-kŭm
Ammonium phosphoricum	ăm-mō′nĭ-ŭm fos-fōr′ĭ-kŭm
Ammonium picricum	ăm-mō′nĭ-ŭm pĭk′rĭ-kŭm
Ammonium valerianicum	ăm-mō′nĭ-ŭm vā-lē-rĭ-ăn′ĭ-kŭm
Amni liquor	**am′ni lik′ōr**
Ampelopsis quinquefolia	ăm-pĕl-ŏp′sĭs qŭin-que-fō′lĭ-a
Amygdalus amara	a-mĭg′da-lŭs a-mā′ra
Amyl nitrosum	ăm′yl nī-trō′sŭm
Anacardium orientale	ăn-a-kär′dĭ-ŭm ō-rĭ-ĕn-tā′lē
Anagallis arvensis	ăn-a-găl′lĭs är-vĕn′sĭs
Anatherum muricatum	ăn-a-thē′rŭm mū-rĭ-kā′tŭm
Angustura	ăn-gŭs-tū′ra
Anilinum	ăn-ĭ-lī′nŭm
Anilinum sulphuricum	ăn-ĭ-lī′nŭm sŭl-fū′rĭ-kŭm
Anthemis nobilis	ăn′the-mĭs nō′bĭ-lĭs
Anthoxanthum odoratum	ăn-thŏx-ăn′thŭm ō-do-rā′tŭm
Antimonium arsenicicum	ăn-tĭ-mō′nĭ-ŭm àr-sĕn-ĭs′ĭ-kŭm
Antimonium crudum	ăn-tĭ-mō′nĭ-ŭm kroo′dŭm
Antimonium iodatum	ăn-tĭ-mō′nĭ-ŭm ī-o-dā′tŭm
Antimonium oxydatum	ăn-tĭ-mō′nĭ-ŭm ŏx-ĭ-dā′tŭm
Antimonium sulphuratum auratum	ăn-tĭ-mō′nĭ-ŭm sŭl-fū-rā′tŭm au-rā′tŭm
Apis mellifica	ā′pĭs mĕl-lĭf′ĭ-ka

Apis virus	ā′pĭs vī′rŭs
Apocynum androsæmifolium	a-pŏs′ĭ-nŭm ăn-dro-sē-mĭ-fō′lĭ-ŭm
Apocynum cannabinum	a-pŏs′ĭ-nŭm kăn-nab′ĭ-nŭm
Apomorphinum muriaticum	ăp-o-mŏr-fī′nŭm mū-rĭ-ăt′ĭ-kŭm
Aralia quinquefolia	a-rā′lĭ-a quĭn-que-fō′lĭ-a
Aralia racemosa	a-rā′lĭ-a răs-e-mō′sa
Aranea diadema	a-rā′ne-a dĭ-a-dē′ma
Argemone mexicana	**är-jem′ō-nē mek′si-kä′nä**
Argentum cyanatum	är-jĕn′tŭm sī-an-ā′tŭm
Argentum iodatum	är-jĕn′tŭm ī-o-dā′tŭm
Argentum metallicum	är-jĕn′tŭm mĕ-tăl′lĭ-kŭm
Argentum muriaticum	är-jĕn′tŭm mū-rĭ-ăt′ĭ-kŭm
Argentum nitricum	är-jĕn′tum nĭ′trĭ-kŭm
Argentum oxydatum	är-jĕn′tŭm ox-ĭ-dā′tŭm
Argentum phosphoricum	är-jĕn′tŭm fŏs-fŏr′ĭ-kŭm
Aristolochia clematitis	**a-ris′tō-lō′ki-ä kle-ma-tē′tĭs**
Aristolochia milhomens	ar-ĭs-to′lō′kĭ-a mĭl′ho-mĕnz
Aristolochia serpentaria	ar-ĭs-to-lō′kĭ-a sur-pĕn-tā′rĭ-a
Arnica montana	är′nĭ-ka mŏn-tā′nä
Arnica montana e radice	är′nĭ-ka mŏn-tā′nä ē ra-dī′sē
Arsenicum album	är-sĕn′ĭ-kŭm ăl′bŭm
Arsenicum iodatum	är-sĕn′ĭ-kŭm ī-o-dā′tŭm
Arsenicum metallicum	är-sĕn′ĭ-kŭm mĕ-tăl′li-ĸŭm
Arsenicum sulphuratum flavum	är-sĕn′ĭ-kŭm sŭl-fū-rā′tŭm flā′vŭm
Arsenicum sulphuratum rubrum	är-sĕn′ĭ-kŭm sŭl-fū-rā′tŭm roo′brŭm
Artemisia Abrotanum	är-te-mĭzh′e-a a-brŏt′a-num
Artemisia Absinthium	[See Absinthium]
Artemisia vulgaris	är-te-mĭzh′e-a vŭl-gā′rĭs
Arum dracontium	ā′rŭm dra-kŏn′she-ŭm
Arum maculatum	ā′rŭm măk-yū-lā′tŭm
Arum triphyllum	ā′rŭm trī-fĭl′lùm
Asafœtida	ăẛ′a-fĕt′-ĭ-da
Asarum canadense	ăs′a-rŭm kăn-a-dĕn′sē
Asarum europæum	ăs′a-rŭm yū-ro-pē′ŭm
Asclepias incarnata	ăs-klē′pĭ-as ĭn-kär-nā′ta
Asclepias syriaca	ăs-klē′pĭ-as sĭ-rĭ′a-ka
Asclepias tuberosa	ăs-klē′pĭ-as tū-be-rō′sa
Asimina triloba	ă-sĭm′ĭ-na trĭ′lō-ba
Asparagus officinalis	ăs-păr′a-gŭs of-fĭs-ĭ-nā′lĭs
Asterias rubens	ăs-tē′rĭ-ăs roo′bĕnz
Athamanta oreoselinum	ăth-a-măn′ta ō-re-o-se-lĭ′nŭm
Atropinum	ăt-ro-pī′nŭm
Atropinum sulphuricum	ăt-ro-pī′nŭm sŭl-fū′rĭ-kŭm
Aurum metallicum	au′rŭm mĕ-tăl′lĭ-kŭm
Aurum muriaticum	au′rŭm mū-rĭ-ăt′ĭ-kŭm

Aurum muriaticum natronatum	au'rŭm mū-rĭ-ăt'ĭ-kŭm nā-trŏ-nā'tŭm
Aurum sulphuratum	au'rŭm sŭl-fū-rā'tŭm
Avena sativa	a-vē'na sa-tī'va
Badiaga	băd-ĭ-ā'ga
Balsamum peruvianum	băl'sa-mŭm pe-roo-vĭ-ā'nŭm
Baptisia tinctoria	băp-tĭzh'e-a tĭnk-tō'rĭ-a
Barosma crenata	ba-rŏz'ma kre-nā'ta
Barosma serratifolia	ba-rŏz'ma sĕr-răt-ĭ-fō'lĭ-a
Baryta acetica	ba-rī'ta a-sĕ'tĭ-ka
Baryta carbonica	ba-rī'ta kär-bŏn'ĭ-ka
Baryta iodata	ba-rī'ta ī-o-dā'ta
Baryta muriatica	ba-rī'ta mū-rĭ-ăt'ĭ-ka
Bebeerinum sulphuricum	bē-bē-rī'nŭm sŭl-fū'rĭ-kŭm
Belladonna	bĕl-la-dŏn'na
Bellis perennis	bĕl-lĭs pĕr-ĕn'nĭs
Benzinum nitricum	bĕn-zī'nŭm nĭ'trĭ-kŭm
Benzoinum	bĕn-zo-ī'nŭm
Berberinum	bur-be-rī'nŭm
Berberis aquifolium	bur'be-rĭs ā-quĭ-fō'lĭ-ŭm
Berberis vulgaris	bur'be-rĭs vŭl-gā'rĭs
Beryllium metallicum	**be-ril'i-um me-tal'li-kum**
Bismuthum oxydatum	bĭz-mū'thŭm ŏx-ĭ-dā'tŭm
Bismuthum sub-nitricum	bĭz-mū'thŭm sŭb-nĭ'trĭ-kŭm
Borax	bō'răx
Bovista	bō-vĭs'ta
Brachyglottis repens	brăk-ĭ-glŏt'tĭs rē'pĕnz
Branca ursina	brăng'ka ŭr-sī'na
Bromium	brō'mĭ-ŭm
Brucinum	broo-sī'nŭm
Bryonia alba	brī-ō'ne-a al'ba
Buthus australis	**bu'thus aus'trā-lis**
Cactus grandiflorus	kăk'tŭs grăn-dĭ-flō'rŭs
Cadmium metallicum	**kad'mi-um me-tal'li-kum**
Cadmium sulphuratum	kăd'mĭ-ŭm sŭl-fū-rā'tŭm
Cadmium sulphuricum	kăd'mĭ-ŭm sŭl-fū'rĭ-kŭm
Caffeinum	kăf-fē-ī'nŭm
Cainca	kā-ĭn'ka
Caladium seguinum	ka-lā'dĭ-ŭm sē-guī'nŭm
Calcarea acetica	kăl-kā're-a a-sĕ'tĭ-ka
Calcarea arsenicica	kăl-kā're-a är-sĕn-ĭs'ĭ-ka
Calcarea bromata	kăl-kā're-a bro-mā'ta
Calcarea carbonica	kăl-kā're-a kär-bŏn'ĭ-ka

Calcarea caustica	kăl-kā're-a kaw'stĭ-ka
Calcarea fluorata	kăl-kā're-a floo-o-rā'ta
Calcarea hypophosphorica	kăl-kā're-a hī-po-fŏs-fŏr'ĭ-ka
Calcarea iodata	kăl-kā're-a ī-o-dā'ta
Calcarea muriatica	kăl-kā're-a mū-rĭ-ăt'ĭ-ka
Calcarea oxalica	kăl-kā're-a ox-ăl'ĭ-ka
Calcarea phosphorica	kăl-kā're-a fŏs-fŏr'ĭ-ka
Calcarea sulphurica	kăl-kā're-a sŭl-fū'rĭ-ka
Calea zacatechichi	ka 'lē-ä zä 'kä-tä 'chĭ-chĭ
Calendula officinalis	ka-lĕn'dū-la ŏf-fĭs-ĭ-nā'lĭs
Calotropis gigantea	ka-lŏt'ro-pĭs jĭ-găn-te'a
Caltha palustris	kăl'tha pa-lŭs'trĭs
Camphora	kăm-fō'ra
Camphora monobromata	kăm-fō'ra mŏn-o-bro-mā'ta
Canna angustifolia	kăn'na ăn-gŭs-tĭ-fō'lĭ-a
Cannabis indica	kăn'na-bĭs ĭn'dĭ-ka
Cannabis sativa	kăn'na-bĭs sa-tī'va
Cantharis	kăn'tha-rĭs
Capsicum annuum	kăp'sĭ-kŭm ăn'nū-ŭm
Carbo animalis	kär'bō ăn-ĭ-mā'lĭs
Carbo vegetabilis	kär'bō vĕj-ĕt-ăb'ĭ-lĭs
Carbonium sulphuratum	kär-bō'nĭ-ŭm sŭl-fū-rā'tŭm
Carduus benedictus	kär'dū-ŭs bĕn-ĕ-dĭk'tŭs
Carduus Marianus	kär'dū-ŭs măr-ĭ-ā'nŭs
Carya alba	kā'rĭ-a ăl'ba
Cascara sagrada	[See Rhamnus purshiana]
Cascarilla	kăs-ka-rĭl'la
Castanea vesca	kăs-tā'ne-a vĕs'ka
Castella texana	kăs 'tĕ-lä tĕks 'ä-nä
Castoreum	kăs-tō're-ŭm
Caulophyllum thalictroides	kaw-lo-tĭl-ĭŭm thăl-ĭk-troĭ'dēz
Causticum	kaw'stĭ-kŭm
Ceanothus americanus	sē-ăn-ō'thŭs a-mĕr-ĭ-kā'nŭs
Cecropia mexicana	sē-krō 'pi-ä mek 'si-kä-nä
Cedron	sē'drŏn
Centruroides elegans	sĕn-trū 'rōi-des el 'ē-gans
Cerasus virginiana	sĕr-ā-sŭs vur-jĭn-ĭ-ā'na
Cereus Bonplandii	sē're-ŭs bŏn-plănd'ĭ-ī
Cerium oxalicum	sē'ri-ŭm ŏx-al'ĭ-kŭm
Chamomilla	kăm-o-mĭl'la
Chelidonium majus	kĕl-ĭ-dō'nĭ-ŭm mā'jŭs
Chelone glabra	kĕ-lō'-nē glā'bra
Chenopodium anthelminticum	kĕn-o-pō'dĭ-ŭm ăn-thĕl-mĭn'tĭ-kŭm
Chimaphila umbellata	kĭm-ăf'ĭ-la ŭm-bĕl-lā'ta
Chininum arsenicicum	kĭ-nī'nŭm är-sĕn-ĭs'ĭ-kŭm

Chininum arsenicosum	kĭ-nī'nŭm är-sĕn-ĭ-kō'sŭm
Chininum muriaticum	kĭ-nī'nŭm mū-rĭ-ăt'ĭ-kŭm
Chininum purum	kĭ-nī'nŭm pū'rŭm
Chininum sulphuricum	kĭ-nī'nŭm sŭl-fū'rĭ-kŭm
Chionanthus virginica	kī-o-năn'thŭs vur-jĭn'ĭ-ka
Chrysarobinum	krĭs-ăr-o-bī'nŭm
Cichorium Intybus	sĭk-ō'ri-ŭm ĭn'tĭ-bŭs
Cicuta maculata	sĭk-ū'ta măk-yū-lā'ta
Cicuta virosa	sĭk-ū'ta vĭ-rō'sa
Cimicifuga racemosa	sĭm-ĭ-sĭf'ū-ga răs-e-mō'sa
Cina	sī'na
Cinchona officinalis	sĭnk-ō'na ŏf-fĭs-ĭ-nā'lĭs
Cinchoninum sulphuricum	sĭnk-o-nī'nŭm sŭl-fū'rĭ-kŭm
Cinnamomum	sĭn-na-mō'mŭm
Cirsium arvense	sŭr'she-ŭm är-vĕn'sē
Cistus canadense	sĭs'tŭs kăn-a-dĕn'sē
Clematis erecta	klĕm'a-tĭs ē-rĕk'ta
Cobaltum metallicum	kō-băl'tum mĕ-tăl'lĭ-kŭm
Cobaltum nitricum	**kō-bal'tum ni'tri-kum**
Coca	[See Erythroxylon coca]
Cocainum muriaticum	kō-ka-ī'nŭm mū-rĭ-ăt'ĭ-kŭm
Cocculus indicus	kŏk'ū-lŭs ĭn'dĭ-kŭs
Coccus cacti	kŏk'kŭs kăk'tī
Cochlearia Armoracia	kŏk-le-ā're-a är-mo-rā'she-a
Codeinum	kō-de-ī'nŭm
Coffea cruda	kŏf'fe-a kroo'da
Colchicum autumnale	kŏl'kĭ-kŭm au-tŭm-nā'lē
Collinsonia canadensis	kŏl-lĭn-sō'nĭ-a kăn-a-dĕn'sĭs
Colocynth	kŏl'o-sĭnth
Comocladia dentata	kō-mo-klā'dĭ-a dĕn-tā'ta
Conium maculatum	kō-nī'um măk-yū-lā'tŭm
Convallaria majalis	kŏn-văl-lā'rĭ-a ma-jā'lĭs
Convolvulus duartinus	kŏn-vŏl'vū-lŭs dū-är-tī'nŭs
Copaiba officinalis	kō-pā'ba ŏf-fĭs-ĭ-nā'lĭs
Corallium rubrum	kō-răl'lĭ-ŭm roo'brŭm
Cornus circinata	kŏr'nŭs sur-sĭ-nā'ta
Cornus florida	kŏr'nŭs flŏr'ĭ-da
Cornus sericea	kŏr'nŭs sĕr-ĭsh'e-a
Cortisone	**kor'dē-sōn**
Cotyledon umbilicus	kŏt-ĭ-lē'don ŭm-bĭl-ī'kŭs
Cratægus Oxyacantha	krā-tē'gŭs ŏx-ĭ-ā-kăn'tha
Creosotum	krē-o-sō'tŭm
Crocus sativus	krō'kŭs sa-tī'vŭs
Crotalus	krŏt'a-lŭs
Croton Tiglium	krō'tŏn tĭg'lĭ-ŭm

Cubeba officinalis	kū-bē′ba ŏf-fĭs-ĭ-nā′lĭs
Cundurango	kŭn-dū-răng′gō
Cuprum aceticum	kū′prŭm a-sĕ′tĭ-kum
Cuprum arsenicosum	kū′prŭm är-sĕn-ĭ-kō′sŭm
Cuprum carbonicum	kū′prŭm kär-bŏn′ĭ-kŭm
Cuprum metallicum	kū′prŭm mĕ-tăl′lĭ-kŭm
Cuprum sulphuricum	kū′prŭm sŭl-fū′rĭ-kŭm
Curare	kū-räh′re
Cyclamen europæum	sĭk′la-mĕn yū-ro-pē′ŭm
Cynara scolymus	sin′ä-rä skŏl′i-mus
Cypripedium pubescens	sĭp-rĭ-pē′dĭ-ŭm pu-bĕs′sĕnz
Cytisus scoparius	sit′i-sus skō-par′i-us
Daphne indica	dăf′nē ĭn′dĭ-ka
Datura arborea	da-tū′ra är-bō′re-a
Dextrum lacticum acidum	deks′trum lak′ti-kum as′id-um
Dictamnus albus	dĭk-tăm′nŭs ăl′bŭs
Digitalis purpurea	dĭj-ĭ-tā′lĭs pur-pū′re-a
Dioscorea villosa	dī-ŏs-kō-rē′a vĭl-lō′sa
Dirca palustris	dur′ka pa-lŭs′trĭs
Dolichos pruriens	dŏl′ĭ-kŏs proo′rĭ-ĕnz
Drosera rotundifolia	drŏs′e-ra ro-tŭn-dĭ-fō′lĭ-a
Duboisia myoporoides	dū-bŏi′sĭ-a mī-o-po-roĭ′dēz
Dulcamara	dŭl-ka-mā′ra
Echinacea angustifolia	ĕk-ĭn-ā′shē-a ăn-gŭs-ti-fō′lĭa
Elaps corallinus	ē′lăps kŏr-ăl-lī′nŭs
Elaterium	ĕl-a-tē′rĭ-ŭm
Epigæa repens	ĕp-i-jē′a rē′pĕnz
Epiphegus Virginiana	ĕp-ĭ-fē′gŭs vur-jĭn-ĭ-ā′na
Equisetum hyemale	ĕk-wĭ-′sē′tŭm hī-e-mā′lē
Erechthites hieracifolia	ĕr-ĕk-thī′tēz hī-e-răs-ĭ-fō′lĭ-a
Erigeron canadense	ĕr-ĭj′e-rŏn kăn-a-dĕn′sē
Eriodictyon glutinosum	ĕr-ĭ-o-dĭk′tĭ-ŏn gloo-tĭn-ō′sŭm
Eryngium aquaticum	ĕr-ĭn′jĭ-ŭm a-quăt′ĭ-kŭm
Eryngium maritimum	ĕr-ĭn′jĭ-ŭm ma-rĭ-tĭ′mŭm
Erythrophlæum judiciale	ĕr-ĭth-ro-flē′ŭm joo-dĭsh-ĭ-ā′lē
Erythroxylon Coca	ĕr-ĭth-rŏx′ĭ-lŏn kō′ka
Eserinum	ĕs-ĕr-ĭ′nŭm
Eucalyptus globulus	yū-ka-lĭp′tŭs glŏb′ū-lŭs
Eugenia Jambos	yū-jē′nĭ-a jăm′bŏs
Euonymus atropurpureus	yū-ŏn′ĭ-mŭs ăt-ro-pŭr-pū′re-ŭs
Euonymus europæus	yū-ŏn′ĭ-mŭs yū-ro-pē′ŭs
Eupatorium aromaticum	yū-pa-tō′rĭ-ŭm ăr-o-măt′ĭ-kŭm
Eupatorium perfoliatum	yū-pa-tō′rĭ-ŭm pur-fō-lĭ-ā′tŭm
Eupatorium purpureum	yū-pa-tō′rĭ-ŭm pur-pū′re-ŭm

Euphorbia corollata	yū-fŏr'bĭ-a cŏr-ŏl-lā'ta
Euphorbia hypericifolia	yū-fŏr'bĭ-a hī-pĕr-ĭs-ĭ-fō'lĭ-a
Euphorbium officinarum	yū-fŏr'bĭ-ŭm ŏf-fĭs-ĭ-nā'rŭm
Euphrasia officinalis	yū-frā'zhe-a ŏf-fĭs-ĭ-nā'lĭs
Eupion	yū'pĭ-ŏn
Fagopyrum esculentum	făg-o-pī'rŭm ĕs-kū-lĕn'tŭm
Ferrum aceticum	fĕr'rŭm a-sē'tĭ-kŭm
Ferrum arsenicicum	fĕr'rŭm är-sĕn-ĭs'ĭ-kŭm
Ferrum bromatum	fĕr'rŭm bro-mā'tŭm
Ferrum carbonicum	fĕr'rŭm kär-bŏn'ĭ-kŭm
Ferrum iodatum	fĕr'rŭm ī-o-dā'tŭm
Ferrum lacticum	fĕr'rŭm lăk'tĭ-kŭm
Ferrum magneticum	fĕr'rŭm măg-nĕt'ĭ-kŭm
Ferrum metallicum	fĕr'rŭm mĕ-tăl'lĭ-kŭm
Ferrum muriaticum	fĕr'rŭm mū-rĭ-ăt'ĭ-kŭm
Ferrum phosphoricum	fĕr'rŭm fŏs-fŏr'ĭ-kŭm
Ferrum sulphuricum	fĕr'rŭm sŭl-fū'rĭ-kŭm
Filix mas	fī'lĭx măs
Fraxinus americana	frăx'i-nŭs a-mĕr-i-kā'na
Frasera carolinensis	frā'ze-ra kär-o-lĭ-nĕn'sĭs
Fucus vesiculosus	fū'kŭs vĕs-ĭk-ū-lō sŭs
Gambogia	găm-bō'jĭ-a
Gaultheria procumbens	gaul-thē'rĭ-a prŏ-kŭm'bĕnz
Gelsemium sempervirens	jĕl-sē'mĭ-ŭm sĕm-per-vī'rĕnz
Genista tinctoria	je-nĭs'ta tĭnk-tō'rĭ-a
Gentiana cruciata	jĕn-she-ā'na croo-she-ā'ta
Gentiana lutea	jĕn-she-ā'na lū'te-a
Geranium maculatum	je-rā'nĭ-ŭm măk-yū-lā'tŭm
GeraniumRobertianum	je-rā-nĭ-ŭm rō-bur-she-ā'nŭm
Geum urbanum	jē'ŭm ŭr-bā'nŭm
Glonoinum	glŏn-ò-ī'nŭm
Gnaphalium polycephalum	na-fā'lĭ-ŭm pŏl-ĭ-sĕf'a-lŭm
Gnaphalium uliginosum	na-fā'lĭ-ŭm yū-lĭj-ĭ-nō'sŭm
Gossypium herbaceum	gŏs-sĭp'ĭ-ŭm her-bā'she-ŭm
Granatum	gra-nā'tŭm
Graphites	grăf-ī'tēz'
Gratiola officinalis	gra-tī'o-la ŏf-fĭs-ĭ-nā'lĭs
Grindelia robusta	grĭn-dē'lĭ-a ro-bŭs'ta
Grindelia squarrosa	grĭn-dē'lĭ-a skwär-rō'sa
Guaco	guā'kō
Guaiacum officinale	gŭā'ya-kŭm ŏf-fĭs-ĭ-nā'lē
Guarea trichiloides	guā're-a trĭ-kĭ-loī'dēz
Guatteria gaumeri	**gu´â-ter´i-a ga-u-mer´i**
Gymnocladus canadensis	jĭm-nŏk'la-dŭs kăn-a-dĕn'sĭs

Hæmatoxylon campechianum	hē-ma-tŏx′ĭ-lŏn kăm-pĕk-ĭ-ā′nŭm
Hamamelis virginica	hăm-a-mē′lĭs vur-jĭn′ĭ′ka
Hecla lava	Hĕk-la lā′va
Hedeoma pulegioides	hë-de-ō′ma pū-lĕj-ĭ-oi′dēz
Hedera helix	**hed′er-a hē′liks**
Hedysarum ildefonsianum	he-dĭs′a-rŭm ĭl-de-fŏn-sĭ-ā′nŭm
Helianthus annuus	hē-lĭ-ăn′thŭs ăn′nū-ŭs
Heliotropium peruvianum	hē-lĭ-o-trō′pĭ-ŭm pe-roo-vĭ-ā′nŭm
Helleborus fœtidus	hĕl-lĕb′o-rŭs fĕt′ĭ-dŭs
Helleborus niger	hĕl-lĕb′o-rŭs nĭ′jer
Helonias dioica	hē-lō′nĭ-as dī-oi′ka
Hepar sulphuris calcareum	hē′pär sŭl′fū-rĭs kăl-kā′re-ŭm
Hepatica triloba	hē-păt′ĭ-ka trĭ′lo-ba
Hippuricum acidum	**hi-pū′ri-cum as′id-um**
Hoitzia coccinea	**hoit-zĭ′a kok-si-nē a**
Hydrangea arborescens	hī-drăn′je-a är-bo-rĕs′sĕnz
Hydrastinum	hī-drăs-tī′nŭm
Hydrastis canadensis	hī-drăs′tĭs kăn-a-dĕn′sĭs
Hydrocotyle asiatica	hī-dro-kŏt′ĭ-lē ā-she-ăt′ĭ-ka
Hydrophyllum virginicum	hī-dro-fĭl′lŭm vur-jĭn′ĭ-kŭm
Hyoscyamus niger	hī-ŏs-sī′a-mŭs nĭ-jer
Hyoscyaminum sulphuricum	hī-ŏs-sī-a-mī′nŭm sŭl-fū′rĭ-kŭm
Hypericum perforatum	hĭ-pĕr′ĭ-kŭm per-fo-rā′tŭm
Iberis amara	ī′bē′rĭs a-mā′ra
Ignatia amara	ĭg-nā′she-a a-mā′ra
Ilex opaca	ī′lĕx o-pā′-ka
Ilex paraguayensis	ī′lĕx pär-a-gwī-ĕn′sĭs
Illicium anisatum	ĭl-lĭsh′e-ŭm ăn-ĭs-ā′tŭm
Indigo	in′dĭ-gō
Indium metallicum	ĭn′dĭ-ŭm mĕ-tăl′lĭ-kŭm
Inula Helenium	ĭn′yū-la hĕl-ē′nĭ-ŭm
Iodium	ī-ō′dĭ-ŭm
Ipecacuanha	ĭp-e-kăk-yū-ăn′a
Ipomea stans cav.	**ip′ō-mē′a stans cav.**
Iridium metallicum	ī-rĭd′ĭ-ŭm mĕ-tăl′lĭ-kŭm
Iris versicolor	ī′rĭs vur-sĭk′o-lŏr
Jacaranda caroba	jăk-a-răn′da kär′o-ba
Jalapa	jăl′a-pa
Jatropha curcas	jăt′ro-fa kŭr′kăs
Juglans cinerea	jū′glănz sĭn-ē′re-a
Juglans regia	jū′glănz rē′jĭ-a
Juncus effusus	jŭnk′ŭs ĕf-fū′sŭs
Juniperus virginiana	jū-nĭp′e-rŭs vur-jĭn-ĭ-ā′na

Kali aceticum	kā′lĭ a-sĕ′ti-kŭm
Kali arsenicosum	kā′lĭ är-sĕn-ĭ-kō′sŭm
Kali bichromicum	kā′lĭ bī-krō′mĭ-kŭm
Kali bromatum	kā′lĭ bro-mā′tŭm
Kali carbonicum	kā′lĭ kär-bŏn′ĭ-kŭm
Kali causticum	kā′lĭ kau′stĭ-kŭm
Kali chloricum	kā′lĭ klŏ′rĭ-kŭm
Kali chromicum	kā′li krō′mĭ-kŭm
Kali cyanatum	kā′lĭ sī-ăn-ā′tŭm
Kali ferrocyanatum	kā′lĭ fĕr-ro-sī-ăn-ā′tŭm
Kali hypophosphorosum	kā′lĭ hī-po-fŏs-fŏr-ō′sŭm
Kali iodatum	kā′lĭ ī-o-dā′tŭm
Kali muriaticum	kā′lĭ mū-rĭ-ăt′i-kŭm
Kali nitricum	kā′lĭ nĭ′trĭ-kŭm
Kali oxalicum	kā′lĭ ŏx-ăl′ĭ-kŭm
Kali permanganicum	kā′lĭ per-măn-găn′ĭ-kŭm
Kali phosphoricum	kā′lĭ fŏs-fŏr′ĭ-kŭm
Kali picricum	kā′lĭ pĭk′ri-kŭm
Kali sulphuricum	kā′lĭ sŭl-fū′rĭ-kŭm
Kali tartaricum	kā′lĭ tär-tär′ĭ-kŭm
Kalmia latifolia	kăl′mĭ-a lăt-ĭ-fō′lĭ-a
Karwinskia humboldtiana	**kär-win′ski-a hum-bōl′ti-ä-nä**
Kino australiensis	kī′nō aus-trā-lĭ-ĕn′sĭs
Laburnum anagyroides	**la-bur′num an′a-jĭ′roid-dēs**
Lachesis	lăk′e-sĭs
Lachnanthes tinctoria	lăk-năn′thēz tĭnk-tō′rĭ-a
Lactuca virosa	lăk-tū′ka vĭ-rō′sa
Lactucarium	lăk-tū-kā′rĭ-ŭm
Lamium album	lā′mĭ-ŭm ăl′bŭm
Lapis albus	lā′pĭs ăl′bŭs
Lappa major	lăp′pa mā′jŏr
Lathyrus sativus	lăth′ĭ-rŭs sa-tī′vŭs
Latrodectus mactans	**lat′rō-dek′tus mak′tans**
Laurocerasus	lau-ro-sĕr′a-sŭs
Ledum palustre	lē′dŭm pa-lŭs′trē
Leptandra virginica	lĕp-tăn′dra vur-jĭn′ĭ-ka
Lilium tigrinum	lĭl′ĭ-um tĭ-grī′nŭm
Linaria vulgaris	lĭ-nā′rĭ-a vŭl-gā′rĭs
Linum catharticum	lī′nŭm kăth-är′tĭ-kŭm
Lippia mexicana	**lip′i-a mek′si-kä′nä**
Lithium benzoicum	lĭth′ĭ-ŭm bĕn-zō′ĭ-kŭm
Lithium bromatum	lĭth′ĭ-ŭm brō-mā′tŭm
Lithium carbonicum	lĭth′ĭ-ŭm kär-bŏn′ĭ-kŭm
Lobelia cardinalis	lō-bē′lĭ-a kär-dĭ-nā′lĭs

Lobelia inflata	lō-bē′lĭ-a ĭn-flā′ta
Lobelia syphilitica	lō-bē′lĭ-a sĭf-ĭ-lĭt′ĭ-ka
Lolium temulentum	lō′lĭ-um tĕm-ū-lĕn′tŭm
Lophophora williamsii	**lo-fof′ō-ra wil-yam′sĭ-ĭ**
Lupulinum	lū-pū-lī′nŭm
Lupulus	lū′pū-lŭs
Lycopersicum esculentum	lī-ko-pur′sĭ-kŭm ĕs-kū-lĕn′tŭm
Lycopodium clavatum	lī-ko-pō′dĭ-um kla-vā′tŭm
Lycopus virginicus	lī′ko-pŭs vur-jĭn′ĭ-kŭs
Magnesia carbonica	măg-nē′she-a kär-bŏn′ĭ-ka
Magnesia muriatica	măg-nē′she-a mū-rĭ-ăt′ĭ-ka
Magnesia oxydata	măg-nē′she-a ŏx-ĭ-dā′ta
Magnesia phosphorica	măg-nē′she-a fŏs-fŏr′ĭ-ka
Magnesia sulphurica	măg-nē′she-a sŭl-fū′rĭ-ka
Magnolia glauca	măg-nō′lĭ-a glău′ka
Mancinella	măn-sĭ-nĕl′la
Mandragora officinarum	**man-drag′ō-ra o-fis′i-nä-rum**
Manganum aceticum	măn′ga-nŭm a-sĕ′ti-kŭm
Manganum carbonicum	măn′ga-nŭm kär-bŏn′ĭ-kŭm
Manganum muriaticum	măn′ga-nŭm mū-rĭ-ăt′ĭ-kŭm
Manganum oxydatum nigrum	măn′ga-nŭm ŏx-ĭ-dā′tŭm nī′grŭm
Medicago sativa	**me′di-kä′gō sa-tĭ′va**
Melilotus alba	mĕl-ĭ-lō′tŭs ăl′ba
Melilotus officinalis	mĕl-ĭ-lō′tŭs ŏf-fĭs-ĭ-nā′lĭs
Menispermum canadense	mĕn-ĭs-pur′mŭm kăn-a-dĕn′sē
Mentha piperita	mĕn′tha pī-pĕ-rī′ta
Menyanthes trifoliata	mĕn-ĭ-ăn′thēz trī-fō-lĭ-ā′ta
Mercurialis perennis	mer-kū-rĭ-ā′lĭs pĕr-ĕn′nĭs
Mephitis mephitica	mē-fĭ′tĭs mē-fĭt′i-**ka**
Mercurius cyanatus	mer-kū′rĭ-ŭs sī-a-nā′tŭs
Mercurius dulcis	mer-kū′rĭ-ŭs dŭl′sĭs
Mercurius et kali iodatus	mer-kū′rĭ-ŭs ĕt kä′lĭ ī-o-dā′tŭs
Mercurius iodatus flavus	mer-kū′rĭ-ŭs ī-o-dā′tŭs flā′vŭs
Mercurius iodatus ruber	mer-kū′rĭ-ŭs ī-o-dā′tŭs roo′ber
Mercurius nitricus	mer-kū′rĭ-ŭs nĭ′trĭ-kŭs
Mercurius præcipitatus albus	mer-kū′rĭ-ŭs prē-sĭp-ĭ-tā′tŭs ăl′bŭs
Mercurius præcipitatus ruber	mer-kū′rĭ-ŭs prē-sĭp-ĭ-tā′tŭs roo′ber
Mercurius solubilis Hahn.	mer-kū′rĭ-ŭs sŏl-ū′bĭ-lĭs Hähn.
Mercurius sublimatus corrosivus	mer-kū′rĭ-ŭs sŭb-lĭ-mā′tŭs kŏr-ro-sī′vŭs
Mercurius sulphuratus **ruber**	mer-kū′rĭ-ŭs sŭl-fū-rā′tŭs **roo′ber**
Mercurius sulphuricus	mer-kū′rĭ-ŭs sŭl-fū′rĭ-kŭs
Mercurius vivus	mer-kū′rĭ-ŭs vī′vŭs
Mezereum	me-zē′re-ŭm
Millifolium	mĭl-lĭ-fō′lĭ-ŭm

Mimosa humilis	mǐ-mō'sa hū'mǐ-lǐs
Mitchella repens	mǐtch-ēl'la rē'pĕnz
Momordica balsamina	mo-mör'dǐ-ka băl-sa-mī'na
Monotropa uniflora	mo-nŏt'ro-pa yū-nǐ-flō'ra
Morphinum	mŏr-fī'nŭm
Morphinum aceticum	mŏr-fī'nŭm a-sĕ'tǐ-kŭm
Morphinum muriaticum	mŏr-fī'nŭm mū-rǐ-ăt'ǐ-kŭm
Morphinum sulphuricum	mŏr-fī'nŭm sŭl-fū'rǐ-kŭm
Moschus	mŏs'kŭs
Murex purpurea	mū'rex pur-pū're-a
Mygale lasiodora	mǐ-gā'lē lăs-ǐ-o-dō'ra
Myrica cerifera	mǐ-rī'ka se-rǐf'e-ra
Myrtus communis	mur'tŭs cŏm-mū'nǐs
Nabalus serpentaria	năb'a-lŭs sŭr-pĕn-tā'rǐ-a
Naja tripudians	nā'ja trǐ-pū'dǐ-ănz
Naphthalinum	năf-tha-li'nŭm
Narceinum	när-sē-ī'nŭm
Narcotinum	när-ko-tī'nŭm
Natrum arsenicicum	nā'trŭm är-sĕn-ĭs'ǐ-kŭm
Natrum bromatum	nā'trŭm bro-mā'tŭm
Natrum carbonicum	nā'trŭm kär-bŏn'ǐ-kŭm
Natrum causticum	nā'trŭm kau'stǐ-kŭm
Natrum fluoricum	**nā´trum flū-or´i-kum**
Natrum hypophosphorosum	nā'trŭm hī-po-fŏs-fŏr-ō'sŭm
Natrum muriaticum	nā'trŭm mū-rǐ-ăt'ǐ-kŭm
Natrum nitricum	nā'trŭm nǐ'trǐ-kŭm
Natrum phosphoricum	nā'trŭm fŏs-fŏr'ǐ-kŭm
Natrum salicylicum	nā'trŭm săl-ǐ-sǐl'ǐ-kŭm
Natrum sulpho-carbolicum	nā'trŭm sŭl-fō-kär-bŏl'ǐ-kŭm
Natrum sulphuricum	nā'trŭm sŭl-fū'rǐ-kŭm
Natrum sulphurosum	nā'trŭm sŭl-fū-rō'sŭm
Niccolum carbonicum	nǐk'o-lŭm kär-bŏn'ǐ-kŭm
Niccolum metallicum	nǐk'o-lŭm mĕ-tăl'lǐ-kŭm
Niccolum sulphuricum	nǐk'o-lŭm sŭl-fū'rǐ-kŭm
Nuphar luteum	nū'far lū'te-ŭm
Nux moschata	nŭx mŏs-kā'ta
Nux vomica	nŭx vŏm'ǐ-ka
Nymphæa odorata	nǐm-fē'a ō-do-rā'ta
Ocimum sanctum	**os´i-mum sangk´tum**
Œnanthe crocata	ē-năn'thē krō-kā'ta
Œnothera biennis	ē-no-thē'ra bǐ-ĕn'nǐs
Oleander	ō-le-ăn'der
Oleum animale	ō'le-ŭm ăn-ǐ-mā'lē

302

Oleum Cajuputi	ō′le-ŭm kăj-ū-pū′tī
Oleum Morrhuæ	ō′le-ŭm mŏr′roo-ē
Oleum Ricini	ō′le-ŭm rĭs′ĭ-nī
Oleum santali	ō′le-ŭm săn′ta-lī
Olibanum	o-lĭb′a-nŭm
Onosmodium virginianum	ō-nŏs-mō′dĭ-ŭm vur-jĭn-ĭ-ā′nŭm
Opium	ō′pĭ-ŭm
Opuntia vulgaris	ō-pŭn′she-a vŭl-gā′rĭs
Osmium metallicum	ŏs′mĭ-ŭm mĕ-tăl′lĭ-kŭm
Oxydendron arboreum	ŏx-ĭ-dĕn′drŏn är-bō′re-ŭm
Pæonia officinalis	pē-ō′nĭ-a ŏf-fĭs-ĭ-nā′lĭs
Palladium	păl-lā′dĭ-ŭm
Pareira brava	par-ā′ra brā′va
Paris quadrifolia	păr′ĭs quŏd-rĭ-fō′lĭ-a
Paronichia illecebrum	**par ′ō-nik ′i-a i-les ′ē-brum**
Passiflora incarnata	păs-sĭ-flō′ra ĭn-kär-nā′ta
Pastinaca sativa	păs-tĭ-nā′ka sa-tī′va
Paullinia pinnata	paw-lĭn′ĭ-a pĭn-nā′ta
Paullinia sorbilis	paw-lĭn′ĭ-a sor′bĭ-lĭs
Penthorum sedoides	pĕn′tho-rŭm **se-doĭ′dēz**
Persea americana	**pur ′sē-a a-mer ′i-kä ′nä**
Petroleum	pē-trō′le-ŭm
Petroselinum sativum	pĕt-ro-se-lī′nŭm sa-ti′vŭm
Phellandrium aquaticum	fĕl-lăn′drĭ-ŭm a-quăt′ĭ-kŭm
Phosphorus	fŏs′fo-rŭs
Phosphorus ruber	fŏs′fo-rŭs roo′ber
Physostigma venenosum	fī-so-stĭg′ma vē-ne-nō′sŭm
Phytolacca decandra	fī-to-lăk′a dĕk-ăn′dra
Picrotoxinum	pĭk-ro-tŏx′ĭ-nŭm
Pilocarpinum muriaticum	pĭ-lo-kär-pī′nŭm mū-rĭ-ăt′ĭ-kŭm
Pilocarpinum nitricum	pĭ-lo-kär-pī′nŭm rĭ′t-rĭ-kŭm
Pilocarpus	pĭl-o-kär′pŭs
Pimpinella saxifraga	pĭmp-ĭ-nĕl′la săx-ĭf′ra-ga
Pinus Lambertiana	pī′nŭs lăm-ber-she-ā′na
Pinus silvestris	pī′nŭs sĭl-vĕs′trĭs
Pinus teocote	**pī ′nus tē ′ō-kō ′te**
Piper methysticum	pī′per me-thĭs′tĭ-kŭm
Piper nigrum	pī′per nī′grŭm
Piscidia erythrina	pĭs-sĭd′ĭ-a ĕr-ĭ-thrī′na
Pituitarum posterium	**pi-tū ′i-ta-rum pos-tē ′ri-um**
Plantago major	plăn-tā′gō mā′jŏr
Platinum et natrum muriaticum	plăt′ĭ-nŭm ĕt nā′trŭm mū-rĭ-ăt′ĭ-kŭm
Platinum metallicum	plăt′ĭ-nŭm mĕ-tăl′lĭ-kŭm
Platinum muriaticum	plăt′ĭ-nŭm mū-rĭ-ăt′ĭ-kŭm

Plectanthus fructicosus	plĕk-tăn'thŭs frŭk-tĭ-kō'sŭs
Plumbago littoralis	plŭm-bā'gō lĭt-to-rā'lĭs
Plumbum aceticum	plŭm'bŭm a-sĕ'tĭ-kŭm
Plumbum carbonicum	plŭm'bŭm kär-bŏn'ĭ-kŭm
Plumbum chromicum	plŭm'bŭm krŏ'mĭ-kŭm
Plumbum iodatum	plŭm'bŭm ī-o-dā'tŭm
Plumbum metallicum	plŭm'bŭm mĕ-tăl'lĭ-kŭm
Podophyllin	pŏd-o-fĭl'lĭn
Podophyllum peltatum	pŏd-o-fĭl'lŭm pĕl-tā'tŭm
Polygonum punctatum	po-lĭg'o-nŭm pŭnk-tā'tŭm
Polyporus officinalis	po-lĭp'o-rŭs ŏf-fĭs-ĭ-nā'lĭs
Polyporus pinicola	po-lĭp'o-rŭs pĭn-ĭk'o-la
Populus tremuloides	pŏp'ū-lŭs trĕm-ū-loĭ'dēz
Pothos fœtidus	pō'thŏs fĕt'ĭ-dŭs
Prinos verticillatus	prī'nŏs vur-tĭs-ĭl-lā'tŭs
Prunus padus	proo'nŭs pā'dŭs
Prunus spinosa	proo'nŭs spĭ-nō'sa
Prunus virginiana	proo'nŭs vur-jĭn-ĭ-ā'na
Ptelea trifoliata	tĕl'e-a trī-fō-lĭ-ā'ta
Pulsatilla	pŭl-sa-tĭl'la
PulsatillaNuttalliana	pŭl-sa-tĭl'la nŭt-tăl-lĭ-ā'na
Pyrus americana	pī'rŭs a-mĕr-ĭ-kā'na
Quassia amara	kwăsh'ĭ-a a-mā'ra
Quillaia saponaria	kwĭl-lā'ya săp-o-nā'rĭ-a
Radium bromatum	rā'dĭ-ŭm brō-mā'tŭm
Rajania subsamarata	**rā-ja´ne-a sub-sam-ä-rä´tä**
Ranunculus acris	ra-nŭn'kū-lŭs ā'krĭs
Ranunculus bulbosus	ra-nŭn'kū-lŭs bŭl'bō'sŭs
Ranunculus repens	ra-nŭn'kū-lŭs rē'pĕnz
Ranunculus sceleratus	ra-nŭn'kū-lŭs sĕl-er-ā'tŭs
Raphanus sativus	răf'a-nŭs sa-tī'vŭs
Ratanhia	ra-tăn'hya
Rauwolfia serpentina	**rō-wol´fi-a sur-pen-të´nä**
Resorcinum	rĕs-or-sī'nŭm
Rhamnus catharticus	răm'nŭs ka-thär'tĭ-kŭs
Rhamnus frangula	răm'nŭs frăn'gū-la
Rhamnus Purshiana	răm'nŭs pur-she-ā'na
Rheum	rē'ŭm
Rhododendron chrysanthemum	rō-do-dĕn'drŏn krĭs-ān'the-mŭm
Rhus aromatica	rŭs ăr-o-măt'ĭ-ka
Rhus glabra	rŭs glā'bra
Rhus Toxicodendron	rŭs tŏx-ĭ-ko-dĕn'drŏn
Rhus venenata	rŭs vĕn-e-nā'ta
Ricinus communis	rĭs'ĭ-nŭs kŏm-mū'nĭs

Robinia pseudacacia	ro-bĭn′ĭ-a sū-da-kā′she-a
Rumex acetosa	roo′mĕx ăs-e-tō′sa
Rumex crispus	roo′mĕx krĭs′pŭs
Ruta graveolens	roo′ta gra-vē′o-lĕnz
Sabadilla	săb-a-dĭl′la
Sabal serrulata	sā′bŭl ser-roo-lā′ta
Sabina	sa-bī′na
Salicinum	săl-ĭ-sī′nŭm
Salix nigra	sā′lĭx nī′gra
Salix purpurea	sā′lĭx pur-pū′re-a
Salol	sā′lŏl
Salvia officinalis	săl′vĭ-a ŏf-fĭs-ĭ-nā′lĭs
Sambucus canadensis	săm-bū′kŭs kăn-a-dĕn′sĭs
Sambucus nigra	săm-bū′kŭs nī′gra
Sanguinaria canadensis	săng-guĭ-nā′rĭ-a kăn-a-dĕn′sĭs
Santoninum	săn-to-nī′nŭm
Sarracenia purpurea	săr-ra-sē′nĭ-a pŭr-pū′re-a
Sarsaparilla	sär-sa-pa-rĭl′la
Sassafras	săs′sa-frăs
Scilla maritima	sĭl′la ma-rĭt′ĭ-ma
Scrophularia nodosa	skrŏf-ū-lā′rĭ-a no-dō′sa
Scutellaria lateriflora	skū-tĕl-lā′rĭ-a lăt-ĕ-rĭ-flō′ra
Secale cornutum	se-kā′lē kŏr-nū′tŭm
Selenium	se-lē′nĭ-ŭm
Sempervivum tectorum	sĕm-per-vī′vŭm tĕc-tō′rŭm
Senecio aureus	se-nē′she-ō au′re-ŭs
Senecio cineraria	**sē-nē′shi-ō sin′e-ra′ri-ä**
Senega	sĕn′e-ga
Senna	sĕn′na
Sepia	sē′pĭ-a
Silicea	sĭl-ĭsh′e-a
Silphium laciniatum	sĭl′fĭ-ŭm lăs-ĭn-ĭ-ā′tŭm
Sinapis alba	sĭn-ā′pĭs ăl′ba
Sinapis nigra	sĭn-ā′pĭs nī′gra
Smilax cordifolia radix	**smī′laks kŏr-di-fō′li-ä rā′diks**
Solaninum	sŏl-a-nī′nŭm
Solanum arrebenta	so-lā′nŭm ăr-re-bĕn′ta
Solanum carolinense	so-lā′nŭm kär-o-lĭ-nĕn′sē
Solanum mammosum	so-lā′nŭm măm-mō′sŭm
Solanum nigrum	so-lā′nŭm nī′grŭm
Solidago Virgaurea	sŏl-ĭ-dā′gō vur′gau′re-a
Spigelia	spī-gē′lĭ-a
Sparteinum sulphuricum	spăr-tē-ĭ′nŭm sŭl-fū′rĭ-kŭm
Spongia	spŭn′jĭ-a

Stannum metallicum	stăn'nŭm mĕ-tăl'lĭ-kŭm
Staphysagria	stăf-ĭs-ā'grĭ-a
Sticta pulmonaria	stĭk'ta pŭl-mo-nā'rĭ-a
Stillingia silvatica	stĭl-lĭn'gĭ-a sĭl-văt'ĭ-ka
Stramonium	stra-mō'nĭ-ŭm
Strontium carbonicum	strŏn'she-ŭm kär-bŏn'ĭ-kŭm
Strophanthus hispidus	strŏ-făn'thŭs hĭs'pĭ-dŭs
Strophanthus sarmentosus	**strŏ-fan´thus sär-men´tŏ-sus**
Strychninum nitricum	strĭk-nī'nŭm nĭ'trĭ-kŭm
Strychninum phosphoricum	strĭk-nī'nŭm fŏs-fŏr'ĭ-kŭm
Strychninum sulphuricum	strĭk-nī'nŭm sŭl-fū'rĭ-kŭm
Sulfanilamide	**sulf´ä-nil´ä-mīde**
Sulphur	sŭl'fur
Sulphur iodatum	sŭl'fur ī-o-dā'tŭm
Sumbul	sŭm'bŭl
Symphoricarpus **racemosus**	sĭm-fŏr-ĭ-kär'pŭs răs-e-mō'sŭs
Symphytum officinale	sĭm-fī'tŭm ŏf-fĭs-ĭ-nā'lē
Syzygium Jambolanum	sĭz-ĭj'ĭ-ŭm jăm-bo-lā'nŭm
Tabacum	tăb'a-kŭm
Tamus communis	tā'mŭs kŏm-mū'nĭs
Tanacetum vulgare	tăn-a-sē'tŭm vŭl'gā'rē
Tanghinia venenifera	tăn-gĭn'ĭ-a vĕn-e-nĭf'e-ra
Taraxacum officinale	ta-răx'a-kŭm ŏf-fĭs'ĭ-nā'lē
Tarentula cubensis	ta-rĕn'tū-la kū-bĕn'sĭs
Tarentula hispana	ta-rĕn'tū-la hĭs-pā'na
Tartarus emeticus	tär'ta-rŭs ē-mĕt'ĭ-kŭs
Taxus baccata	tăx'ŭs băk-kā'ta
Tellurium	tĕl-lū'rĭ-ŭm
Terebinthinæ oleum	tĕr-e-bĭn'thĭ-nē ō'le-ŭm
Teucrium marum verum	tū'krĭ-ŭm mā'rŭm vē'rŭm
Thaspium aureum	thăs'pĭ-ŭm au're-ŭm
Thea sinensis	thē'a sĭ-nĕn'sĭs
Theridion	the-rĭd'ĭ-ŏn
Thlaspi Bursa pastoris	thlăs'pī bur'sa păs-tō'rĭs
Thuja occidentalis	thū'ya ŏk-sĭ-dĕn-tā'lĭs
Thymol	**thī´mŏl**
Thymus Serpyllum	thī'mŭs ser-pĭl'lŭm
Thyroidinum	thī-roi-dĭ'num
Glandulæ thyroidæ	glăn'dū-la thē-roi'dē-a
Tongo	tŏng'gō
Tradescantia diuretica	trăd-ĕs-kăn'she-a dī-yū-rĕt'ĭ-ka
Trifolium pratense	trĭ-fō'lĭ-ŭm pra-tĕn'sē
Trifolium repens	trĭ-fō'lĭ-ŭm rē'pĕnz
Trillium	trĭl'lĭ-ŭm

306

Triosteum perfoliatum	trī-ŏs'te-ŭm per-fō-lĭ-ā'tŭm
Triticum repens	trĭt'ĭ-kŭm rē'pĕnz
Tussilago petasites	tŭs-sĭ-lā'gō pĕt-a-sī'tēz
Urtica dioica	ur-tī'ka dī-oi'ka
Urtica urens	ur-tī'ka yū'rĕnz
Usnea barbata	ŭs'ne-a bär-bā'ta
Ustilago Maidis	ŭs-tĭ-la'go mā'ĭ-dĭs
Uva ursi	yū'va ur'sĭ
Uranium nitricum	yū-rā'nĭ-ŭm nĭ'tri-kŭm
Valeriana officinalis	va-lē-rĭ-ā'na ŏf-fĭs-ĭ-nā'lĭs
Venus mercenaria	**vē´nus mur´sēn-nâr´i-ä**
Veratrinum	vĕr-a-trĭ'nŭm
Veratrum album	ve-rā'trŭm ăl'bŭm
Veratrum viride	ve-rā'trŭm vĭr'ĭ-dē
Verbascum Thapsus	vur-băs'kŭm thăp'sŭs
Verbena hastata	vur-bē'na hăs-tā'ta
Verbena officinalis	vur-bē'na ŏf-fĭs-ĭ-nā'lĭs
Veronica beccabunga	ve-rŏn'ĭ-ka bĕk'ka-bŭng'ga
Viburnum Opulus	vĭ-bur'nŭm ŏ'pū-lŭs
Viburnum prunifolium	vĭ-bur'nŭm proo-nĭ-fō'lĭ-ŭm
Vinca minor	vĭn-ka mĭ'nŏr
Viola odorata	vī'o-la ō-do-rā'ta
Viola tricolor	vī'o-la trī'ko-lŏr
Viscum album	vĭs'kŭm ăl'bŭm
Wyethia helenioides	wī-ē'thĭ-a hĕ-lĕn-ĭ-oī'dēz
Xanthoxylum fraxineum	zăn-thŏx'ĭ lŭm frăx-ĭn'e-ŭm
Yucca filamentosa	yŭk'ka fĭl-a-mĕn-tō'sa
Zincum aceticum	zĭng-kŭm a-sĕ'tĭ-kŭm
Zincum bromatum	zĭng-kŭm bro-mā'tŭm
Zincum carbonicum	zĭng-kŭm kār-bŏn'ĭ-kŭm
Zincum cyanatum	zĭng-kŭm sī-ăn-ā'tŭm
Zincum iodatum	zĭng-kŭm ī-o-dā'tŭm
Zincum metallicum	zĭng-kŭm mĕ-tăl'lĭ-kŭm
Zincum muriaticum	zĭng-kŭm mū-rĭ-ăt'-ĭ-kŭm
Zincum oxydatum	zĭng-kŭm ŏx-ĭ-dā'tŭm
Zincum phosphoratum	zĭng-kŭm fŏs-fo-rā'tŭm
Zincum sulphuricum	zĭng-kŭm sŭl-fū'rĭ-kŭm
Zincum valerianicum	zĭng-kŭm vă-lē-rĭ-ăn'ĭ-kŭm
Zingiber officinale	zĭn'jĭ-ber ŏf-fĭs-ĭ-nā'lĭ

307

A DICTIONARY OF HOMEOPATHY*

by Benjamin C. Woodbury, Jr., M. D.
Boston, Mass.

The title of this paper was originally intended to read: "A Dictionary *for* Homeopathy." After several attempts, however, to impress this idea upon the mind of our diligent and industrious chairman, the writer was finally brought to the cold realization that the paper should be called "A Dictionary *of* Homeopathy"; and so it must stand.

Its subject-matter is offered by way of suggestion for future consideration and makes no claim toward finality.

Hence to paraphrase the now justly-famous phrase of Abraham Lincoln, whom a recent American poet has apostrophized as

"The quaint figure that men love,
The prairie lawyer, master of us all;" —

the writer's original concept was "A Dictionary *of* Homeopathy," "*for* Homeopathy," and written or compiled "*by* a representative body of the Homeopathic profession."

The idea of a volume of comprehensive and current homeopathic terminology must have occurred to many another, yet so far as the writer's personal knowledge is concerned no such compilation has ever been made, if proposed or attempted.

It is, therefore, with no little degree of trepidation that I venture to suggest the very pressing need of such a work.

It is true that throughout Hahnemann's writings certain terms appear, which it was the author's endeavor to elucidate in an adequate manner; yet with what measure of success but brief reference to early homeopathic literature will suffice to show how far afield were many of the applications of these definitions by his professed followers.

It is likewise true that the late Dr. Bernhardt Fincke made a more or less abortive attempt in his volume on High Potencies to introduce into general homeopathic parlance a variety of terms which were of only particular application to his own explanation of the *modus operandi* of the homeopathic cure.

A limited number of those terms found practical application and have been retained in common usage.

During the early part of the nineteenth century Dr. John H. Clarke, of London, presented to the profession his admirable and classical *Dictionary of the Homeopathic Materia Medica*. This, however, is quite a different thing

*From the *Journal of the American Institute of Homoeopathy,* Vol. 14, #3, Sept. 1921.

from a Dictionary of Homeopathy, i.e., an encyclopedia, which in addition to the explanation of homeopathic terms,[1] might include in a general way a description of homeopathic drugs, with a brief account of their action, dosage and usage, much in the same way as is to be found in any standard medical lexicon.

And in the early seventies Dr. Timothy Field Allen published his exhaustive and painstaking *Encyclopedia of Pure Materia Medica.*

All these and similar works deal with homeopathic materia medica but are not encyclopedias of general information relative to homeopathy as a distinctive method in practice or as a separate school of medicine.

The idea of a volume compiled with this specific intention occurred to the writer not long since on noting the painstaking and careful manner in which the author of a recent medical dictionary[2] has prepared his data regarding homeopathic terminology and the preparation, dose and usage of homeopathic medicines.

We have already at hand the nucleus of such a compendium in the compilation of Dr. Carmichael[3], as representative of the committee appointed by the American Institute on Nomenclature.

Why could not the data already collected by this committee be elaborated into an adequate volume to include similar data as already is becoming current in regular medicine through the editorship of such careful writers as Gould, Lippincott, Dunglinson, Stedman and others, and especially compiled and edited as a companion volume to the authorized treatise on Homeopathy issued under the official sanction of the Institute?

The Glossary proposed for separate publication by Dr. W. B. Hinsdale[4] is virtually this sort of a compendium so far as homeopathic terminology is concerned. Let us go further and make the Dictionary of Homeopathy a volume which shall contain in addition to the definitions of homeopathic terms, brief and concise data upon homeopathic medicines, their preparations, dosage and indications.

Medical lexicons and encyclopedias of regular medicine have in the past made little if any reference to Homeopathy, save the briefest definition. Nor does Hahnemann shine with any great luminosity in orthodox medical traditions, if the following reference in a history of medicine published recently is to

---

[1] Homeopathic Nomenclature, T.H. Carmichael, M.D., Philadelphia, *Journal of the American Institute of Homeopathy,* December, 1917.

[2] *A Practical Medical Dictionary,* Thomas Lathrop Stedman, A.M., M.D.

[3] Pharmaceutical Catechism, *Journal of the American Institute of Homeopathy,* February, March, June, November, 1919. *Vide* also: 'The Dose', *Hahnemannian Monthly,* January 1920.

[4] Report of Committee on Nomenclature, *Journal of the American Institute of Homeopathy,* April 1917.

[5] *An Introduction to the Study of Medicine,* Fielding H. Garrison, M.D., W.B. Saunders Co., 1917.

be taken as a criterion.

For we find that Garrison[5] makes reference to Homeopathy as "really one of the many isolated theoretic systems of the preceding century... The extreme popularity of Hahnemann's doctrines is probably due to the fact that they lessened the scale of dosage of drugs in practice. He was in fact, the introducer of the small dose. Otherwise his system is but an offshoot of eighteenth century theorizing. He died a millionaire in Paris in 1843."

Dr. Stedman states in his Preface that "the sectarian lines which have divided medical practitioners are, happily, gradually fading away. Homeopathic and eclectic physicians no longer ignore the discoveries of modern experimental medicine, but rather *are doing their part to advance true science* [italics added]. On the other hand, therapeutists of all schools are learning that there is virtue in Homeopathy and Isopathy, as well as in Enantiopathy and Allopathy, that, in fact, there is but one science of medicine, and they are ready to apply any one of these healing principles in suitable cases. Prejudice and antagonism are often based largely upon misunderstanding and to promote unity among practitioners of the therapeutic art I have defined the terms peculiar to Homeopathic and Eclectic Therapeutics."

It would be a waste of valuable time to rehearse all the various definitions given by the author on subjects dealing with Homeopathy. The common terms and a few likewise of those not ordinarily found may suffice for our purpose. Let us consider them alphabetically.

Passing such universally used remedies as *Aconitum, Actaea r., Adonis v.,* etc. —and undoubtedly many of us will do well to read carefully even between the lines to refresh our failing memories—we come to:

Agaricus Muscarius. Fly agaric, poison mushroom; a tincture from the fresh fungus is employed in Homeopathy in the irregular heart action of coffee and tea drinkers and tobacco-smokers, in doses of the third to thirtieth potency.

Apis Mellifica. A homeopathic remedy, made by shaking a number of bees together in a bottle to make them angry, then pouring alcohol over them; employed in nephritis complicating scarlet fever; in erysipelas, conjunctivitis with smarting of the eyes, and to control night screaming of children; dose third to thirtieth potency.

Apium Virus. Bee poison; a homeopathic remedy prepared by extracting bee stings (see *Apis Mellifica)* and triturating them with sugar of milk; employed for the same purposes and in the same doses as *Apis.*

Autotherapy. 1. Self-treatment. 2. Spontaneous cure. 3. Autosero-therapy. 4. Treatment of disease by the administration of the patient's own pathological excretions, as for example, the swallowing of the discharge from a wound or the subcutaneous injection of the filtered sputum in the case of tuberculosis; Duncan's method.

Auto-Tuberculin. Tuberculin prepared from cultures made from the patient's own sputum.

Bacillinum. A homeopathic nosode prepared from tuberculous lung tissue.

Calcarea carbonica. A homeopathic preparation from the white middle layer of the oyster shell, given in scrofula, sweating of the feet, rickets, acid dyspepsia, gall stone, colic and night sweats, in doses of the 6th to 200th potencies.

Calcarea Fluorica. A homeopathic preparation of fluor-spar used in bone tumors, cataract, and varicose veins in doses of the 3x to 12x potencies.

Calcarea Ostrearum. Calcarea carbonica.

Calcarea Phosphorica. Precipitated calcium phosphate, a homeopathic preparation, recommended in bone diseases, rickets, tuberculosis, leucorrhea, and rheumatism in doses of 3x to 12x potencies.

Carbo-nitrogenoid constitution. In Homeopathy, one of von Grauvogl's three constitutional groups, the one in which there is too slow an oxidation of the blood, anoxemia.

Causticum. A homeopathic remedy prepared by mixing recently slaked lime with potassium bi-sulphate and distilling; employed in various neuroses and paralysis, chronic rheumatism and catarrhal troubles.

Centesimal. (L. *Centesimis,* Hundredth). Relating to or divided into hundredths, *c. scale.* In Homeopathy, the system of potentization in which each succeeding trituration or dilution contains 1/100 as much as the preceding one; *i.e.,* one drop or one grain of any given potency is mixed with 99 drops or grains of the menstruum to make the next higher potency.

Cina. The homeopathic tincture from the dried flowers of worm-seed *Artemisia Santonica;* employed as an anthelmintic, and in other conditions marked by itching of the nose or anus, night crying, and grinding of the teeth during sleep, in doses of the 1st, 6th, or 30th potency.

Collinsonia canadensis. Citronella, stonewort, the herb, employed in eclectic practice in the treatment of Clergyman's sore throat, digestive and urinary disorders, and hemorrhoids, in doses of mx* 10-15 (0.6-1.0 g.) of the specific preparation in syrup or water.

Crotalus. A homeopathic preparation of the venom of the rattlesnake, *Crotalus horridus,* triturated with milk sugar; employed in ecchymosis, oozing of blood, hemorrhagic measles, etc., in doses of the sixth to thirtieth potency.

Crotalin. Trade name of a preparation made from rattlesnake virus, which has been recommended in the treatment of epilepsy.

Diphtherin. Diphtheria toxin. The toxin of diphtheria.

---

*minim; approximately 1 drop.

Drug Disease. 1. Morbid symptoms caused by a drug and by the disease for the cure of which that drug is given. 2. In Homeopathy the aggregate of symptoms noted in the proving of a drug, which symptoms, when caused by a natural disease, are indications for the administration of small doses or high potencies of the same drug.

Dose. The quantity of a drug or other remedy to be taken or applied all at one time or in fractional amounts within a given period.

Dose. In Homeopathy, the dilution or attenuation of the remedy, and the number of times the remedy is taken.

Dynamic. D. School, a group of theorists founded by Stahl, who professed the belief that all vital action is the result of an internal force independent of anything external to the body.

Dynamization. In Homeopathy the increase of potency of a medicine by trituration or by dilution in water with succussion; see POTENCY.

Dynamize. To increase the potency of a medicine by trituration or by succussion in water.

Echinacea. In homeopathic practice the tincture from the fresh root is employed in septic conditions in doses of mx 5-10 (0.3-0.6 g.) of the mother tincture. In eclectic practice it is employed as an alterative and in septic conditions in doses of mx 5-30 (0.3-2.0 g.) of the specific preparation.

Fluoride calcium F. Fluor-spar.

Glonoin. Trinitro-glyceryl. $C_3H_5(NO_3)_3$. Nitroglycerin.

Hahnemannian. (Samuel Christian Frederic *Hahnemann.* German physician, the founder of the doctrines of Homeopathy, 1755-1843.) Relating to Hahnemann or to the doctrine he taught.

Hepar. Hepar sulphuris calcareum, impure calcium sulphide (calc. sulphurata) triturated with sugar of milk. Employed in homeopathic therapeutics in boils, pustular eruptions, quinsy, etc., in the sixth to the thirtieth potency.

Heteropathy. (G. *heteros,* other, + *pathos,* suffering) allopathy.

Homeopathy. Homeopathy. Homeopathist.

Homeopathic. Homeopathic, relating to homeopathy.

Homeopathist (or Homeopathist). A medical practitioner of the homeopathic school.

Homeopathy (or Homeopathy). (G. *homoios,* like, similar, + *pathos,* suffering (disease). A system of therapeutics founded or developed by Samuel Hahnemann based upon the *observation* that certain drugs, when given in large doses in health, will produce certain conditions similar to those relieved, when occurring as symptoms of disease, by the same drug in small doses. This is called the law of similia, from the aphorism, *similia similibus curantur,* like is cured by like. Included in the homeopathic doctrine is the theory of dynamization which is that by repeated trituration, or dilution with agitation, the potency or power of a drug is enormously increased, certain substances, such as lycopodium and common salt, which are inert in appreciable doses even acquiring therapeutic properties when so treated.

Homeotherapeutic, or (Homeotherapeutic). 1. Homeopathic. 2. Relating to homeotherapy.

Homeotherapeutics, or (homeotherapeutics). 1. Homeopathy, 2. Homeotherapy.

Homeotherapy. (G. *homoios,* like + *therapia,* treatment). Treatment or prevention of a disease by means of a product similar to, but not identical with the active causal agent, as in Jennerian vaccination.

Hydrogenoid. Constitution. In Homeopathy one of von Grauvogl's three constitutional groups, the one in which there is too great an amount of fluid in the blood and tissues, hydremia. See OXYGENOID and CARBO NITROGENOID.

Hydrophobinum. A homeopathic nosode prepared from the virus of rabies.

Idiopathic disease. A disease for which no cause is found.

Isopathy (G. *isos,* equal + *pathos,* suffering). Theory or system of treatment of disease by means of the causal agent of a product of the same disease; also the treatment of a diseased organ by an extract of the same organ from a healthy animal.

Isoserum treatment. Therapeutic employment of serum taken from a person having or having had the same disease as the patient under treatment; also called isoserotherapy.

Isotherapy. (L. *isos,* equal + *therapeia,* treatment). Treatment or prophylaxis of a disease by means of the active causal agent, as in the preventive inoculations against rabies or in the use of bacterial vaccines.

Isotoxin. (G. *isos,* alike). A toxin in the blood active against an animal of the same species.

Keynote. In Homeopathy, one of the characteristic symptoms of a drug, serving as a guide for the exhibition of the remedy when a similar symptom occurs in disease.

Lachesis (G. *lachesis,* destroy, fate). The venom of *Lachesis mutus,* the bushmaster snake of South America, employed in homeopathic practice in the treatment of septicemia, varicose veins, diphtheria with great prostration, and peritonitis, in doses from the 6th to the 30th potency.

Law of similars. See SIMILIA SIMILIBUS CURANTUR.

Lycopodium. In homeopathic practice it is employed for pyrosis, constipation, brick-dust in the urine, jaundice, and impotence, in the thirtieth potency.

Lyssin. 1. The virus of rabies. 2. Hydrophobinum.

Materia Medica Pura. A treatise by Hahnemann embodying the results of his provings, or the records of the drug pathogenesis of sixty-one drugs, the basis of the homeopathic materia medica.

Maximum dose. The largest dose of a drug that can be taken without danger of poisoning.

Mercurius iodatus flavus. Yellow iodide of mercury, employed in sore throat, faucial ulceration and syphilis in doses of the third decimal trituration.

Mercurius iodatus ruber. Red iodide of mercury, employed in ulcerated sore throat and diphtheria in doses of the 3d trituration.

Mercurius vivus. Metallic mercury triturated with sugar of milk, employed in bromidrosis, cough with a ropy expectoration, and syphilis, in doses of the sixth to thirtieth potency.

Miasm, miasma. (G. *miasma,* 'stamp'). 1. Noxious effluvia or emanations formerly regarded as the cause of malaria and of various epidemic diseases. 2. Hahnemann's term for the infectious principle, a virus, which when taken into the organism may set up a specific disease.

Miasmatic. Relating to or caused by miasma.

Milk Sugar. Lactose.

Minimum. (L) The least, or smallest possible.

Morbific. (L. *morbus,* disease, + *facere,* to make). Disease producing, pathogenic.

Myrica. The bark of *Myrica cerifera,* bayberry, wax myrtle; in eclectic practice it is employed in sore throat.

Natrum. The official homeopathic name for sodium.

Natrum muriaticum. Sodium chloride, one part of common salt dissolved in nine parts by weight of distilled water; used in anemia, watery coryza, cold sores, cracked lips, marasmus, intermittent fever, headache, constipation and mental depression, in doses of the thirtieth to two hundredth potency.

Natrum phosphoricum. Sodium phosphate; used in cases of general acidity, in rheumatism, heart burn, acid dyspepsia, and acid diarrhea, in the 3x to 12x trituration.

Natrum sulphuricum. Sodium sulphate; used in bilious states, influenza, jaundice, diabetes, asthma and renal disorders, in doses of the 3x to 12x trituration.

Nux moschata. The homeopathic term for a tincture made from powdered nutmeg, myristica; employed in mental troubles, uncontrollable sleepiness, nervous aphasia and flatulence, in dose of the 6th, 30th and 200th potencies.

Nux vomica. Employed in homeopathic practice for the relief of hyperesthesia, the constipation of the sedentary, dry catarrh, and alcoholism, in doses of the mother tincture up to the 30th potency.

Oenanthe. (G. *oinos,* wine + *anthe,* flower). The root of *Oenanthe crocata,* water hemlock, an herb of western Europe; the tincture of the fresh root is employed in homeopathic practice in epilepsy and tetanic and other convulsions in doses of the 1st decimal to the 6th potency.

Oligodynamic. Active in very small quantity; noting for example, the germicidal effect of an exceedingly dilute solution (such as one to one hundred million) of copper in distilled water.

Oxygenoid constitution. In Homeopathy one of von Grauvogl's three consti-tutional groups, the one in which there is too great oxidation of the blood. See CARBONITROGENIOID and HYDROGENOID.

Pathogenesis. Drug Picture. 1. The production of morbid symptoms by drugs; 2. In Homeopathy, the record of all the symptoms observed in the proving of a drug on persons of all ages and both sexes, as well as of the effects of a poisonous dose of the same drug, or the toxicological record.

Pathogenetic. Pathogenic (G. *pathos,* suffering, disease, + *gennao,* to pro-duce) causing disease, morbific.

Pathognomonic. Characteristic or indicative of a disease, noting certain typi-cal symptoms.

Pathognomy. Diagnosis by means of a study of the typical symptoms of a disease, or of the subjective sensations of a patient.

Pathognostic. Pathognomic.

Pharmacodynamic. (G. *pharmakon* drug + *dynamis,* force). Relating to drug action.

Pharmacodynamics. The science of the physiological and therapeutic action of drugs.

Pharmacology. The branch of science which has to do with drugs in all their relations.

Pharmacotherapy. Treatment of disease by means of drugs.

Phytolacca. Given in eclectic practice in the treatment of sore nipples, the sore mouth of nursing infants, in sore throat, and subinvolution of the uterus.

Placebo. (L. 'I will please'). An indifferent substance, in the form of a medi-cine given for the moral or suggestive effect.

Potency (L. *potentia,* power). 1. Power, force, strength. 2. In Homeopathy, (a) the therapeutic efficacy of a drug as increased by succussion or trituration with alcohol or sugar of milk, respectively; (b) the degree of dilution or attenuation of a drug by which its therapeutic efficacy is increased. There are two degrees or systems of potency, the decimal and the centesimal. In the decimal system one part of the crude drug is triturated with nine parts of sugar of milk to make the first decimal potency. To make the second decimal potency one part of the first potency is triturated with nine parts of the sugar of milk; and so on. In the case of drugs, of which tinctures can be made, one drop of the mother tincture is added to nine drops of alcohol (in larger amounts but in the same proportion) and the mixture is strongly shaken (succussed) to make the first decimal dilution or potency; one drop of this succussed with nine drops of alcohol makes the second decimal dilution or potency, and so on.

The centesimal potencies are made in the same way, except that one grain or one drop is triturated or shaken with 99 grains or drops of the diluent to make the first centesimal potency; and one part of this again is mixed with 99 parts of the diluent to make the second centesimal potency. The centesimal potencies are indicated by numbers from 1 to 30 (usually, though not always, the highest potency used); the decimal potencies are indicated by the signs 1x, 2x, 30x, etc.

Potential. (L. *potentia,* power). 1. Capable of doing or being, though not yet doing or being; possible but not actual.

Potentialization. The rendering potent; in Homeopathy the increase in potency of a drug through dilution or attenuation.

Potentialize. To render potent; specifically, in Homeopathy, to increase the potency or therapeutic efficacy of a drug by dilution or attenuation; potentize.

Potentiation. Potentialization.

Potentize. In Homeopathy to render potent, potentialize, said of the dynamization of drugs by dilution or attenuation.

Fluxion potency. A dilution or potency made with a machine, water being used as a vehicle, and pushed to an extreme degree—as high, it is stated, as the 1/1000 or even 1/1000000 dilution.*

High potency, the Homeopathic preparation of a drug above the 30th dilution.

Prove. In Homeopathy, a test of the action of a drug upon a healthy person in order to obtain the therapeutic range of the same.

Proving. In Homeopathy, a test of the action of a drug upon the healthy body; a record of all the unusual sensations, or deviations from normal health, experienced by one taking the drug.

Psora. (G.) 1. Scabies. 2. Psoriasis. 3. Hahnemann's term for the itch dycrasia: defined as the parent of all chronic diseases, skin diseases, neoplasms, insanity, etc.; it was similar to, though of more extended application than, the "herpetic diathesis" of French writers.

Psoric. Relating to or suffering from scabies, psorus.

Psorinum. A homeopathic nosode prepared from the contents of the itch vesicle; it is employed in cases marked by profuse sweating, in offensive odor from the body, or headache with hunger.

Psoroid. Resembling scabies.

Psorous. Psoric.

Remedy. An agent which cures diseases or alleviates its symptoms. *Concordant remedies.* In Homeopathy, remedies of dissimilar origin whose actions are similar, and which may therefore be given in succession; *Inimical remedies,* in Homeopathy, remedies whose actions are dissimilar or antagonistic and which therefore may not be given in succession: *Tissue*

---

*I believe what is meant here is the number of times the remedy has been diluted. 1/1,000 would mean 1M ... 1/1,000,000 would mean MM. —*Editor.*

remedies, see under TISSUE.

Repercussive. Driving in or away, repellant.

Repertory. (L. *repertorium,* list, inventory). In homeopathic practice an index of symptoms peculiar to a special disease, with the name of the remedy or remedies having the same symptom, i.e., producing the same symptom when given in a proving.

Rhus. A genus of trees of the order of *anacardiaceae,* several species of which are employed in medicine.

Rhus toxicodendron. Poison oak, poison ivy, climbing sumach, picry, the leaf-lets of *Rhus radicans;* a volatile acid contained in the leaves of this plant causes in susceptible individuals a violent dermatitis; it is employed in eclectic practice in the exanthemata and erysipelas; in Homeopathy in erysipelas, eczema, sprains, lumbago, and rheumatism in the 6th to the 30th potency.

Saccharum Lactis (U. S. Br.). Sugar of milk, lactose, a sugar obtained from the whey of cows' milk $C_{12}H_{22}O_{11} + H_2O$, occurring as a gritty powder of moderately sweetish taste; diuretic in daily doses of 1-6 oz. (30 to 180g.), but employed chiefly in pharmacy in the making of triturations and other preparations.

Self-limited. Noting a disease which tends to cease after a definite period, as a result of its own processes; pneumonia is a typical example of a self-limited disease.

Senecio. The herb and root of *Senecio aureus,* squaw-weed, ragwort, a common weed of the eastern United States; 2. A tincture from the fresh flowering plants of *Senecio aureus* employed in homeopathic practice in dysmenorrhea and other menstrual disorders in doses of the 1st to the 6th potencies.

Sepia. 1. A black secretion of the cuttle fish, from which a pigment is made 2. In homeopathic practice, a tincture prepared from dried and powdered sepia, used in leucorrhea, dyspepsia, chronic nasal catarrh, and facial neuralgia in pregnant women, especially when associated with sallowness or a slight degree of jaundice; dose 6th and 30th potencies.

Sepsine. A ptomaine formed in putrefying animal matter.

Septicine. A ptomaine from decaying animal matter.

Silica. Dioxide of silicon, silicic anhydride SiO_2.

Silicea. The homeopathic preparation of silica triturated with sugar of milk; employed in the treatment of boils, and carbuncles, rickets, chronic headache, and bromidrosis of the feet, in doses of the 6th to the 200th potency.

Similia Similibus Curantur. (L. 'likes are cured by likes'). The homeopathic formula expressing the law of similars, or the doctrine that any drug which is capable of producing morbid symptoms in the healthy will remove similar symptoms occurring as an expression of disease. Another rendering of the formula, the one employed by Hahnemann, the founder of Homeopathy, is *Similia Similibus Curentur,* 'let likes be cured by likes'; this is called by homeopathic writers a rule of art, the other being regarded as expressing a law of nature.

Similimum, Simillimum. (L. *Simillimus,* most like). In homeopathy, the remedy indicated in a certain case because the same drug, when given to a healthy person, will produce the symptom complex most nearly approaching that of the disease in question.

Spongia. (G) Sponge. In homeopathic practice roasted sponge, spongia tosta, triturated with sugar of milk; employed in the treatment of croup and of chronic hoarseness in doses of the 3d to 30th potency.

Spongia Tosta. Turkish sponges cut into small pieces and heated in an apparatus like a coffee roaster; employed in Homeopathy, see SPONGIA.

Stannum. (L) Tin, a metallic element, symbol Sn, atomic weight 119. A trituration of the precipitated metal with sugar of milk is employed in Homeopathy in chronic catarrhal and other conditions marked by extreme weakness; dose, 6th to 15th decimal potency.

Sticta. Lungwort, a lichen *Sticta pulmonaria;* employed in eclectic practice for chronic coughs and rheumatism, especially when there is pain between the shoulders shooting up to the back of the head; employed in Homeopathy in the treatment of catarrhal troubles with dryness of the mucous membranes and in hard, dry coughs.

Subjective. Perceived by the individual only and not evident to the examiner, noting certain symptoms such as pain.

Succuss. (L. *succutere,* to shake up). To make succussion.

Sulphur (U. S. Br.). 1. Brimstone, an element, symbol S. atomic weight 32.07, occurring in native state in bright yellow color and occurs in volcanic countries. 2. In homeopathic practice a trituration of sublimed sulphur with sugar of milk, employed as an antipsoric*, to control the psora or underlying hereditary constitutional taint which interferes with the effect of otherwise well indicated drugs; dose 1x to 30th potency.

Sycosis. 1. Pustular folliculitis of the beard. 2. Hahnemann's term for the constitutional effects of the gonorrheal virus.

Symptom. (*symptoma; sym,* 'with' + *ptoma (pipto)* 'I fall'). Any morbid phenomenon or departure from the normal in function, appearance, or sensation experienced by the patient and indicative of disease.

Characteristic symptom, in Homeopathy a symptom peculiar to or specially characteristic or pathognomonic of any drugs.

Concomitant symptom, accessory symptom.

Antipsoric(G. *anti,* against, + *psora,* the itch). Curative of scabies, or the itch. A *remedy,* in Homeopathy, one which is especially serviceable in the treatment of psora or of chronic diseases in general.

Drug symptom, in Homeopathy, one of the unusual sensations or deviations from normal health experienced by a person who is proving a drug; it offers an indication, according to the doctrines of similars, for the therapeutic employment of the drug.

Guiding symptoms, characteristic symptoms.

Keynote Characteristic symptom.

Objective symptom, one which is evident to the observer.

Pathogenic symptom, in Homeopathy, one observed in the proving of a drug, and also one of the symptoms of poisoning by a drug.

Subjective symptom, one apparent only to the patient himself.

Symptomatic. Relating to a symptom or symptoms, indicative.

Symptom-complex. Complex (1) syndrome.

Symptom-group. Symptom-complex, syndrome.

Syndrome (G. *syndromos,* a running together, a meeting). The aggregate of symptoms associated with any morbid process, and constituting together the picture of the disease.

Syndromic. Relating to a syndrome.

Syphilinum. A homeopathic attenuation of the syphilitic virus.

Tablet. A small disc, usually of sugar of milk, impregnated with a tincture or other fluid form of some medicament (tablet saturate) or containing a finely powdered drug incorporated with it (tablet triturate); each tablet contains a dose, or a fraction of a dose, of the remedy, and is taken internally or dissolved in water and administered hypodermically.

Tarantula. One of a number of poisonous spiders around the shores of the Mediterranean and in tropical and sub-tropical America. *Tarantula cubensis,* a tincture made from the live Cuban tarantula, employed in homeopathic practice in the treatment of carbuncles, felons, and malignant diphtheria, in doses of the 6th to 30th potency.

Tartar Emetic. Antimonii et potassii tartras.

Tincture. The pharmacopoeial name of an alcoholic solution or extract of a non-volatile vegetable substance being called *Spiritus Hahnemannian Tincture.* In Homeopathy a preparation of equal parts by weight of alcohol and of the expressed juice of a plant; this is allowed to stand eight or ten hours and is then filtered. *Mother Tincture,* the standard Homeopathic tincture of any drug, made by macerating or dissolving the drug in alcohol or water; the attenuations or dilutions are made from this: its sign is q, the Greek TH; the mother tincture of an acid is the first decimal dilution, or one part of acid to nine parts of distilled water but in a few cases it is the centesimal dilution, and in the case of phosphorus it is the third decimal dilution.

Tissue remedies. Twelve salts especially used in the biochemical school of Homeopathy; these are *Kali sulphuricum, Natrum sulphuricum,*

Calcarea fluorica, Silicea, Calcarea sulphurica, Natrum muriaticum, Kali muriaticum, Calcarea phosphorica, Magnesia phosphorica, Ferrum phosphoricum, Natrum phosphoricum and *Kali phosphoricum.*

Toxicology. The science of poisons, their source, chemical composition and action, test, and antidotes.

Treatment. Therapeutics, therapy; the medical or surgical care of a patient; the institution of measures or the giving of remedies designed to cure a disease. *Symptomatic treatment,* expectant. *Similar treatment,* Homeopathy.

Triturate. (L. *triturare,* to rub, grind, triturate). Trituration, a term in homeopathic pharmacy, adopted by the U.S.P. to denote a powder prepared by triturating together definite quantities of a medicinal substance and sugar of milk. In homeopathic pharmacies the triturations are in the proportion of one part of the drug to nine parts of sugar of milk (decimal), or of one of the drug to ninety-nine of sugar of milk (centesimal trituration); in the U.S.P. the general formula is 10 parts of the drug to 90 of sugar of milk.

Trituration. (L. *trituratio.*) 1. Trituratio. 2. The act of reducing a drug to a fine powder, and at the same time incorporating it thoroughly with sugar of milk, by rubbing the two together in a mortar.

Trombidium. (*Trombidium,* a genus of mites). In homeopathic practice a trituration made from the parasitic red acarus of the fly. *Trombidium muscae domesticae,* employed in the treatment of dysentery, especially when the symptoms are made worse by eating and drinking, in doses of the 6th to the 30th potency.

Tuberculine. A ptomaine derived from cultures of the tubercle bacillus.

Tuberculinum. A homeopathic trituration of dried tuberculous sputum.

Vaccinin. A homeopathic attenuation of the virus of cow pox, vaccininum.

Vaccininum. A homeopathic attenuation of the virus of cow pox.

Variolinum. A homeopathic or isopathic preparation of the contents of a small-pox postule, potentized by trituration or succussion.

Vial. Phial, a small bottle for holding liquid medicines.

Vis. (L. *force*). Force, energy, power. *Vis medicatrix naturae,* the natural curative power, the power inherent in the organism of overcoming disease without the aid of medicaments or other therapeutic agencies.

Vitalism. The theory that all animal functions are dependent upon a special form of energy or force, the vital force, distinct from any other physical force.

Vitalist. One who adheres to the doctrines of vitalism.

Wood-charcoal. Carbo ligni.

As a final word on this subject I may say that a possible criticism of previous epitomes of homeopathic nomenclature are by the therapeutist and not by the lexicographer. Dr. Stedman's definitions which have been quoted are at once accurate and are stamped with the true hall marks of professional lexicography.

It is a curious fact that in the second century of homeopathic history we find that there are two distinct movements in the medical world; one of them in the regular school toward the recognition and investigation of the homeopathic method; the other equally as distinctive, perhaps, within our own ranks in the direction of allopathy.

When these two therapeutic poles are so obviously being reversed, and we find such a growing tendency toward the recognition of Hahnemannian principles among regular medical writers, does it not behoove those of us who are still desirous of seeing Homeopathy become the dominant therapeutic method to arouse from our post-prandial lethargy—is that they have for the most part been compiled by we who have been feasting lavishly upon the bounty of our fathers—cast off our half-homeopathic encumbrances and stand undefiled before the world?

Our colleagues of the old school are many of them "already in the field; why stand we here idle?" Contrast this store-house of therapeutic truth now placed before the regular profession with the attitude assumed a half century ago, when the very name of Homeopathy was a by-word, almost, and a hissing, and we can with but a slight degree of perspicacity* predict what the trend will be fifty, or even twenty years hence.

Reference to Homeopathy in these notes alone—and I have undoubtedly overlooked some definitions in my hurried review of this lexicon—is made no less than seventy times.

It is the spirit of the times to go forward. The harvest to be gleaned in the near future in the therapeutic field is great, but the workers are all too few. When shall we see the truly curative, instead of the substitutive method the vogue in therapeutics? We need many recruits in the great army of medical reconstruction.

---

*acuteness of perception or understanding.

A GLOSSARY OF ALTERNATIVE AND HOLISTIC HEALTH CARE THERAPIES

For quite some time now I have debated whether or not to include this section in my dictionary. Finally, with this the fourth edition, I decided to do so if I could keep it brief and succinct. I wanted to provide some information for the homeopath on health alternatives without creating another dictionary within a dictionary. That would be fodder for another, separate tome. I chose rather to offer a few brief descriptive sentences. This way the reader can garner a quick and hopefully effortless understanding of the particular therapy in question.

In making decisions as to what to define, I decided to restrict this glossary to holistic health modalities rather than individual treatments such as colloidal silver, melatonin, kombucha tea, spirulina (popularized by Christopher Hills, 1926-1997), etc. I also decided not to include separate entries for astrology, numerology, etc. as these are largely 'intuitive arts'. Whether or not the above-mentioned subjects have validity or health benefits, I had to draw lines and be clear on my intent.

Another issue I had to wrestle with was whether or not to give individual entry status to copyrighted technique-names. Take for example the bodywork entry. I decided to include those therapies within the bodywork entry as it is the intent of all to increase an individual's freedom by relieving muscular/skeletal tension, decreasing pain and increasing blood and lymph, circulation, etc. Each has developed their own methodology based on respective phenomenologies and each seems to recognize the value inherent in the emotional connection. So, with that in mind, I decided to group these intensive touch therapies into one entry, **bodywork**.

Let me state for the record that I am not advocating, recommending, nor negating, but educating. One may visit the library or bookstore, physician or therapist to delve deeper, if that is not already obvious.

---

*If one does not find a technique listed in the following pages it may be found in the dictionary proper. The description of therapies in this section or in the dictionary proper is not to be construed as medical advice nor as a replacement for competent medical opinion and services. Seek the appropriate health care professional.

abreaction the release or elimination of tension which has accumulated as a result of conflict or repressed emotions. It is done by a conscious examination, reflection, and acting out.

acupressure the application of pressure by a blunt object (finger tip, blunt tool) to points along the body to treat tension, pain, and disease. It is similar to acupuncture but no needles are employed. Shiatsu is traditional Japanese acupressure or finger massage.

acupuncture the insertion of needles into points of the body to regulate *chi* and energies in the various bodily meridians in order to treat disease.

Alexander Technique a hands-on instructional technique developed by F.M. Alexander (1869-1955) to improve the posture, coordination, and movement and eliminate unhealthy habits of movement.

ambient music a pleasant, non-intrusive, non-melodic music designed for relaxation or meditation. It may also be used for visualization exercises or to arouse energies.

anma an ancient form of Japanese deep therapeutic massage (it originated in China some 4,000 years ago), used primarily to stimulate the flow of blood. A non-oil massage, it preceded shiatsu. The following are Japanese systems of massage: Ko Ho Anma (traditional), Zoku Shin Do (traditional East Asian foot reflexology), Gen Ko Anma (modern), Sei Tai (structural alignment), and Keiraku Shiatsu (meridian shiatsu).

anointment oil anointment has become more and more popular recently. Not only does massaging a good oil into the skin provide nutrients, it addresses health issues and the spiritual life as well.

anthroposophical medicine developed by Rudolf Steiner (1861-1925), this medical philosophy stresses the importance of spiritual and physical components of the individual both in disease and in health. Many remedies are utilized: art and movement therapy, counseling, dietary and nutritional therapy, homeopathic, herbal, and anthroposophical remedies, rhythmical massage, and hydrotherapy, etc. See entry in dictionary proper.

apitherapy the use of injected bee venom and/or actual stings of bees to cure or alleviate a variety of illnesses, especially arthritis and multiple sclerosis.

applied kinesiology the application of kinesiology (the study of the muscles and their movements) to assess muscle function, posture, etc. and analyze substances which may enhance or inhibit the functioning of the body. It was developed in the 1960s by George Goodheart, D.C. One may test whether a substance (food, medicine, remedy, etc.) is beneficial or harmful for the patient by assessing muscular strength when that substance is held and pressure is applied to a test muscle. If the muscle goes weak, that substance is assumed to have a weakening effect on the health/body. See

TOUCH FOR HEALTH.

Arica a self-development training technique developed by Oscar Ichazo. It includes movement and breathing exercises in combination with what Ichazo calls the nine levels of consciousness.

aromatherapy the therapeutic use of essential oils, primarily to treat emotional disorders (stress, anxiety, etc.). The oils may be inhaled, massaged into the skin or used in baths.

art therapy the use of painting, sculpture, and drawing to help patients reconcile their emotional conflicts, gain heightened self-awareness, and express unspoken and unconscious concerns. It can also be used to diagnose and then assess progress which the client is making towards a new level of health.

auric healing the psychic diagnosis and healing of a person's aura or auric field. The aura is an energy field which every living thing has. This energy field acts as a medium for the interaction of other energies present in the environment. The aura is believed to be made up of seven colors, with a healthy aura indicative of a healthy body.

auricular acupuncture acupuncture carried out on any of the two hundred points on the ear. The whole body can be treated in this way.

autogenic training a method of self-regulation or meditation to calm the body and mind developed by J.H. Schultz in the late 1920s. He created six standard phrases to induce a state of deep relaxation.

auto-suggestion the use of suggestion to bring about physical and/or psychological changes in the person. Suggestions are often affirmations or positive thoughts intended to enhance self-esteem or do away with fears. Emile Coue (1857-1926) was the inventor, and his affirmation 'Every day, in every way, I am getting better and better' was quite popular in the late 1960s and early 1970s.

aversion therapy a behavioral therapy which helps one to learn new behavioral patterns through the use of punishment.

ayurvedic medicine a medical philosophy derived from the Vedas (Indian sacred scriptures) which includes a great variety of traditional Indian remedies combined with yogic breath work, bathing, enemas, mantras, fasting, and cleansing diets. "Practitioners treat the patient as a whole, advising on personal life-style habits, diet and choice of sexual partner, as well as taking into consideration astrological factors and evaluating the quality of urine (pulse, tongue, too), sweat and the voice."—Drury, p. 111. Maharishi Ayur-Veda is a modern reformulation of ayurveda as proposed by Maharishi Mahesh Yogi.

Bach Flower Remedies 38 flower essences developed by Dr. E. Bach (1886-1936) in the mid 20th century. These essences treat primarily emotional and temperamental imbalances, yet physical problems may often be resolved as well. They are not homeopathic remedies. See entry in dictionary proper.

Barbara Brennan Healing Technique a spiritual healing system whereby the practitioner attempts to balance the client's energy field after clearing it of blocked and unhealthy energies.

Bates Method a method developed by American ophthalmologist W.H. Bates (1881-1931), which utilizes eye, memory, and imaginative exercises in concert to improve vision. Palming and sunning are among the therapeutic techniques that he devised.

bee venom therapy see APITHERAPY.

Bier's Hyperaemic Treatment a hot air (144-230⁰F) treatment recommended for sciatica, arthritis, and varicose veins. Devised by the late Dr. med. A. Bier.

Billings Method (cervical-mucus method) a method of natural birth control developed by Drs. John and Evelyn Billings, based on observing the menstrual cycle patterns.

biochemic remedies see dictionary entry.

Biodynamic agriculture/gardening "...applies a unique and sustainable approach to agricultural practice which takes into consideration the ecology of the Earth as a whole and its relationship to the workings of the universe. Biodynamic agriculture is distinct from organic farming in two fundamental ways. It employs a unique set of herbal preparations which, when applied to plants, compost, and fields in homeopathic dilutions, enliven and harmonize the soil. And, biodynamic farmers look at *processes* rather than *substances* or *organisms.* They seek to *stimulate* processes which are the source of the problem rather than addressing the symptoms." - *Lilipoh,* Summer/Fall, p. 15, 1997. It was founded by Dr. Ehrenfried E. Pfeiffer (1899 •), who also did seminal work in a sensitive crystallization testing method for cancer. There are nine biodynamic preparations. See ANTHROPOSOPHICAL MEDICINE entry in dictionary.

bioenergetic medicine (vibrational medicine) a relatively new field which encompasses healing modalities based on energetics rather than material doses (see MATERIAL DOSES in dictionary proper). For example, the use of penicillin to treat bacterial infections is not energetics but rather the pitting of material versus material. A homeopathic remedy given to treat a bacterial infection is an example of energetic therapy because there is no material substance left in the remedy when it is dissolved in the patient's mouth. When the remedy hits the moist mouth, vibrational energy is liberated which affects the person's innate curative abilities, and healing occurs.

bioenergetics (core energetics) the use of physical exercises/movements in combination with breathing techniques and verbal psychotherapy to release repressed emotions which limit the healthy functioning and freedom of the individual. It was developed by Alexander Lowen (1910-) and has its roots in Reichian therapy.

bioenergy   the flow of energy/life-force/*chi* in the body.

biofeedback   a technique for influencing bodily functions by visualizing, re-laxing, and/or imagining while observing metered sound or light. By direct-ing one's awareness to how the body feels in comparison to metered feed-back, one can adjust one's own biology. In other words, when the body receives feedback on its performance it can adjust itself to accentuate or inhibit that performance.

biofield therapeutics   a generic term which describes any of the many thera-pies which attempt to manipulate the massless energetic field (*chi?*, aura?) which surrounds and permeates living things.

biological dentistry   dentistry which realises the importance of using non-toxic restoration materials for dental procedures and addresses the un-recognized impact which dental toxins and hidden dental infections have on health.

Bio-Magnetic Touch Healing a simple hands-on magnetic healing tech-nique using the index and middle fingers of each hand to touch specific points on the body. Healing takes place as the combination of correct points and light touch activates the inherent healing ability of the body.

biorhythms   the concept that life is a flow of ups and downs and that these cycles can be charted. There are three cycles: physical (23 days), emo-tional (28 days), and intellectual (33 days). With this in mind, one may chart the rhythms and plan one's activities appropriately.

Bircher-Benner System   a dietary method based upon the work of Dr. Bircher-Benner, based on a raw foods diet supplemented with cereals. Eggs and cheeses are allowable.

Blackmore's celloids   see dictionary entry.

Blood Type Diet   a diet regimen based upon one's blood type. The origina-tor of this interesting concept is Peter D'Adamo, N.D. *(Eat Right For Your Type*, 1996). His extensive research reveals that O types should eat meat, eliminate most grains, and exercise vigorously; A types should be vegetarians, do mild, gentle exercise and meditate; while B types should have a varied diet, including dairy, and engage in moderate exercise. A-B types blend the characteristics of A and B, and should engage in calming exercise. Types O and A should avoid dairy products.

body armor   a concept in Reichian therapy which says that musculature has memory ('cellular memory') of previous traumatic events. As a result, energy does not flow as freely throughout the body as it could. Addition-ally, those muscles 'armor' themselves against the recall of those painful experiences.

bodywork/massage techniques   a variety of techniques designed to improve range of motion, alleviate muscular and skeletal tension and pain, and increase circulation. These goals are accomplished by the selected use of energetic and cathartic (breath and muscular release) work, rhythmical movement, and massage. Bodywork therapies acknowledge that there is 'cellular memory' (see BODY ARMOR). Ultimately treatments are intended to create a new physiological, structural, emotional and energetic balance in the recipient (often in the practitioner, too). There are many, many such techniques, including:

Alchemical bodywork a deep bodywork technique which uses hypnosis in order to access emotional aspects of bodily tension.

Aston Patterning a process similar to Feldenkrais in that it combines movement education, fitness, ergonomics and hands-on structural bodywork.

Bonnie Prudden Myotherapy a type of trigger point therapy developed by Ms. Prudden.

Bowen technique a deep bodywork technique consisting of gentle, dynamic moves to the muscle and connective tissue. It balances the body and stimulates energy flow. It was developed in the 1950s by Tom Bowen. According to its proponents, it helps other ailments such as asthma, migraines, and difficult digestion, often in only two sessions.

Breema Bodywork a deep bodywork therapy, which may be done alone or with a practitioner, originating with the Kurds (Breemava is a Kurdish village).

Chi Nei Tsang (Internal Organ Massage) a Taoist massage technique which concentrates on the abdomen and navel area. It strives to balance energies of the internal organs.

Cranial-Sacral Therapy/Technique developed most recently by John Upledger, but pioneered in the 1930s by W.G. Sutherland, it consists of very gentle pressure to massage the bones, membranes and fluids that support and envelop the cranium and spine.

Deep Tissue Massage utilizes deep pressure both in specific areas and with long strokes to release pain and chronic tension. It too is a generic term, like structural integration (SI) or postural integration (PI).

Hakomi Integrative Somatics (Hakomi Bodywork) a body-centered psychotherapy which incorporates bodywork, movement work, and inner work. Its main thrust is to dis-create beliefs established in childhood which inhibit health and adult life.

Hellerwork a technique much like Rolfing, developed by Joseph Heller, combining deep-tissue muscle therapy and movement reeducation. A dialogue is carried out as well to access emotional issues which may be present.

Meir Schneider Self-Healing Method a bodywork technique combining elements of Feldenkrais and Alexander.

Myofascial Release this therapy seeks to free the body from fascia (connective tissue) which has become stuck to itself and other tissues, thus freeing up all related structures for greater movement.

Neuromuscular Therapy (Myotherapy) uses a concentrated pressure to irritated areas in the muscles. Trigger point therapy, biomechanical postures, strain/counter strain techniques are also employed.

Postural Integration see STRUCTURAL INTEGRATION.

Rolfing a method of deep manipulative techniques of the muscles and connective tissues to improve posture, body alignment, and joint function; developed by Ida Rolf.

Rosen Method a method developed by Marion Rosen, much like Ilana Rubenfeld's method. See RUBENFELD SYNERGY METHOD.

Rubenfeld Synergy Method bodywork with the specific incorporation of psychotherapy. It uses touch, movement, verbal promptings, and imagination to allow the client to become aware of emotions and memories stored in the body. Ilana Rubenfeld developed this technique, incorporating elements from the Alexander Technique, gestalt therapy, Feldenkrais, and hypnosis.

Soma (Soma neuromuscular integration) a body alignment technique much like Rolfing. It is deep manipulation of the muscular and connective tissues to improve posture, joint function, and body alignment.

St. John Method a technique developed by Paul St. John. See NEUROMUSCULAR THERAPY.

Structural Integration a generic term for any bodywork therapy which attempts to do deep, profound work in order to realign the musculature and skeletal systems often affecting posture.

Trigger Point Myotherapy the application of pressure to specific points ('trigger points') on the body to relieve tension and pain. Trigger points are tender and congested areas which often radiate pain to other areas. It is similar to shiatsu.

Tui Na one system of Traditional Chinese massage. *Tui* means pushing, often with slight vibratory effect, and *Na* means moving while performing *ning* (*ning* is another technique—there are eight major ones—which means pinching and lifting, or grasping, in a stationary position). Conscious manipulation of energy is paramount here and practitioners are encouraged to cultivate their *chi* via Chi Kung in order to better serve their clients.

There are many other techniques including the following: Kripalu Bodywork, Body Insight Therapy, Hanna Somatic Education, Rebalancing, Active Muscular Relaxation Technique, Awareness-Oriented Structural Therapy, Benjamin System of Muscular Therapy, Cross-Fiber Friction Massage, Deep Compression Massage, Laban Movement Analysis, Lomilomi Massage (Hawaiian massage), LooyenWork, Myofascial Release Therapy, Parasympathetic Massage, Pfrimmer Technique, Proprioceptive Neuromuscular Facilitation (PNF Stretching), Thai Massage, Visceral Manipulation, and Cayce/Reilly Massage.

bo-shin a traditional Chinese method of facial and ear analysis. Clues to the health of the body can be seen in the face and ear. The nervous system corresponds to the area above the eyes, the circulatory to the area from the eyes to the top of the lips, and the digestive system to the mouth and chin areas. The entire body is represented in the ear.

botanical medicine see HERBAL MEDICINE.

Brazilian toe massage massage of the toes to stimulate the acupuncture meridians. Using specific fingers in combination with the thumb, the practitioner massages particular toes.

brief strobic phototherapy the use of rhythmic light and color to diffuse negative emotional/psychological patternings. Light stimulation with facilitation of verbal expression helps to resolve and shift emotional and cognitive states which can have a positive effect on the physical health.

Bristol Diet a cleansing and preventative diet developed by Alec Forbes which prohibits coffee, tea and salt and eliminates smoked, bottled, preserved, canned, and artificially flavored/colored foodstuffs.

Burton Treatment (immuno-augmentative therapy, IAT) a method of cancer treatment devised by L. Burton which attempts to restore the immune system's natural ability of hunting and destroying cancer cells. In his research, Dr. Burton found that the immune system needs four specific proteins in order to function optimally. Therapy consists of injecting one or more of these proteins into the patient, based on blood tests to determine which of these proteins the patient is deficient in.

calisthenics light gymnastic exercises often done on mats with no equipment, such as push-ups, jumping jacks, and stretches.

Callanetics a system of exercising the largest and deepest muscles of the body by using gentle movements and deep muscular contractions. Callan Pickney, the founder, maintains that one hour of Callanetics is equivalent to seven hours of conventional exercises.

Cascade Treatment (J.B.L. Cascade Treatment) a method of colonic irrigation advocated by Charles A. Tyrell. 'J.B.L.' stands for 'Joy-Beauty-Life'.

Cayce Therapy a method of healing using a vast number of therapies and remedies recommended by Edgar Cayce (1877-1945) to thousands and thousands of clients. The 'Sleeping Prophet', as he was known, went into a trance state and, after accessing his 'higher self', made specific suggestions for herbs, homeopathics, hydrotherapy, osteopathy, nutritional therapy, color therapy, and other therapies including conventional ones to the client. His diagnosis and treatment suggestions were remarkably accurate. In his career he gave over 30,000 readings.

cell salts see dictionary entry.

cellular repatterning see NEURO-CELLULAR REPATTERNING.

cellular therapy (live cell therapy) the implantation of healthy cells into human beings for a variety of therapeutic purposes, including reversing degenerative diseases and revitalizing the body. See *Live Cell Therapy* (W. Kuhnau).

cervical mucus method see BILLINGS METHOD.

chakras (Sanskrit, 'wheels') energy centers in the body. Some say there are these energy centers in the aura as well. There are seven major chakras (lst-root/base of spine, 2nd-genitals, 3rd-solar plexus, 4th-heart, 5th-throat, 6th-third eye/between the eyebrows, 7th-crown of head) situated along the channels of energy which run up and down the spine. There are many others situated in other parts of the body (hands, feet, etc.). Chakra Balancing is a technique based on laying-on of hands, which clears energy blocks and harmonizes the chakras.

channel someone who tunes into either healing energies or verbal guidance from a spiritual source (angel, soul, cosmic consciousness) and then makes it accessible to others by speaking, writing, touching an ill person, etc..

chelation therapy a series of intravenous (IV) injections of EDTA, a chelating chemical, which binds to toxic metals in the body. The bound EDTA is then removed, resulting in less toxic tissues. EDTA binds the so-called toxic heavy metals (lead, mercury, cadmium, nickel, copper, etc). As it binds calcium, it is also used to remove from plaque formations within the arteries. EDTA is ethylene diamine tetra-acetic acid, a synthetic amino acid. Chelation therapy is an alternative to coronary bypass surgery.

chi (qi) the energy that flows in meridians throughout the body. In Chinese systems, martial arts and medicine, this concept is essential in understanding the functioning of the body.

chi kung a series of simple exercises, often with little physical movement, which cultivate (enhance and store) *chi* in the individual.

Chinese/Oriental Medicine (Traditional Chinese Medicine, TCM) the traditional system of medicine developed in China, in which practitioners utilize tongue and pulse diagnosis to ascertain the imbalances in the client. Then, accordingly, they administer therapies, i.e., acupuncture, herbs, moxibustion, massage, and nutritional and lifestyle counseling.

chiropractic (Gr., 'done with hands') a system of healing based on the belief that health problems stem from misalignment in the skeletal system. Chiropractors, as well as naprapaths, naturopaths, myopractors, and osteopaths, etc., using their own specific manipulatory techniques, adjust those misalignments allowing bodily energies to move uninhibited and imbalances to be removed. Chiropractic was developed by Daniel David Palmer (1845-1913). D.C. is the appellation for chiropractors. See also

CHIROPRACTIC, OSTEOPATHY in dictionary proper.

chromotherapy see COLOR THERAPY.

clay and mud therapy see MUD BATH.

clinical ecology (environmental medicine) treatment based on the connection between illness and environmental factors (including food and chemical allergies).

co-counseling a form of peer counseling in psychotherapy, in which one person acts as therapist and the other as patient; then they exchange those roles in a counseling session.

colon therapy/irrigation (colonics) the cleansing of the large intestine by the injection of quantities of water and/or other substances. In turn, the intestinal walls are cleansed of impacted material, resulting in a decrease in absorbed toxins into the body and a more healthy functioning waste removal system.

color therapy the use of color in the treatment of disease and imbalances in the body (emotional, mental, physical, spiritual). The patient may not only be exposed to colored lights, but also advised to eat certain colored foods, breathe colors, wear different colored clothing or wear colored eyeglasses.

complementary medicine alternative medicine. See dictionary entry.

copper apparently the metal copper, when worn for example in a bracelet, can alleviate aches and pains associated with arthritis and rheumatism.

core energetic therapy a therapy quite similar to bioenergetics which attempts to break down client defenses so that one may reach a core level of consciousness. Counseling and bodywork techniques are used to allow the client to have cathartic releases. A more vibrant, loving, creative person is the intended result.

Coueism see AUTO-SUGGESTION.

cranial-sacral therapy see BODYWORK.

cryotherapy (ice therapy) the use of ice or other methods of applying cold to the body in order to relieve illness. It is very helpful in cases of traumatic injury.

cupping a technique for drawing blood to the surface of the skin, by placing a cup on the skin (with or without a cut beneath) with a burning/smoldering tuft of herb or cotton inside. Once extinguished, a partial vacuum is created within and blood is drawn into the cup. A technique used in Traditional Chinese Medicine; also one of the bloodletting techniques of 19th century allopathic medicine.

curative eurythmy see EURYTHMY.

cybernetics see PSYCHOCYBERNETICS.

cymatics a vibrational therapy using sound waves to restore healthy functioning to the cells. A type of sound therapy originally developed in the 1960s by Peter Manners.

dance therapy   an intimate and profound medium of therapy which directly expresses the mind and body. In the early 1940s psychiatrists found that patients felt tangible benefits after receiving dance classes. Like art therapy, clients are encouraged to feel, gain insights, have fun, and be free to create. Music, rhythm, and synchronous movement promote healing by altering mood states, establishing rapport, and reducing isolation.

deep tissue muscle therapy   see BODYWORK/MASSAGE.

dermo-optical perception (skin-sight, DOP)   the ability to see or perceive without the use of the eyes. One passes the fingers over the person or image or presses a photo against the skin in order to sense or diagnose what is going on with the client.

DMSO (dimethylsulfoxide) therapy   DMSO is a chemical which penetrates the skin and enters the body. Surpisingly, substances which are dissolved in it are also carried right through the skin. For example, it is possible to dissolve aspirin in DMSO and apply the mixture to arthritic joints. DMSO will act as a carrier for other healing substances to target areas of the body.

Do-In   a form of self-shiatsu. One stimulates acupuncture points or meridians using the hands or assuming postures or movements.

Dong diet   an anti-arthritic diet developed by Colin Dong. It is a low fat diet consisting of fish, rice, small portions of chicken, and vegetables.

dowsing   a way of divining by the use of a pendulum or rod. It is called radiesthesia when used in the therapeutic sense (medical radiesthesia). The different movements of the pendulum will indicate to the dowser information as to the patient's health. Dowsing can be used in many, many ways. You may be most familiar with 'dowsing for water' by using a y-shaped stick or piece of metal wire.

dowsing chart/map   see W.O. WOOD CHART.

dream therapy   the analysis of dreams in order to get perspective on the psyche and on one's life. Dreams are often composed of unconscious feelings. Often symbolic of our emotional state or life-condition, upon analysis one may solve problems through dream analysis.

ear coning   the use of slender cones of wax-covered muslin or gauze cloth. The small end of the cone is gently inserted in the ear, the other end lit. The gentle vacuum created by the slowly burning cone causes ear wax and other deposits to be drawn up into the cone, which is then discarded.

Egoscue method   a treatment method for musculoskeletal pain and training techniques for athletes, developed by P. Egoscue, who believed that people do not move enough. Individualized hour-long workouts are performed daily.

Ehret's mucusless diet   a health regimen which attempts to eliminate all mucus-producing foods from the diet. A. Ehret also advocated fasting, vegetarianism and increased physical activity. See dictionary.

electrical muscle stimulation (EMS) the stimulation of deep muscle contractionsby low-amperage electricity to promote muscular relaxation, increased circulation and the elimination of waste products.

electro-acupuncture stimulation of acupuncture points and meridians using minute electrical currents It has been used for the treatment of pain using a TENS unit (Transcutaneous Electrical Nerve Stimulation). See TENS.

electro-therapy the therapeutic use of electricity applied to the surface of the body or by placing the body into an electrical or electro-magnetic field or ultrasonic field. Examples include galvanism, faradism, high frequency currents, interferential therapy, sinusoidal current, diathermy, ultrasonics, endogenous endocrinotherapy, pulsed high frequency therapy, and microwave diathermy.

encounter therapy a group psychological therapy in which participants perceive each other in truthful and genuine ways, expressing their feelings honestly and openly, either verbally or physically. Participants report a greater awareness and comfortableness with themselves and others.

Enneagram a psychological and spiritual tool/therapy designed to identify which of nine personality types the person is. It is based on an ancient Sufi system of understanding personality. With this self-awareness one can change undesirable aspects and enhance one's strengths. It helps a person see the trance they are in, transcend it and become liberated in the process.

environmental medicine see CLINICAL ECOLOGY.

Esalen massage a relaxing massage much like Swedish massage but done slowly and rhythmical. If done properly the client often falls asleep.

eurythmy a concept based on Steiner's anthroposophy where healing occurs using movement in combination with the sounds of speech. Exercises have been developed for the digestive tract, the kidney and urinary systems, rheumatic illnesses, and heart and circulatory systems, etc.

expressive therapies art-centered therapies such as dance therapy, drama therapy, music therapy, psychodrama, art therapy, and poetry therapy.

Exultation of Flowers flower essence healing which operates on the basis of radiations flowing through the body and raising the general vitality. Developed by Alick McInnes, this method transfers flower radiations to water and uses no preservatives. Blossoms are held close to the water but not immersed. Radiations are intensified by the action of butterflies, bees and other insect activities.

Eye Movement Desensitization and Reprocessing (EMDR) a method of reducing or eliminating stored emotional trauma by using NLP in combination with hand-led eye movements. This complex model was developed by Francine Shapiro. She her book by the same title.

eye-robics a method of eye exercises combining Dr. Bates' methods with other aspects dealing with the mental, physical, emotional, and spiritual self-growth techniques.

faith healing basically prayer therapy, done alone or with a healer, in which an appeal is made to a spiritual authority (God, angel, ancestral spirit, etc.).

Feldenkrais method a movement therapy developed by Israeli Moshe Feldenkrais which combines verbal instruction/dialogue, movement training, and touch guidance to create freer and more efficient movement. Breathing and body alignment are addressed and balance and coordination improved.

feng shui an ancient Chinese practice of adjusting home and work environments to improve health, prosperity, and happiness. Color, furniture arrangement/placement, etc. all have effects on the flow of *chi*, vital energy.

flotation tank see samadhi tank.

flower essences liquid extractions of flowers which are used in healing. It is a general term applied to the essences prepared by Bach as well as others. There are a variety of essences which treat primarily negative emotional states. These essences are not homeopathic, although they are frequently confused with homeopathic remedies. See BACH FLOWER REMEDIES.

focusing a self-help, psychological counseling method developed by Chicago therapist E.T. Gendlin. It is based on the belief that information about issues in a persons life can be accessed through *focusing* on how those issues feel in the body. The individual in turn gets in greater contact and experiences increased clarity with distressing issues and how to go about dealing with them.

food allergy muscle test an applied kinesiology test which tests the subject's allergic/sensitive response to foods. The tester stands in front of the testee and presses down on the extended arm while asking the testee to resist. Then the tester places the food item on the testee's tongue and again presses down on the arm. If the arm goes weak it is generally assumed that the person cannot tolerate that food. (Nutritional supplements and other items can be tested in this manner besides foods.)

food combining the combining of foods in order to enhance nutrition. For instance, beans and rice do not offer a complete source of protein when eaten separately. However, when they are combined, all of the essential amino acids are supplied. Food combining also means knowing which foods should not be eaten together. For example, melons should be eaten alone to avoid fermentation; meat and carbohydrates should not be combined.

Food combining can be seen in other health systems as well. Ayurveda believes matter is made up of three *doshas* (Vata, Pitta and Kapha). Knowing which of these energies foods are composed of allows one to combine them into meals which support the overall energy of the body. For example, whole fresh milk contains all three *doshas* and thus maintains the body. Bananas (Vata) eaten with walnuts (Pitta, Kapha) nourish the whole body.

G-Jo Acupressure ('first aid' acupressure) a system of acupressure using a limited number of acupressure points to quickly relieve acute health situations. For example G-Jo Point #10 (*nei quan* or pericardium meridian point 6) refers to a point located 2 inches from the wrist up the inner forearm. Stimulation of this point treats blockages or oppression in the chest (heart attacks, respiratory problems, the breast and shoulder, etc.)

gem therapy   the therapeutic use of gems and semi-precious stones for healing purposes. Different gems have different healing qualities.

Gerson therapy   see dictionary entry, which also includes references to other cancer therapies.

Gestalt therapy a psychotherapeutic technique developed by Fred (Fritz) Perls to increase self-awareness. It says that an analysis of parts does not allow one to understand the whole. He urged patients to be aware of how they were experiencing the now. He cut through the niceties of the person to find out who the person really is. He used role-playing and strict self-observation. Gestalt means 'whole'.

grape cure   a method of cure (eating massive quantities of grapes and even grape juice) for many diseases, particularly cancer. Developed by Johanna Brandt: "After the nine years' battle with death, I discovered almost accidentally that fresh grapes, when taken alone, answered the three requirements of dissolving, eliminating and building." Two pounds of red grapes are eaten on the first day, adding one pound daily until a maximum of 12 pounds is reached.

graphology   analysis of handwriting. Some practitioners of this method can ascertain minute details about the health and personality of persons.

Guelphe fast   a type of fast, usually for one day, based on fresh fruit and vegetable juices. Sometimes just one type of juice is consumed during the day. Herbal teas are allowed.

guided imagery   the use of mental pictures to promote physical or psychological healing. Practitioners lead patients through specific exercises in order to use a subconscious programming of the mind to alleviate stress, decrease high blood pressure, enhance the immune system, etc. It is very similar to hypnosis and progressive relaxation.

Gyrotonics (GXS)   an exercise system carried out on low-impact specially designed equipment. Exercises are carried out with particular breathing patterns as well.

hair analysis   an analytical technique designed to determine the level of minerals in hair. It can be a guide for examining toxic substances in the body and can be used to assess nutritional imbalances, etc.

hara the focus of one's being, the vital center located just below the navel. It is an essential concept in many bodywork and spiritual practices.

Hay diet a diet developed by Wm. H. Hay based on food combining and understanding the acid-base balance of foods.

heat therapy see THERMOTHERAPY.

herbal medicine the art and science of restoring health in an ill person by the use of plants and their extracts. The American Botanical Council (ABC), P.O. Box 201660, Austin, TX 78720 is an excellent resource for herbal information and reference materials.

heliotherapy exposure to the sun to cure or heal disease.

high colonic irrigation see COLON THERAPY.

holistic health the concept of health which states that freedom from disease stems from the balance of body, mind and spirit.

Holotropic Breathwork a form of therapy which aims to integrate the physical, psychological, and spiritual aspects of the client by combining intense breathing, powerful music and bodywork. It attempts to dissolve negative blockages which the client may have, helping him to achieve greater freedom in his life. It was developed by Stanislov Grof.

homeopathy a therapeutic medical science which holistically treats illnesses and inherent constitutional problems with the 'like cures like' principle, using minute doses of specially prepared potentized substances from the mineral, animal, and plant kingdoms. See also the introductory essay to this volume.

Hoshino therapy the use of acupressure on the 250 points that relate to the biomechanical functioning of the body. These points are located on muscles, tendons, and ligaments and the combination of finger pressure and warmth from the practitioner's hands work to decrease the hardening of soft tissue. It was developed by T. Hoshino.

Hoxsey treatment an anti-cancer therapy. See dictionary entry.

hydrochloric acid therapy a treatment for some cancers, angina pectoris, and anemia by giving hydrochloric acid solution in order to supply the mineral potassium. This method of therapy, developed by Ferguson and Guy in the 1930s, supposedly enhanced the proper absorption of minerals during the digestive process.

hydrotherapy the therapeutic use of water to heal sickness. This is a vast subject, and the healing power of water can not be overstated. Sitz baths, sweating baths, douches, steaming, cold/hot packs, compresses, fomentations, enemas, steam inhalation, colonic irrigation, and mineral water therapy are just some of the ways of employing the healing properties of this ordinary substance we call water, H_2O.

hyperbaric oxygen therapy (HBOT) a form of oxygen therapy which exposes the client to 100 percent pure oxygen under pressures greater than atmospheric pressure in a special chamber. It forces oxygen into all of the tissues of the body and has been shown to be of benefit in heart disease, gangrene, stroke, circulatory problems, etc.

hypnosis (Gr. *hypnos*, 'sleep') an altered state of consciousness combining relaxation, suggestion, and an enhanced awareness. Hypnotherapy is hypnosis used therapeutically or in the clinical situation. The person is progressively relaxed and then once in an altered state, suggestions of a helpful nature are give to the person to help him/her overcome emotional difficulties, heighten abilities, or treat a wide range of medical conditions (migraine, obesity, alcoholism, etc.).

hypnotherapy see HYPNOSIS.

imagery see GUIDED IMAGERY.

impact therapy a pressure wave treatment designed to mobilize joints, relieve pain, and alleviate stiffness, congestion and tenderness in and around joints. There are three types: static, mobile, and spinal. It involves releasing a bag of sand from a short height onto the indicated joint or area. It is maintained that this small amount of pressure helps to adjust and realign tissues allowing normal function to return.

intuitive arts a general term used to describe techniques involving psychic abilities, intuition, and divination, such as numerology, astrology, tarot, runes, and psychic readings.

iridology (irido-diagnosis) a therapeutic science which uses maps of the iris to discern the health of the individual. Certain areas of the iris relate to certain areas of the body. For instance, at approximately 2:30 on the outer edge of the right iris can be found the thyroid area. If that area is colored, or of an unusual shape it may mean there is something wrong with the thyroid gland or function. This, too is a vast subject and quite complex, especially as reflected in the work of the German physician, Deck.

isolation tank see SAMADHI TANK.

isometric exercise a type of exercise which involves exerting one muscular group against another in order to strengthen them both. It may also be employed against a wall or other solid entity.

Jin Shin Do a technique created by Iona M. Teeguarden using acupressure, Reichian segmental theory and Taoist yogic breathing methods to release emotional and physical armoring. It tries to create a peaceful trance state so the client can see his emotional problems more clearly.

Jin Shin Jyutsu/Jitsu a Japanese therapy which attempts to harmonize the flow of energy through the body through some physical manipulation of musculature. The practitioner releases trapped energy in the body's 26 safety energy locks to bring about deep relaxation and awaken innate abilities toward mental, physical, emotional, and spiritual balance.

journaling a rapid and uncensored method of writing down one's feelings in order to unburden or clear oneself from debilitating or harmful emotions.

kampo traditional Japanese medicine, similar to TCM (traditional Chinese medicine), but including traditional medicines from Japanese folklore. Despite being very modern, 43 percent of Japan's Western-trained medical practitioners use *kampo* medicines, and Japan's national health insurance pays for them.

Kempner rice diet see RICE DIET.

ketogenic diet a diet specifically designed for epileptics to help eliminate or reduce seizures. It is a diet very high in fat and very low in carbohydrates, forcing the body to burn fat instead of carbohydrates. This causes ketosis which helps to control seizures. It requires medical supervision.

Kirlian photography/diagnosis the use of a special camera to photograph halos or coronas of light surrounding the subject. These auras, according to some, indicate the vitality or life-energy of the subject being photographed. Semyon and Valentina Kirlian developed the method.

kundalini that spiritual/psychic energy, associated with the first/root chakra, found at the base of the spine. It is often represented as a coiled snake which, when awakened, rises up the spine to the top of the head as a rush of energy and spiritual power.

Laban method a method of analyzing movement, based on the work of R. Laban, to increase awareness of what movement communicates and attempts to express. Once analyzed, the client is given suggestions to improve movement. It is especially effective for dancers, actors, and athletes.

labyrinth walking the practice of walking in a labyrinth, in the belief that it can have health benefits.

Lakhovsky oscillatory coils coils which can send balancing frequencies into the ill person in order to reestablish health, based on the work of French engineer Lakhovsky, who regarded living organisms as made up of high frequency oscillating circuits.

laying-on of hands spiritual or faith healing in which the healer actually places his/her hands on or near the subject and prays for healing to occur.

light therapy (chromotherapy) the use of light in all its varieties to heal illness.

live cell therapy see CELLULAR THERAPY.

Livingston/Wheeler regimen/diet a cancer regimen consisting of vaccines, bacterial reagents, IV-administered vitamins, long-term antibiotic use and a modified Gerson diet with coffee enemas. See dictionary entry for GERSON THERAPY.

logotherapy a method of psychotherapy developed by Victor Frankl. It is a meaning-centered psychotherapy which focuses on the future and man's 'will to meaning'. "*Logotherapy* is education to responsibility, and with this responsibility the patient must push forward independently towards a concrete meaning of his own personal existence, must choose it on his own. In this system, as Frankl himself says, "The Existential questions of value and meaning in life are raised but not solved." - *The Layman Speaks,* 13:6, p. 190, 1960.

lohan kung Buddhist yoga techniques, animal movements, and fitness exercises designed to improve or activate the bodily energies.

lunar phase cycle a complex method of natural, rhythmic birth control dependent upon the sun-moon angle present at the woman's moment of birth.

Luscher color test a method of personality testing developed by Max Luscher. He theorized that a person's preference for or dislike of certain colors is indicative of a particular state of mind and/or glandular balance.

lymphatic drainage massage a special form of massage designed to stimulate the flow of lymph to move and remove sluggish fluids, cellular toxins and other wastes. See dictionary entry.

macrobiotics healthy-living concepts developed by George Ohsawa, who wrote *Zen Macrobiotics* (1962), and popularized by Michio Kushi. Some people just practice the dietary aspect of macrobiotics (synchronizing eating habits with nature's cycles, balancing yin and yang foods, etc.). However it is an all-encompassing way to balance the health and to look at the world and universe. Balance is achieved through knowledge of the interplay between yin and yang.

magnetic field therapy (magnetic therapy, bio-magnetic therapy) the use of magnetism (as generated by magnets, pulsed magnetism and electromagnetic frequency generators) to treat health conditions.

massage 'to knead'. Massage therapy is the scientific manipulation of the soft tissues of the body by applying pressure (usually with the hands) and/ or causing movement of the joints. In addition to the healing power of touch, massage enhances blood and lymphatic flow, induces relaxation and reduces stress, increases joint range of motion, and enhances personal vitality.

McDougall diet a vegan diet. Only whole, unprocessed foods of plant origin are permitted.

meditation a technique to control the mind which leads to feelings of inner tranquility and can result in transcendental experiences of self-realization and improved self-awareness. There are many, many meditation techniques.

megavitamin therapy the use of high doses of vitamins to heal disease and improve the functioning of the body. See ORTHO-MOLECULAR THERAPY.

mental ataraxis a meditative technique. The person once into the meditative state is helped by a therapist who verbally makes suggestions to release anxieties and stressors. It differs from imagery because no visualization is used.

mesmerism   see HYPNOSIS.

metamorphic technique   a form of foot manipulation similar to reflexology (originally called prenatal therapy). Developed by Robert St. Johns, it stimulates energy to enable the client to reach his full potential. It is especially useful for relationship problems, chronic illnesses and mental illness and to help restore emotional balance. ('Metamorphic' because each of us is capable of metamorphosing, or changing, into something better).

microwave resonance therapy   a low-intensity (continuous or pulsed) sinusoidal microwave radiation to treat various conditions, such as arthritis, chronic pain, hypertension, and wound healing. It can also be applied at acupuncture points.

moxibustion   the burning of a dried herb or tuft of cotton (moxa) on or near an acupuncture point on the body. This gentle heat affects the *chi* and is useful in certain forms of illness (such as asthma, chills, and arthritic conditions).

mucusless diet   see EHRET'S MUCUSLESS DIET.

mud bath   the use of wet warm (100^0 F) clays applied to the body or the person immersed in the bath or wrapped in a cotton sheet or canvas. This is not only good for skin health but is generally accepted to be rejuvenating to the whole body, for example by removal of toxins and stimulation of lymph flow.

muscle testing   see APPLIED KINESIOLOGY.

music therapy   the use of a variety of musics and/or sounds to lead one to liberate emotions or to experience transcendental or transpersonal states of consciousness. It has many uses, among them in handicapped children to attempt to overcome disabilities or personal limitations.

myopractics   a manipulative technique much like those practiced by chiropractors, naturopaths, and osteopaths. Especially important to the myopractor is the pelvic region and the structural problems that often arise from imbalances in that area which in turn effect the back.

naprapathy   see dictionary entry.

natural birth control   any method of birth control which does not depend upon artificial means. Often called the 'rhythm method', in which the woman charts her fertile days depending upon subtle changes in her body temperature.

naturopathy   see dictionary entry.

negative ion   negative ions have a positive and healing effect on the body. One may experience the negative ion effect by being outdoors during or after rainfall as opposed to being in the middle of a city where positive ions outnumber negative ions and have a draining effect on ones energy. Machines are available which generate negative ions.

Network Chiropractic a network of chiropractors who use the Network Spinal Analysis technique, a method which applies chiropractic adjustments in specific sequences. Gentle taps and touches to the spine can produce dramatic physical and emotional releases. It was started in 1979 by Donald Epstein. The major difference between Network and other chiropractic is the sequence or timing in which adjustments are introduced.

neuroceuticals natural compounds which supply the components that brain cells need to maintain structural and electrical activity. They also enhance the utilization of oxygen by the brain, protect nerve cells from damage and provide basic chemical components for the production of neurotransmitters. Included in this category would be phosphatidyl serine, taurine, magnesium, vitamin C, glutamine, CoQ10, ginkgolides, acetyl L-carnitine, GABA, and L-pyroglutamic acid. See NUTRACEUTICALS and PHYTOTHERAPY in the dictionary.

neuro-cellular repatterning a technique for releasing negative traumatic energies from the body based on the recognition that love is the true healer.

neuro-linguistic programming (NLP) a method of reprogramming a client's habitual behavioral and speech patterns to help him go beyond personal limitations to achieve heightened levels of awareness and effectiveness in life. By conversing with the client the practitioner observes his posture, breathing, language, eye movements and gestures in order to detect and then alter negative and limiting unconscious patterns.

neuromuscular therapy (NMT) a bodywork therapy which treats the neuromuscular components of pain by locating its origins. Soft-tissue release work is essential to loosen unbalanced muscles and allied tissues to restore circulation and normal physiological functioning. Structural homeostasis is restored by restoring normal physiological functioning in nerve and the musculoskeletal systems. See BODYWORK.

NLP see NEURO-LINGUISTIC PROGRAMMING.

nutraceutical see dictionary entry.

Ohashiatsu a personalized method of Shiatsu developed by Wataru Ohashi. The client's center or *hara* is assessed and then worked on, using stretching and pressing movements all over the body and working in flow with the client's breathing patterns.

Option Method a personal growth technique which uses a question-and-answer format to help the client see his self-defeating or limiting beliefs.

Ortho-bionomy see BODYWORK.

orgone therapy therapy using 'orgone' (a term used by W. Reich (3-24-1897 • 11-3-1957) to describe 'life energy', or *prana,* or *chi)* to enhance the client's life energy. Through experimentation Reich developed apparatus to accumulate 'orgone' and then transfer it to the client.

Oriental diagnosis the study of biological change, through one of four commonly used forms of diagnosis: *Bo-Shin* (observation or seeing), *Bun-Shin* (sounds, hearing), *Mon-Shin* (questioning), *Setsu-Shin* (touch).

Ornish diet a diet very similar to the Pritikin diet, but which also calls for stress reduction practices and emphasizes emotional social support systems. It requires stretching daily and an hour walk three times a week. The diet allows no added fat; naturally occuring fat in foods must amount to less than 10 percent of calories from fat.

ortho-bionomy an empowerment technique (rather than a physical healing technique per se) which uses non-invasive, gentle touch along with verbal communication to enhance awareness through body movement.

orthomolecular therapy/medicine a term coined by Linus Pauling, Ph.D., referring to a therapeutic approach which tries to adjust the environment of the body's cells to improve their functioning. "The preservation of good health and the treatment of disease by varying the concentrations in the human body of substances that are normally present in the body and required for health." A similar field is megavitamin therapy, an approach developed by Abram Hoffer and others.

osteopathy a system of healing based on the belief that misalignment in the skeletal system causes disease or imbalances in energy flow in the body. Osteopaths use the designation D.O. and today are equivalent in stature to MDs. This theory was formulated by Andrew T. Still (1828-1917).

oxygen therapy the therapeutic use of oxygen in all its many forms, e.g., hydrogen peroxide, ozone, and hyperbaric oxygen therapy (HBOT). See HYPERBARIC OXYGEN THERAPY.

ovulation birth control method see BILLINGS METHOD.

past-life therapy a therapy which attempts to release traumatic past life events from the subconscious energy fields of the body in order to resolve current illnesses.

Pathwork a psychotherapeutic technique using verbal dialogue to assist the client in transforming his shadow self or dark side. The goal of this (and of course many of these psychotherapeutic techniques) is to create integration, inner peace, and help one connect to a greater degree with the purpose of the soul.

phonotherapy sound therapy. See MUSIC THERAPY.

photocognitive therapy (PCT) the use of light directed onto areas of the head to stimulate remembrance of life trauma in order to recognize it and disperse the negative energy associated with it. It is also useful in past life regression therapy.

phrenology see dictionary entry.

physiatric medicine the evaluation and non-surgical treatment of diseases and disabilities of the nerves, muscles, joints, brain, spinal cord, etc. It uses physical, occupational, and speech therapists in various capacities for client rehabilitation. A physiatric physician is a physician who uses primarily physical medical treatments in his/her practice.

phytotherapy see dictionary entry.

Pilates a gentle, balanced and harmonious method of exercising using floor calisthenic-type exercises and machine-assisted ones. It emphasizes correct body alignment, mental concentration, and awareness of the breath. It is quite beneficial because there is no or little pressure on joints and the exercises are symmetrical. It was developed by a German, Joseph Pilates.

PNF stretching see PROPRIOCEPTIVE NEUROMUSCULAR FACILITATION.

point holding a technique designed to allow emotional release. It requires multiple practitioners who hold acupressure points (determined by applied kinesiology and iridology), sometimes for up to two hours, to help the client achieve emotional release.

polarity therapy a system of balancing energy in the body. The body is an electric field and its electricity must flow unimpeded in order for optimal health to result. R. Stone and Pannetier developed four areas in which energy flow can be balanced: diet, exercise, self-awareness, and bodywork. Essentially the therapist balances the positive and negative poles of the body. The theory of polarity maintains that life is in a dynamic state of flux between opposite poles of energy. Different sides of the body represent different poles or electromagnetic charges and circuits can be established when the body is touched or parts of the body are touched.

polarizing treatment (GKI) the use of potassium chloride, glucose, and small amounts of insulin to treat cancer and other degenerative diseases by re-establishing proper levels of potassium in the cells. It also helps relieve pain. GKI stands for glucose, potassium (element abbreviation 'K'), and insulin.

postural integration see BODYWORK.

postural reeducation therapies consist of three major systems, Alexander, Feldenkrais, and Trager.

pranic healing any healing technique which combines the meditative use of breath and the subsequent direction of *prana (chi)* to cause healing. Pranic healers use this technique to scan, cleanse, energize, and stabilize the energies of the body, especially of the etheric body.

primal therapy a psychological therapeutic approach which attempts to liberate the client from longstanding emotional pain. Originated by Arthur Janov, who developed this therapy to dismantle neurotic barriers built by an unreal self to shield the client from pain and painful experiences. 'Primal scream therapy' is an allied term.

Pritikin diet basically a vegetarian diet high in complex carbohydrates and fiber, low in fat developed by Nathan Pritikin. It also requires 45 minutes of walking daily.

proliferation therapy see PROLOTHERAPY.

prolotherapy (TILT, proliferation therapy, sclerotherapy, reconstruction therapy) a type of medical treatment that regrows tendons and ligaments. It is a technique of injecting irritant solutions into the tissues for the purpose of proliferation of new fibrous tissues at their attachment points on the bone. This in turn adds new strength to that area. The most common proliferant solution used is Hackett's solution: dextrose (25%), glycerine (25%), and phenol (2.4%) in water. Other proliferants include quinine, urea, Hemwall's solution, sodium morrhuate, and Gedney's solution. Physician G.S. Hackett coined the term 'prolotherapy' (short for 'proliferation therapy'). *Pain, Pain Go Away* (Wm. Faber) is a good reference.

proprioceptive neuromuscular facilitation (PNF Stretching) a technique which improves one's muscular strength and flexibility if performed on a regular basis. It involves stretching with the application of resistance at various points in the stretch. This fools the muscular proprioceptors into thinking they aren't stretching that much, thus allowing for even more stretch. It is often employed in physical therapy.

psionic therapy/medicine combines elements of the paranormal, dowsing, and energy flow concepts in the treatment of illness. Practitioners usually use the W.O. Wood dowsing chart to diagnose imbalances in the body and to detect patterns of potential disease. The practitioner takes into consideration hereditary and miasmatic influences and often uses homeopathic remedies. 'Radiesthesia' is an allied term. See W.O. WOOD CHART.

psychic or spiritual massage a type of massage in which the practitioner psychically feels energies and magnetic currents about the body and 'massages' them.

psychocybernetics the concept that the brain must transmit healthy concepts into the cells before any state of illness can be eliminated. This method relies heavily on the concept of positive thinking, emphasizing that a positive state of mind is part and parcel of healing. Cybernetics deals with the analysis of the flow of information occurring in biological systems.

psychodietetics the relationship between diet and one's emotional life. Emotional disorders can have their origin in faulty nutrition; one's nutrition can be modified into order to have a more positive impact on emotional health.

psychometry divination of the state of health (or any other information) by using objects from an absent person. The practitioner receives psychic impressions from objects which the person once held or owned.

psychoperistalsis a method to 'dissolve and discharge residual metabolic waste products of psychosomatic origin'. It is an aspect of biodynamic psychology. As the body reflects the mental state, effective bodywork can cause emotional release. This technique influences the intestines by massaging rigid flexor muscles which hold onto negative emotional feelings. Release of this 'body armor' results in increased peristaltic sounds and abreaction (the release of repressed emotions). This method has its origins with the Norwegians Boyesen, Braatoy, and Bulow-Hansen.

psychosynthesis a comprehensive approach to psychotherapy developed out of dissatisfaction with Freud's psychoanalysis by Assagioli, an Italian psychiatrist. It is similar to transpersonal psychology and concentrates on five main areas: psychotherapy, personal integration/actualization, education, and social and interpersonal relationships.

psychic surgery surgery carried out using no surgical instruments, only fingers and hands (mainly found in Brazil and in the Philippines).

psychodrama an action-oriented therapy which encourages one to act out problems or conflicts by spontaneously creating those situations, either from the past, present, or future, real or imagined. Aside from abreaction, it allows one to look at life as it is and as one would like it to be. See ABREACTION.

psycho-muscular release therapy (PRMT) a system developed by P. Blythe, based upon the idea that most chronic, persistent psychoneurotic conditions are due to an inability to relax certain muscles. It concentrates on releasing dammed-up emotions held in the body.

psychosynthesis a type of psychotherapy which recognizes personal integration and a transpersonal integration of self, e.g., altruistic love, cooperative spirit, and a global perspective.

pyramid energy an unusual energy supposedly found inside an equilateral pyramid constructed with the Egyptian Cheops pyramid as a model. It has been found that items placed in the pyramid benefit from that energy: polluted water is purified, meditation improves inside the pyramid, foods don't spoil but dehydrate, water placed in or under the pyramid takes on healing and tonic powers, etc.

Qi Gong see CHI KUNG.

radiance technique an energetic healing technique similar to Reiki. It involves the use of symbolism to generate universal light vibration.

radiesthesia see DOWSING and related entries in the dictionary proper.

radionics see entry in the dictionary proper.

radix a neo-Reichian therapy which works from the ocular segment to the pelvic segment utilizing bioenergetic techniques to release fear, anger, and pain.

rapid eye therapy (RET) a therapy based on neurolinguistic programming which relies on the release of emotional tension through the eyes. Often combined with hypnosis, the client is brought to focus upon painful emotional trauma which is then released through rapid eye movements and blinking.

rebirthing the use of hyperventilation to induce states of emotional climax and transcendence. One reexperiences and releases emotional pain of all sorts. This therapy was developed by Leonard Orr and modified, with music, by Stanislov Grof. When one finishes a rebirthing session one feels lighter, less tense, and profoundly relaxed. Wet rebirthing (rebirthing in warm water) is a variation and tends to enhance the rebirthing experience. It allows for an experience resembling that of a fetus in the womb.

reconstruction therapy see PROLOTHERAPY.

reflexology the science of foot and hand massage. There are hundreds of points on the hands and feet which reflex to different areas of the body. Thus it is possible to treat the bladder or sinuses, for example, by applying firm pressure on the associated points on the feet. Reflexology helps to release blocks in the body's energy zones, bringing relief of pain and bodily tension.

Reichian therapy a therapy which involves dismantling layers of 'trauma' through the seven different zones (segments) of the body (ocular, oral, cervical, thoracic, diaphragmatic, abdominal and pelvic), based on a concept, developed by W. Reich, of body and character armoring. He felt that repression of emotions and the sexual instincts could lead to physical and energetic blockages in the body and behavior. Deterioration of health is the result.

Reiki (pronounced 'ray-key') transmission of energy by the Reiki practitioner holding their hands close to or lightly on the body. It is used for mental, emotional, physical, and/or spiritual healing. There are three levels of Reiki training. Supposedly discovered in Tibetan scriptures by M. Usui and introduced to the West by Saichi Takata. 'Reiki' means 'transcendent or universal energy' and involves the use of sounds and symbols to tap into universal healing energies.

Reiki Plus traditional Reiki plus psychotherapeutic Reiki. Here the placement of the hands on the head is used to tap into the collective unconscious.

rice diet (Kempner rice diet) a high carbohydrate, high fiber, low fat and low sodium diet which consists of brown rice, fruit, tea, and fruit juices. Other grains and vegetables may be added at some point as well as nonfat dairy products. It is similar to the Pritikin, macrobiotic, McDougall, and reversal diets.

Rolfing see BODYWORK.

Robert Jaffe Advanced Energy Healing a technique developed by physician R. Jaffe using heart-centered awareness, intuitive perceptions and energetic healing techniques to transform energy patterns that cause disease.

Rosen method a psychotherapeutic technique developed by Marion Rosen which combines verbal and touch communication to create a space of relaxation and self-awareness. Past or buried feelings/memories are often brought up and the client assisted in clearing those emotional blockages.

Rubenfeld Synergy Method see BODYWORK.

Ryoduraku a variant of acupuncture which uses an instrument to diagnose and treat illness. Developed by Y. Nakatani.

samadhi tank a sensory deprivation tank designed for deep relaxation or personal reflection. The individual floats in a sound- and light-deprived salt bath. As stillness settles in the individual has only a sense of mind.

sanjeevini a prayer-based medical therapy used widely in India. It combines the power of prayer with sacred yantra-mandala templates. When a placebo is placed within the template (much like Rae potency cards) it becomes infused with healing energy which the recipient then ingests.

Schuessler cell salts see dictionary entry.

sclerotherapy see PROLOTHERAPY.

sensitivity training (T-group training) a group psychotherapy method which explores the effects which an individual's behavior has on other individuals. This interplay of relationships assists all in understanding the self and others.

sensory isolation/deprivation tank see SAMADHI TANK.

Sentic cycles a method of classifying emotions based on the work of M. Clynes. He says that emotions have dynamic forms of expression which are coded into the central nervous system. There are seven emotions (anger, hate, grief, love, sex, joy, and reverence) and the client is taught to express these emotions in sequence while listening to the therapist or a guidance tape.

shamanism/shamanic healing a shaman is a medicine man who is able to enter a trance state and 'journey' to other realms, another reality, in order to access healing energies/messages for his client. The shaman usually calls on his spirit helpers/power animals to assist him in his healing tasks. Soul retrieval and power animal retrieval are other aspects of shamanism.

SHEN Therapy (Specific Human Energy Nexus, or SHEN Physio-Emotional Release Therapy) the use of light hand placements to release deeply embedded negative emotional states and energies. The practitioner uses his energy flow to unblock dammed energies.

shiatsu (acupressure) a Japanese bodywork therapy which stimulates acupuncture points *(tsubo)* not with needles but with pressure from blunt objects or fingers. Thumb pressure is the most common and is applied for about 2 to 10 seconds. Various massage strokes are often employed to enhance blood and lymph fluid circulation. One advantage of this therapy is that it can be self-administered. Barefoot shiatsu is a variant and uses foot pressure to stimulate the meridian points.

Shintaido an approach to human movement which emphasizes the holistic aspect of body, mind, and spirit and combines physical exercise with poetic physical expression. It is not a martial art but when practiced may appear that way. Formulated by H. Aoki, a Japanese educator.

Silva Healing Method (Silva Mind Control) a meditation/visualization technique developed by Jose Silva to resolve difficulties and deepseated problems in one's life.

Soma a neuromuscular integrative technique. See BODYWORK.

somatoemotional release with gentle touch the therapist encourages the client to assumes positions the client was in when he/she was traumatized. As this occurs, the negativity associated with that trauma is released (usually in the form of heat) and the client can re-experience the pain and associated emotions. Based upon the work of John E. Upledger and Z. Karni.

somatography a system of therapy based on inner and outer body work to help the client become more in tune with himself and get to know himself more intimately.

sound therapy see MUSIC THERAPY.

spirit releasement therapy a hypnotic technique designed to release spirits or nonphysical entities that are attached to the client. The practitioner engages the entities (ghosts? etc.) in dialogue, attempting to convince them that they are misplaced and need to go to their proper place, namely 'the light'. Past-life therapy techniques may also be used.

spiritual healing see FAITH HEALING.

sports massage massage which focuses on the muscles associated with a particular athletic activity. It incorporates stretching and heavy pressure.

St. John's neuromuscular therapy see BODYWORK.

strain-counterstrain therapy a complex method of neuromuscular pain relief developed by osteopathic doctor L. Jones. It involves trigger point work to locate an area of referred pain. The client is then positioned so that there is no more referred pain and holds that position for a minute and a half. Then the body is moved back into the original position, the trigger point is released and the referred pain is gone.

structural integration see BODYWORK.

subliminal therapy a form of audio or visual therapy which impacts the subconscious in such a way as to influence the individual's behavior. In the audio use of this technique, strongly stated positive messages are recorded on the tape and music is recorded over them. Thus, consciously one hears just music, but the unconscious hears the messages, too. One may purchase all sorts of audio tapes for purposes ranging from improving one's golf game to enhancing self-esteem and confidence.

supraluminal phototherapy the use of special lights to correct the relationship between human consciousness (supraluminal space-time) and the electromagnetic field which controls bodily structure and physiology.

Swedish massage a form of massage known for its long strokes, kneading and friction. It also incorporates active and passive joint movement. It was developed by a Swedish physician, Per Henrik Ling (1776-1839) and originally called Swedish Movement Cure.

T-group see SENSITIVITY TRAINING.

TENS (transcutaneous electrical nerve stimulation) an electrical device which provides a low voltage, low amperage current to relax muscles and relieve chronic pain. A 'TENS unit' is usually worn and the wearer can adjust the current to a necessary level in order to provide pain relief. See ELECTRO-ACUPUNCTURE.

Thai massage a sacred form of massage with roots in Ayurvedic medicine and Hatha yoga. It is done with clothing on and utilizes techniques similar to shiatsu, acupressure, reflexology and yoga. It is primarily done with the client lying on his back.

thalassotherapy seashore therapy. The belief that being by the sea, swimming, walking, etc., has therapeutic effects and benefits.

Therapeutic Touch a non-invasive laying-on of hands healing technique rediscovered by Dolores Krieger, RN. It is based on human energy transfer and inspired by research demonstrating the effectiveness of psychic healing. It is usually practiced by nurses in hospitals.

thermotherapy the therapeutic use of heat to treat illness. This would include any method which uses heat as its main therapeutic means, including sauna and steam baths, hot blankets, infra-red and radiant heat, and wax baths.

Thought Field Therapy (TFT) a variation of applied kinesiology (AK), developed by Callahan, which harmonizes destructive emotional states in the client. It combines gentle tapping on acupuncture points and meridians on the face, upper body and left hand, in a set pattern to dissipate negative emotional states. Consult *Thought Field Therapy and Trauma* (R.J. Callahan). Callahan says his technique bypasses cognition.

Three In One A type of therapy attempting to enhance brain-body integration when it has been severely hampered by early emotional trauma and patterning. 'Precision Muscle Testing' is used to diagnose emotional trauma and blockages; then 'One Brain' techniques are used to diffuse negative emotional patterns.

toning a meditative technique designed to change or enhance the energy in oneself and/or the environment. A toning session is often combined with rhythmic breathing, meditation, and visualization. It can relieve tension and blockages. Typically one stands erect, and vocally sounds out a tone which comes up from the Earth through the feet. As the voice and energy build one may feel releases on a variety of levels.

Touch for Health a therapy similar to applied kinesiology in that gentle pressure is applied to contracted muscles as well as other points of the body in order to balance bodily energy. This therapy maintains that changes in body posture and muscular tone affect the position and functioning of internal organs and their energy. The practitioner uses acupuncture meridians, relating them to an 'indicator' or 'test muscle' (usually arm or leg). Weakness in such test muscle relates to the body as a whole and all sorts of factors (physical, mental, emotional, nutritional) can be diagnosed as either good or harmful for the system. It was developed by John Thie, D.C.

Trager therapy (passive joint massage) a movement re-education approach to seek out mental and emotional aspects of muscular tension. It employs rocking, cradling, and other movements to help the client see that physically restrictive patterns can be altered. It is based on the work of Milton Trager (1909 • 1-20-1997). He wrote *Trager Mentastics*.

Transactional Analysis a method developed by E. Berne to allow patients a quick way to understand how their personality was formed and how they interact with others. Interactions are thus analyzed as modes of functioning: parent, adult and child.

Transcendental Meditation (TM, japa yoga) a form of mantra yoga taught by Maharishi Mahesh Yogi. One repeats, silently, over and over a mantra which has a meditative effect on the mind and in turn on the physiology of the body. It relieves stress, lowers the basal metabolic rate, and blood pressure in addition to increasing self-awareness and eventually experiencing transcendental consciousness.

transpersonal psychology (fourth force psychology) a type of psychology which focuses on self-transcendence, health and well-being rather than devoting so much attention to neurosis and disease patterns. One aim is to help transcend the ego and one's association with it. It is closely associated with the human-growth potential movement. Classical Freudian psychoanalytical theory is considered 'first force', behavioristic 'second force', and humanistic 'third'.

Trauma Touch Therapy specially designed to help clients with trauma and abuse histories. Combining psychotherapeutic techniques the therapist encourages empowerment and choice in getting more in touch with bodily sensations.

Traumatic Incident Reduction (TIR) a technique developed by Frank Gerbode which arose out of Scientology and is similar to the process of 'auditing'. It basically involves guiding the client through his traumatic experiences allowing him to gain insights and then clarity on those issues.

trichology the science of hair or hair-parts. The practitioner of this science treats thinning hair, problems of the scalp, and hair loss.

TILT (Trigger injection of ligament and tendon therapy) see PROLOTHERAPY.

trigger point therapy see BODYWORK.

trophology the science of combining foods to obtain the best nutritional value from them.

tsubo a type of acupressure very similar to shiatsu. Both rely on the sequential application of pressure applied from one end of the meridian to the other.

underwater birthing a form of natural childbirth in which the mother delivers the child in warm or body temperature water. Adherents of this method maintain that it is a nonviolent way for a being to enter the world. Mayol, Odent, Charkovsky, and LeBoyer are the main popularizers of this method.

urine therapy the therapeutic use of one's urine. Urine may either be imbibed or applied externally. John W. Armstrong wrote *The Water of Life: A Treatise on Urine Therapy,* and is the most recent popularizer of this traditional system of treatment.

Usui system of natural healing a system of Reiki healing. See REIKI.

vegetarianism the belief that eating flesh foods is not beneficial to health and/or amoral. There are varying degrees of vegetarianism, for example ovo-lacto vegetarian (eggs and milk may be consumed) and veganism (foods of plant origin only).

visceral manipulation a manipulative technique of the visceral connective tissue and abdominal organs, designed to normalize position and balance of function in those areas.

Visual Kinesthetic Dissociation (VKD) this method for resolving emotional problems is based on NLP but adds the element of 'dissociation from trauma', to it. It helps the client to observe from a distance rather than being subjectively overwhelmed by it.

visualization the creation of mental visual forms which in turn can have a profoundly positive effect on one's health. Continually visualizing oneself as a strong, self-confident, potent person gradually creates that reality.

Vita Florum a selection of flower essences in water created by Elizabeth Bellhouse, who was led to flowers-for-healing by divine guidance. According to Bellhouse, the 'potentized' water contains the radiations of the Creator, the flowers are merely the vehicle. These essences heal the body, as opposed to Bach remedies which act more on the emotional/mental aspects, and Exultation of Flowers which acts on the psyche. See BACH FLOWER REMEDIES, EXULTATION OF FLOWERS.

vitamin therapy the therapeutic use of vitamins or specific combinations of vitamins to heal. For example, most of us know that ascorbic acid (Vitamin C) is used to prevent scurvy; less well known is the use of vitamins B6, B3, and C to treat schizoprenia.

voice dialogue a method of psychotherapy with Jungian influences which attempts to increase self-awareness in the client by uncovering a client's 'sub-personalities' and archetypes. Each of these has its own way of thinking, perceiving, feeling, and behaving. Here the client sits in a circle of empty chairs and, in turn, moves to chairs assuming another personality as it surfaces and vocalizing that personality. The therapist/facilitator offers subtle suggestions and later offers observations.

watsu (water shiatsu) shiatsu massage conducted in warm water, i.e., jacuzzi tub. The client is guided through a series of movements and stretches while receiving a shiatsu treatment.

wet rebirthing see REBIRTHING.

wheatgrass diet the use of wheatgrass juice to detoxify the body, increase energy, and provide essential enzymes. The benefits were discovered by A. Wigmore, also popularizer of this powerful food supplement. One starts with 1 oz of juice and gradually increases to 4 oz. It may also be applied to wounds, placed into bath water, and used as an enema.

whole foods diet a nutritional system developed by Bernard Jensen and others, which stresses the use of whole, natural, pure foods. Dr. Jensen, of iridology fame, suggests the natural diet be composed of 60% vegetables, 20& fruits, 10% starches, and 10% protein. Of these, 60% should be eaten raw and 40% cooked. This diet will then maintain a healthy 80/20 ratio of alkaline to acid.

Wigmore diet a diet/nutritional outlook based on the work of Ann Wigmore. It consists of seed sprouts, wheat grass juice, and raw vegetables and fruits.

W. O. Wood Chart (dowsing chart/map) a chart developed by dowser W.O. Wood to help dowsers to register their pendulum readings. It is primarily used in treating disease and can be used with the client present or at a distant (absent). In the latter, a 'witness' is necessary so that the dowser can tune into the client's vibrations. The witness could be a lock of hair, blood specimen, handwriting, piece of unwashed clothing, etc.

yin and yang the polarities of life as espoused by Chinese theorists. Yin is dark, passive, negative, inward and feminine. Yang is bright, active, positive, outward and masculine. Yin relates to the hollow organs and Yang to the solid organs. Yin relates to absorption and excretion, yang to regulatory functions.

yoga from the Sanskrit which means 'to unite or bind together' as in what one hopes to accomplish while practicing any of the great variety of yogic spiritual techniques to reach union with God. There are many reasons to practice yoga but perhaps the one which is common to all is a goal of spiritual progress and enlightenment. Hatha, Iyengar, kundalini, japa, Oki, Kripalu, bhakti, karma, are just a few of the many, many yogas. Asanas are positions which one assumes in any of the varieties of yoga. Mudras are hand/finger positions one assumes during yoga postures or meditations.

zero balancing a touch method often used for stress reduction, much like acupressure, for aligning body structure and energy. It is similar to acupressure and the practitioner attempts to reduce imbalances in the body's 'structure/energetic relationship'. It was developed by F.F. Smith, an osteopath.

Zone Diet a complex diet based on pioneering work done by B. Sears (The Zone, Mastering the Zone). His diet seeks to balance the hormonal responses to the digestion of food. He recommends three meals consisting of a moderate serving of low-fat protein with a large amount of vegetables (with olive oil or sliced almonds) and fruit for dessert. In addition to these three meals he strongly suggests two well-timed snacks. The 'zone' really refers to a zone of optimal insulin levels controlled by the diet. It is excess insulin that makes one fat, and the body produces excess insuline when one eats either (1) too much fat-free carbohydrates, or (2) too many calories at a meal.

zone therapy see REFLEXOLOGY. Though different, during the turn of the 20th century, Fitzgerald and Bowers described 'zone therapy' which advocated various forms of touch and physical manipulation to cure disease. They also recommended various accessories and electrical devices in applying their theories.

REFERENCES

The American Holistic Health Association's Complete Guide to Alternative Medicine (1996, Collinge)

Alternative Healing: The Complete A-Z Guide to More Than 150 Alternative Therapies (1996, Kastner and Burroughs)

The Medical Advisor: The Complete Guide to Alternative and Conventional Treatments (1996, Time/Life Books, 1200 pp)

The Self-Health Handbook (1996, Dachman and Kinnan)

Alternative Healthcare: A Comprehensive Guide to Therapies and Remedies (1996, Bradford, ed)

The Complete Family Guide to Alternative Medicine: An Illustrated Encyclopedia of Natural Healing (1996, C.N. Shealy, editor)

Alternative Healing (1996, A. Fox and B. Fox)

Alternative Medicine: What Works (1996, A. Fugh-Berman) is a basic no-frills, well-referenced and very affordable book. Its thirty pages of references is a shining feature.

The Encyclopedia of Alternative Medicine (1996, J. Jacobs, editor)

New Choices in Natural Healing (1995, Bill Gottlieb, editor)

The Alternative Health and Medicine Encyclopedia (1995, J.E. Marti)

Alternative Medicine: The Definitive Guide (1995, B. Goldberg Group, Ed.)

A Consumers Guide to Alternative Health Care (1995, Clayton and McCullough)

Natural Therapies: The Complete A-Z of Complementary Health (1994, M. McCarthy, editor)

World Medicine: The East-West Guide to Healing Your Body (1993, Monte, et al, editors)

Reader's Digest Family Guide to Natural Medicine (1993, Guinness, ed.)

The Complete Handbook of Natural Healing (1991, M. Starck)

Alternative Healing and Your Health (fully illustrated) (1991, J.M. Pilkington)

Encyclopedia of Natural Medicine (1991, Murray and Pizzorno)

The Manual of Natural Therapy (1989, Olshevsky/Noy/Zwang)

Holistic Health Promotion: A Guide for Practice (1989, B. Dossey, Keegan, Kolkmeier, Guzzetta)

The Complete Handbook of Holistic Health (1983, Moore and Moore)

The Alternative Health Guide (1983, Inglis and West)

A Visual Encyclopedia of Unconventional Medicine (1978, Ann Hill, Ed.)

Alternative Medicine Yellow Pages (1995, Bonk)

Alternative Medicine: Expanding Medical Horizons (1994, Berman, Larson)

Reader's Guide to Alternative Health Methods (1993, Hafner, editor)

A Consumers Guide to Alternative Medicine (1992, Butler and S. Barrett)

The Illustrated Dictionary of Natural Health (1989, Drury)

Alternative Medicine: A Bibliography of Books in English (1985, West and Trevelyan)

The Complete Illustrated Guide to Chinese Medicine (1996, T. Williams)

The Encyclopedia of Medicinal Plants (1996, Chevallier)

Racketeering in Medicine: The Suppression of Alternatives (1992, J.P. Carter)

The Visual Encyclopedia of Natural Healing (1991, Prevention Magazine)

The Other Medicines (1985, R. Gross)

Studies in the History of Alternative Medicine (1988, Roger Cooper)

Alternatives in Healing (1988, Mills and Finando)

Guide to the New Medicine: What Works, What Doesn't (1982, H. Pizer)

The Complete Book of Natural Therapies (1980, Carroll)

The Grosset Encyclopedia of Natural Medicine (1980, Robert Thomson)

Dimensions in Wholistic Healing: New Frontiers in the Treatment of the Whole Person (1979, Otto and Knight)

Natural Medicine (1978, Robert Thomson)

Wholistic Dimensions in Healing (1978, L.J. Kaslof)

A SELECTED HOMEOPATHIC OBITUARY

Dates were obtained through obituaries in Bradford's Scrapbook at Hahnemann Archives in Philadelphia, and the IHA, AIH, *Homoeopathic Physician,* and other journals. Research by Chris Ellithorp, Julian Winston, and Jay Yasgur with thanks to Mary Gooch at the Glasgow Homeopathic Library. Thanks also to Maesimund Panos, Wilfried Stock, and especially to Thierry Montfort and the Boiron Co. for their help with the French personages. Cleave references from his *Biographical Cyclopaedia of Homeopathic Physicians and Surgeons.*

> *But we all pass off with a task undone,*
> *Sudden and silent, and one by one.*
> *But the tasks we leave unfinished here*
> *We will finish up in another sphere.*

—T.L. Bradford
Transactions of AIH, 1908

Adams, Elizabeth S. (1821 •) an orphan at 15, she became a nurse and public school teacher. She had a peculiar fitness for the care of the sick' so she took up medicine under CS Lozier and graduated from the NY Med Coll for Women in 1869. She was a skilled homeopathician.

Adams, Myron Howell (1-7-1846 • 6-6-1929) An 1870 graduate of Hahnemann (Phil.) and author of *A Practical Guide to Homeopathic Treatment* ... (1913).

Aegidi, Karl Julius (•) Influential German homeopath who lived in the late 18th and early 19th centuries. He was physician to Princess Frederica of Prussia.

Allen, Henry C. (10-2-1836 • 1-22-1909) Author. Born in Canada. Ran the Hering Medical College in Chicago. President IHA 1886. Editor of *Medical Advance*. Graduated Cleveland 1861. Taught at Homeo. Dept. of the University of Michigan and at Cleveland Homeopathic Med. Coll. He wrote a number of books: *Keynotes of Leading Remedies, Materia Medica of the Nosodes*, etc. He was a descendent of Ethan Allen on the paternal side.

Key to abbreviations:

CHQ *Classical Homeopathic Quarterly*
HP *Homoeopathic Physician*
HR *Homoeopathic Recorder*
HT *Homeopathy Today*
JAIH *Journal of the American Institute of Homeopathy*

AFH American Foundation for Homeopathy
AIH American Institute of Homeopathy
IHA International Hahnemannian Assoc

Allen, John Henry (1854 • 8-1-1925) Author of *Chronic Diseases* and *Diseases of the Skin*. Pres. of IHA 1900. Prof. at Hering Medical College (Chicago).

Allen, Timothy Field (4-24-1837 • 12-5-1902) Taught materia medica and therapeutics at NY Hom. Med. Coll. and was Dean of the college for some 11 years (1882-1893). Co-editor of *US Medical and Surgical Journal* 1867-70; *NY Journal of Homeopathy* 1873-74. Graduated Amherst College and NYU Medical 1861. Director of New York Botanical Gardens. Compiled the massive *Encyclopedia of Pure Materia Medica*, 12 Vol., and wrote a number of other books as well, i.e., *Ophthalmic Therapeutics, Characeae of America,* etc. He had a son, Paul Allen (9-4-1863 •) who graduated from NY Hom Med Coll in 1889. He taught materia medica at his alma mater. He was an active force in NY homeopathy for more than 40 years.

Alexander, Elsie H. (1834 •) an 1854 graduate of the Western Homeopathic Coll. of Med. (Cleve), she filled the Chair of Demonstrator of Anatomy for two years as well. She was also an 1857 graduate of the Eclectic Coll. of Cinn.

Altschul, Elias (1812 •) German homeopath and author of *Homoopathischer Reise-Almanach* (1862).

Ameke, Wilhelm (1847 • 1-22-1886) Died age 39. Author, *History of Homeopathy.*

Angell, Henry (1-27-1829 • 5-28-1911) Author of *Diseases of the Eye* (1870). Editor of *New England Medical Gazette* established in 1866. He was an 1852 graduate of the Homeo. Med. Coll. of Pa. (Phil.) and wrote an important and controversial paper entitled 'Diet' in the *North American Journal of Homeopathy.* He became an expert in ophthalmology having studied with some of Europes best eye specialists.

Anshutz, Edward Pollock (3-23-1846 • 1-31 or 2-1-1918) Author and compiler for B&T. Honorary degree from Hering Medical College in 1909. Editor: *Homoeopathic Envoy* and *Homoeopathic Recorder.*

Armstrong, Wilbur Price (1860-1940) graduate in 1884 from Cleveland.

Arndt, Hugo Emil Rudolph (1845 •) Author of *A System of Medicine Based upon the law of Homeopathy* (1885).

Atkins, Edward Babcock (1851 • 1-8-1908) An 1877 graduate of NYU and friend of homeopathy. He wrote *The Relation of Homeopathy to Natural Science* (1889).

Aurand, Samuel Herbert (1854 •) Homeopath and author of *Botanical Materia Medica and Pharmacology* (1899).

Austin, Alonzo E. (6-1-1868 • 6-20-1948) Pupil of Kent. Doctor to John D. Rockefeller, Jr.

Bach, Edward (1886 • 1936) the developer of the 38 Bach flower remedies. He was influenced by Hahnemann's seminal work. His approach to healing the ill can be summarized as follows: It is not the disease which needs to be treated but the moods, characteristics and personality of the patient. "As the herbs heal our fears, anxieties, our worries, our faults, our ills will leave us."

Bachas, Irene Dimitriadou (9-13-1930 • 1985) learned homeopathy under Vithoulkas in the mid-1960s and later under M. Blackie. Dr. Blackie described Dr. Bachas as the best student she ever had. She helped establish homeopathy in Greece and Vithoulkas decribed her as "the diamond of homeopathy and a source of strength." She was president of the Hellenic Homeopathic Association and vice-president of the LIGA for several years.

Baehr, Bernhard (4-17-1828 • 10-21-1884). German physician and author of *The Science of Therapeutics...* (1875).

Baer, Oliver Perry (8-25-1816 • 8-10-1888). Wrote on diphtheria. He was educated by the Jesuits, later studied medicine and homeopathy eventually settling in Indiana. He was president of the Indiana State Institute of Homeopathy.

Ball, Alonzo S. (2-11-1800 • 12-17-1893). Early homeopath and one of the original members of the AIH.

Ballard, E.A. (3-8-1838 • 11-9-1891).

Barnes, Geo. W. (12-9-1825 • 1890) An 1851 graduate of Cleveland Homeo. College; later taught there as well.

Bartlett, Abner R. (1812 • 12-26-1862) 1856 grad. of Western Coll of Hom. (Cleveland), where he taught for a short period of time.

Bartlett, Clarence (5-22-1858 • 8-26-1935). Graduate of Hahnemann (Phila.) in 1879 and taught at his alma mater and authored many texts on the practice of medicine. He was intimately involved with the journal *Hahnemannian Monthly,* working with Dudley and Van Lennep. He edited and published *Farrington's Clinical Materia Medica* (1887).

Bassett, John Samuel (4-23-1830 • 8-1-1912) He began his homeopathic practice in Paterson, NJ, then later moved to NYC, where he garnered much respect especially among the wealthy and influential of that city. Many times he was solicited to teach but he refused. He was considered to be a first-rate diagnostician.

Bastyr, John Bartholomew (1912 • 6-29-1995). Naturopath and chiropractor, he helped found the National College of Naturopathic Medicine (Portland, OR) and the Naturopathic College (Seattle, WA) which later changed its name to Bastyr College of Naturopathic Medicine.

Bayard, Edward (3-6-1806 • 9-28-1889). Brother-in-law of Elizabeth Cady Stanton. Founder of the IHA. Secretary of AIH 1845-8. Co-editor, *North American Journal of Homoeopathy* 1860-62. 1851 grad. of Cleveland

Homeo. Med. College.

Bayes, William (1823 • 1882) British homeopath and author of *Applied Homeopathy; or, specific restorative medicine* (1871).

Beakley, Jacob (7-20-1812 • 8-6-1872) Author. Teacher. Surgeon. Dean of New York Homeopathic Medical College. Prof and Dean of the Homeo. Med. College of Pa.

Becker, Alexander Christian (1815 • 1849) Wrote *Diseases of the eye treated homeopathically* (1847).

Beckwith, David Herrick (2-13-1826 • 11-19-1909) professor at Cleveland Homeo. Med. College and Pulte in Cincinnati. Important figure in the history of the Cleveland college and 1851 graduate. Intimately associated with the Huron Street Hospital, Cleveland. A grad. of the Eclectic Med. Inst. (Cinn.) and the first class of the Western College of Homeopathy (Cleve.) 1871 Pres. of AIH.

Beckwith, Seth R. (1830 • 1-20-1905) 1853 graduate and professor at Cleveland Homeopathic Med. College and instrumental in the functioning of that institution. He became associated with Pulte Med. Coll., serving that institution for many years. VP of AIH in 1864. He also authored *A new therapeutics for the cure of disease by sending ozone, oxygen, and medicine into diseased tissues* (1899). He was President Garfield's family physician at the time of his assassination in 1881.

Bell, James Bachelder (2-21-1818 • 9-26-1914). Author of *Homeopathic Therapeutics of Diarrhoea* President IHA 1892. 1859 graduate of Hom. Med. Coll. of PA. "In medicine he is Hahnemannian; in religion Evangelical; and in politics, Republican."

Bellows, Howard Perry (1852 •) Supervised the Ophthamological, Otological and Laryngological Society in its proving of Belladonna: *A Reproving of Belladonna...* (1906).

Benjamin, Alva (1884 • 1975) A British homeopath who worked at the Royal London Homeo. Hospital for many years. He was president of the LIGA.

Berjeau, Jean Philibert (1809 • 1891) French homeopath and author of *The Homeopathic Treatment of Syphilis, Gonorhhea...* (1870).

Bernard, Henri (1895 • 1980) Great French homeopath and author. He developed constitutional theories of homeopathic treatment. He wrote four books (*Nouveau Traite d'Homeopathie*, 1947, *La Reticulo-endotheliose chronique ou sycose*, 1950, *Traite de Medecine Homeopathique*, 1951, and *Doctrine Homeopathique*, 1966) as well as many journal articles.

Berridge, Edward W. (c.1878 • c.1929).One of the founders of the IHA. Editor of *The Organon*. 1869 graduate of Hahnemann (Phil.). He was a British homeopath and adherent of high potency prescribing. He was mentor to Thomas Skinner. Author of *Complete Repertory on the Diseases of the Eye.*

Bettely, G.W. (• 1865) An expert on materia medica, he taught for several years at Western Coll. of Homeopathy (Cleve.) Student of S.R .Beckwith.

Betts, B. Frank (12-1-1845 •) A graduate of Hahnemann Med. Coll. in 1868, he also became intimately involved with homeopathic education at his alma mater, his specialties being gynecology, hygiene and dietetics.

Beuchelt, Hellmuth (1895 •) German author of *Homoopathische Konstitutions...* (1956).

Beurgi, Emil (1872 •) German homepath and author.

Bhaduri, Behari Lal (c.1840 • 3-27-1891) Noted Indian homeopath who was in the vanguard of Indian homeopaths at the turn of the 20th century, and started the *Indian Homoeopathic Review*.

Biddle, Isabel (5-24-1884 • 12-5-1970). A graduate of Chicago Coll. of Osteopathy (1905); in 1940s took the AFH Post-Graduate School in Homeopathy.

Bidwell, Glen Irving (•). Still practicing near Rochester, NY in 1951. Pupil of Kent. Author of *How To Use the Repertory* (1915) Graduate of Hering College 1905.

Biegler, Joseph A. (1832 • 12-21-1907). President IHA 1890.

Bier, August Karl Gustav (1861 • 1949) German author and though not a homeopath was supportive of it. He wrote *Homoopathie und harmonische Ordnung der Heilkunde* (1949) and *What Should be our Attitude toward Homeopathy?* (B & T, 1925).

Biggar, Hamilton Fisk (3-15-1839 in Canada • 11-29-1926) Graduated from Cleveland, 1866, and became intimately associated with his alma mater in teaching and performing surgical work. Doctor to John D. Rockefeller Sr. "As a clear, concise instructor he had but few equals." He had a son who took up homeopathy, H.F., Jr.

Bigler, Wm. H. (6-10-1840 •12-10-1904) He was an 1871 graduate of Hahnemann (Phila.) and became a professor of physiology there for a number of years.

Bittinger, Rev. Benjamin Franklin (1824 • 1913) Compiled the book on the creation of the Hahnemann Monument (Wash., D.C.) from materials collected by H.M. Smith.

Blair, A. O. (3-13-1806 • 1882 or 3). One of the founders of Cleveland Homeopathic College and taught there for some 25 years.

Blackie, Margery Grace (2-4-1898 • 8-24-1981). Became physician to the Queen of England and the royal family in 1969, succeeding Sir John Weir. She was president of the British Homeopathic Society in 1949 and Dean of the Faculty of Homeopathy for 17 years. Babington-Smith wrote a biography, *Champion of Homeopathy: The Life of Margery Blackie*. James Compton-Burnett was her uncle. Blackie wrote the popular *The Patient, Not The Cure* (1977).

Blackwood, Alexander Leslie (7-28-1862 • 12-31-1924). Author of *A*

Manual of Materia Medica... (2nd ed., 1925). Professor at Hahnemann Medical College (Chic.)

Bodman, Francis Hervey (1900 • 1980) British homeopath and scholar. He lived much of his life in Bristol, wrote *Insights into Homeopathy* (1990) and was president of the Faculty of Homoeopathy (London) during the mid 1950s.

Boenninghausen, Clemens Maria Frans von (3-2-1785 • 1-26-1864) Wrote the first repertory. Author. Lawyer. Lay practitioner. Discovered homeopathy when he was cured of tuberculosis by a pupil of Hahnemann's. He had a son, Karl, who was also a physician. See entry in dictionary.

Boericke, Felix A. (7-2-1857 • 2-23-1929) 1890 graduate of Hahnemann (Chic.). Son of Francis E. Boericke.

Boericke, Francis Edmund (6-3-1826 • 12-17-1901) Founder of the Boericke & Tafel pharmacy in 1869 along with Adolph Tafel. They also ran a publishing branch called Hahnemann Publishing House. He invented a hand-cranked machine to manufacture high potency remedies. Graduated Homeopathic Medical College of Pennsylvania in 1857 where he lectured. He had two sons, Frank and Felix. F.E. had two brothers, Francis Oscar and Anton.

Boericke, Garth Wilkinson (8-12-1893 • 1-8-1968) Son of William. Last teacher of homeopathy at Hahnemann in Philadelphia. He was pres. of the AIH and taught materia medica at the AFH Post-Graduate Course. Graduated from U. of Michigan Med. Dept. in Ann Arbor, 1918.

Boericke, Oscar Eugene (•) 1898 grad. of Hahnemann (Phil.) Brother of William. Wrote the repertory as contained in Boericke's *Materia Medica* (1906).

Boericke, William (11-26-1849 Austria • 4-1-1929). Author of *Boericke's Materia Medica* (1901) and *The Principles of Homeopathy* (1874). Nephew of F.E.Boericke. Editor of *California Homeopath* and founded the *Pacific Coast Journal of Homoeopathy* in 1880 (edited it until 1915). He also co-founded the Pacific Homoeopathic Medical College (1881). Also wrote *A Compendium of the Principles of Homoeopathy* (1912) and *Twelve Tissue Remedies of Schuessler* (1888). 1880 graduate of Hahnemann (Phila.). Son of F.O. Boericke.

Boger, Cyrus Maxwell (5-13-1861 • 9-2-1935). Author from Parkersburg, WV. President IHA 1904. Graduated from Hahnemann (Phil.) in 1888. He was an expert of Boenninghausen's repertorial system and wrote *Boenninghausen's Characteristics and Repertory* (1937), *A Synoptic Key of the Materia Medica* (1915), *Times of the Remedies and the Moon Phases*, etc.

Boiron, Henri (12-4-1906 • 3-24-1994). Established Laboratoires Boiron in Lyon along with his twin brother Jean in 1932. He was Chairman of the

French Homeopathic Pharmacists' Trade Assoc. for some thirty years. In 1992 at the annual Boiron shareholders meeting, Henri described one of the most important events for him: "For me, after years of effort carried out with the French administration for Public Health, it was obtaining the inclusion of homeopathy in the *French Pharmacopoeia, 8th Edition,* in 1965."

Boiron, Jean (12-4-1906 • 7-25-1996) Twin brother of Henri. Together they created Laboratoires Boiron (Lyon, France) in 1932. He said, "The guiding light of my life was to have homeopathy known."

Bojanus, Karl (1818 • 5-28-1897) Russian homeopath. Presented a paper in Phila. 1876 and came to World Homeopathic Congress in Chicago in 1893.

Bonqueval, J.G. de (•) Swiss homeopath who concentated on electro-homeopathy, writing, in 1885, *Theory and Practice of Electro-homeopathy.*

Boone, Joel T., Lt. Commander (8-29-1889 • 4-2-1974) Graduate of Hahnemann, Phila. Winner of Congressional Medal of Honor WWI. White House Physician to President Herbert Hoover. Appointed medical director of Veterans' Administration in the early 1950s.

Borland, Douglas (1885 Glasgow • 11-29-1960) Pupil of Kent in 1908. He wrote a number of monographs: *Children's Types, Digestive Drugs, Pneumonias,* etc.

Borneman, John Alexander I (1879 • 4-8-1955) was professor emeritus of pharmacy at Hahnemann Medical College and Hospital (Phil.) and at the Philadelphia College of Pharmacy and Science. He founded Borneman Laboratories in 1907. He emigrated from Germany when he was 11. He was a pharmacy graduate of the Philadelphia College of Pharmacy in 1902. "Was noted for his work in botany and kept a nursery at his home where he grew belladonna and digitalis and many other homeopathic plants. Hahnemann Med. Coll. conducted provings in the 1920s and he supplied the school with raw materials and remedies. Graduates of Hahnemann will recall their freshman year trip to the Borneman Labs. in Norwood to observe the manufacture of homeopathic remedies."—*JAIH,* 1955.

Borneman, John Anthony Jr. (5-16-1904 • 4-6-1996) Continued in his father's footsteps and essentially ran the pharmacy for many years becoming president in 1955 when his father J.A. Borneman I died. He lectured on medicinal plants at the NCH Summer School during the Millersville years.

Boyd, Linn John (1895 •) Homeopath and author of *A Study of the Simile in Medicine* (1936). He spoke to the Cleveland Homeopathy Medical Society on 11-11-1941.

Boyd, Wm. Ernest (1891 Scotland • 1955) Eminent British homeopath, developer of the Emanometer and of Boyd's Drug Groups. The emanometer could measure the 'force' in different homeopathic potencies and could match the vibrations of the remedy with the vibrations of the ill person, thus aiding in the proper selection of the remedy. See BOYD'S DRUG GROUP in dictionary.

Boyle, Francis Wade (1945 • 10-3-1993) A minister, naturopathic physician, homeopath and author. He was an expert in botanical medicine. He taught at NCNM and CCNM.

Boynton, S.A. (2-24-1835 •) Physician to President Garfield just after he was shot. He was a relative of Mrs. Garfield and treated her for quite some time. Professor of Physiology at the Cleveland Homoe. College.

Boyson, Wm. A. (1894 • 4-23-1972). Served as dean of the AFH Post-Graduate School in Homeopathy for some 17 years. A 1930 graduate of Hahnemann (Phil.). President of the AIH 1964/4. He was active in homeopathic provings.

Bradford, Thomas Lindsley (6-6-1847 • 12-3-1918). Author and compiler of homeopathic historical materials. Librarian at Hahnemann, Philadelphia. Graduated in 1871 from the Homeopathic Med. Coll. of Missouri. His major books were: *Homoeopathic Bibliography of the United States* (1892), *The Pioneers of Homoeopathy* (1898), *The Logic of Figures* (1900), and *Index to Homoeopathic Provings* (1901). His clinical love was pediatrics.

Brahde, Carl V.J. (1836 • 9-x-1881) Early Danish homeopath.

Brainard, Jehu (~1806 • 3-10-1878) Though never graduating from any formal institution he occupied many professorships in a variety of institutions during his life. He was a founding member of the Cleve. Homeo. Med. Coll. and served there until 1860. Later upon moving to Wash. D.C. he helped establish the Homeopathic Medical Association and was president of that body in 1872.

Breyfogle, William LaMartine (1845 • 6-15-1915) Author of *Epitome of Homeopathic Medicines* (1869). Graduate of Hahnemann (Phil.) in 1868. His son, Jr., graduated from Chic. Homeo. Med. Coll. in 1882.

Brown, Mary Belle (3-1-1846 • 7-13-1924) A grad. of the NY Homeopathic Med. Coll. for Women and served as dean of that institution for several years. She practiced for 30 years in NYC.

Budlong, Jonathan C. (8-28-1836 • 7-24-1907). Surgeon general of the state of Rhode Island, 1875-94.

Buck, Jirah D. (11-20-1838 •) 1890 Pres. of the AIH. Grad (1864) and professor at Cleveland Homeopathic College. He became involved with Pulte Med. College as well. He wrote three books: *A Study of Man and the Way to Health* (1888), *Mystic Masonry*, and *Paracelsus and Other Essays*.

Burgher, John C. (11-1-1822 •) an 1854 grad of Homeo. Med. Coll of Pa

(Phil.) and noted Pittsburgh, PA homeopath. He studied under and then became partners with J.P. Dake. Burgher first proposed the founding of the Homeo. Med. Soc. of Allegheny city/county and served as it's president for three years. He was Vice Pres. of the AIH in 1872. He had a son who became a homeopath, J.C., Jr.

Burnett, James Compton (7-10-1840 • 4-2-1901). British. Author of many short treatises including *50 Reasons for Being a Homoeopath, Diseases of Spleen and Their Remedies, The New Cure for Consumption, Curability of Tumors,* and *Gold as a Remedy.* Great-uncle of Margery Blackie. He was primarily an organopathic clinician supporting the works of Rademacher. He was the first to study vaccinosis. Known as "Dr. Gout" for his successful treatment of gout with his secret remedy, *Urtica urens,* which he refused to reveal during his lifetime.

He took his medical degree from Glasgow and "...the Professor of Anatomy specially congratulated him on his brilliant examination and later implored him not to ruin a promising career by going in for Homoeopathy - which the young man had by then decided on. Burnett replied that he could not buy worldly honours at the cost of his conscience." (*Layman Speaks,* 1963, 16:11, p. 373)

Burt, William H. (2-25-1836 • 1-27-1897 reported also as Feb. 2). Author. First prover of *Collinsonia* and other remedies. Graduate of Cleveland, 1858.

Bute, George Henry (5-27-1792/3 • 2-13-1876). Came from Germany to Philadelphia in 1819. First prover of *Rhus tox., Alum, Cistus canadensis, Sanguinaria, Chimiphila, Rhus ven,* and *Rhus glab.* among others. He became a friend and student of Hering while serving as a missionary in Paramaribo (in what is now Suriname) as Hering cured him of spotted fever with homeopathy. Later he moved to Nazareth, PA and then implored Hering to join him. Hering came to Philadelphia in 1833 and the two both developed large practices in that city.

Butler, Clarence Willard (5-1-1848 • 12-20-1904). Graduated NY Homeopathic 1872. Member of the "Unanimous Club", a classical group.

Cailleux, Roland (1908 •) French homeopath and author. He wrote *La Doctrine homoeopathique et ses critiques* (1946).

Carleton, Bukk J. (11-11-1856 • 10-20-1915). Author of *Urinary Diseases* (1905). Member of the "Unanimous Club", a classical group.

Carleton, Edmund (12-11-1839 • 6-15-1912). Author of *Homeopathy in Medicine and Surgery* (1913). Graduated NY Hom. 1871. President of IHA 1894.

Carleton, Spencer (ca. 1874 • 7-11-1939). Son of Edmund.

Carmichael, Thomas H. (1-27-1858 • 10-9-1942) An 1888 graduate of Hahnemann (Phila.) and lecturer at his alma mater on pharmaceutics and materia medica. He was president of the AIH in 1911-12 and was involved in the revision of the Homoeopathic Pharmacopoeia of the United States (HPUS). He wrote the Preface to the HPUS in 1936.

Cartier, Francois (1864 • 1928) Author and President of the French Homeopathic Society in 1906.

Caruthers, R.E. (• 3-1885). Practiced in Allegheny County, Pa.

Case, Erastus Eli (5-28-1847 • 10-27-1918). B.A. Yale (1872). Graduated NY Hom. (1874). IHA President 1901-2. Practiced in Hartford, CT. Author of one of the first clinical texts on classical homeopathy, *Some Clinical Experiences of E.E. Case, M.D.*

Caspari, Carl Gottlob (1798 • 1828) Author of *Caspari's Homeopathic Domestic Physician* (1852, from the German 8th ed.). See dictionary under MESMERIZED.

Chapman, Millie J. (7-23-1845 •) Donated her library to the Huron Road Hospital, Cleveland. She was an 1874 grad. of Cleveland Hom. Med. Coll. Served as VP of the AIH. She practiced in Pittsburgh, PA.

Charlton, Callie Brown (1851 • 1934) first woman to practice homeopathy in Oregon. She was an 1886 grad. of Hahnemann (Chic.) and practiced in Portland until her retirement in 1912. After being widowed in 1872 she became determined to study medicine. She taught school for a number of years in order to acquire the necessary funds to attend medical school.

Chase, Sarah Blakelee (1-18-1837 •) along with her husband, Hayard D., they preceptored with Dr. Bosler of Dayton, OH and entered Cleve. Homeo. Med. Coll. and graduated in 1870. She was the first woman admitted to the Med. Soc. of Cleveland and the Homeo. Assoc. of OH.

Chavanon, Paul (12-8-1898 • 11-21-1962) Famous French homeopath, author and Laureat de la Faculte de Medecine de Paris. His true interest lay in otolaryngology and immunization. He is considered the father of homeopathic otorhinolaryngology as encapsulated in his *Therapeutique O.R.L. homoeopathique* (1935).

Chepmell (•) Homeopath and author of *A Domestic Homeopathy...* (1849).

Clapp, Herbert Codman (1-31-1846 •) Practiced with Samuel Gregg, the pioneer of homeopathy in New England. He was a prominent homeopath in Boston and at the Boston U. School of Medicine. He had a great interest in tuberculosis, wrote chapters in Arndt's *System of Medicine* and a book, *Auscultation and Percussion* (1878).

Clapp, Otis Sr. (• 9-19-1886). An early homeopath in Boston. Founded the first homeopathic pharmacy in Boston.

Clark, George Hardy (1860 •) Author of *The ABC Manual of Materia Medica and Therapeutics* (1901).

Clark, Lucy Swanton (3-15-1906 • 11-6-1991) She did an internship and residence at the homeopathic institutions Huron Road Hospital in Cleveland and Flower and Fifth Avenue Hospital in NYC, respectively. She taught for several years at the AFH post-graduate school. "Lucy will long be remembered for her contributions to the education of other physicians ... and for her kindness and her contributions to building peace on earth."— *JAIH* 84:4, p. 119.

Clarke, John Henry (1853 • 11-24-1931). The pre-eminent British homeopath. His major works were *The Dictionary of Practical Materia Medica* (1900), *A Clinical Repertory of the Dictionary of Materia Medica* (1904), and *The Prescriber* (1885). It is said he had a writing desk in his carriage so he could work on his books between calls. He presided over the 1906 World's Homoeopathic Congress.

Cleveland, Charles Luther (• alive in 1929) 1883 graduate of Cleve. Homeo. Med. Coll. He wrote *Salient Materia Medica and Therapeutics* (1888).

Close, Stuart M. (11-24-1860 • 6-26-1929). A graduate of the NY Homeo. Med. Coll. Pupil of B. Fincke and P.P. Wells. Taught homeopathic philosophy at NY Homeopathic 1909-1913. Teacher of H.A. Roberts. President of IHA 1906. Founded Brooklyn Hahnemannian Union in 1896. Editor of the "Department of Homeopathic Philosophy" for the *Homeopathic Recorder.* He authored *The Genius of Homeopathy: Lectures and Essays on Homeopathic Philosophy.* He was an accomplished musician.

Cloud, J. A. (•) Homeopath and author of *Homoeopathy: its difficulties and some of the principal ...* (1869).

Cogwell, Charles Herbert (8-14-1844 •) One of the founders of the State University of Iowa Homeopathic Medical Dept. He was professor and Dean, too. This college was founded in 1877 and closed its doors 47 years later in 1921. During that period it had just two materia medica professors and three Deans (G. Royal, WH Dickinson, and Cogswell).

Collet, Fr. Denys (1824-1909) French homeopath and author who concentrated his researches on isopathy. In 1898, he published *Isopathie: Methode Pasteur par voie interne*. He initiated the isopathic movement in France c. 1865. He was one of the first to employ isopathics, using dynamizations of diphtheria secretions, pneumonia mucus, saliva, urine, pus, and blood.

Comellas, Ramon (•) came from Barcelona, Spain and, in 1850, introduced homeopathy into Mexico.

Comstock, Thomas Griswold (7-27-1829 •) An 1852 graduate of the Homeo. Med. Coll. of Pa. He was professor of obsterics at the Missouri Homeo. Med. Coll. and as a homeopathic practitioner was regarded as among the foremost in the West.

Cookinham, Franklin H. (1881 • 5-9-1977). A beloved physician who, for many years, helped keep homeopathy alive during its 'lost years' (1930s–1970). He sat with Grimmer and Smith in Kent's lectures. He practiced in San Francisco and was secretary of the Cal. State Homeopathic Assoc.

for 25 years. He went by the nickname of 'Cookie'. His father, Dorwin A. (1850 • 4-14-1923) was a homeopathic physician who graduated in 1889 from Kansas City Homeo. Med. Coll. He practiced in Topeka, KS.

Cooper, Jack (1917 • 6-4-1987) Like Cookinham and Renner, helped to keep homeopathy alive during its dark years. He was President of the AIH.

Cooper, Robert T. (6-2-1844 • 9-14-1903). English. Contemporary of Burnett, Hughes, and Skinner. Wrote a treatise on cancer.

Copeland, Royal S. (11-7-1868 • 6-17-1938). Graduate of U. Michigan Homeo. Med. Coll., 1889. Professor of Ophthalmology and Otology at his alma mater (1895-1908) before moving to NYC in 1908 to become Dean of NY Homeo. Med. Coll. and director of Flower Hospital for ten years, until 1918, when he became the NYC Public Health Commissioner (until 1923). He was elected to the US Senate in 1922, serving until his sudden death in 1938. As Senator, he was responsible for the bill authorizing the Homeopathic Pharmacopeia of the U.S. He was an adroit politician (Mayor of Ann Arbor, MI 1901-1903). Author of *Refraction, Diseases of the Ear*, and *The Scientific Reasonableness of Homeopathy*.

Cowperthwaite, Allen Corson (5-3-1848 • 3-1-1926). He authored several books, the most important being *Text-Book of Materia Medica and Therapeutics* (1891). Teacher at the San Francisco Homeopathic Med. Coll., Hahnemann (Chic.), and the Homoeopathic Med. Dept. at the U. of Iowa, where he was professor of materia medica and dean for 15 years, 1877-1892. He was a poet and litterateur. He was president of the New England, Iowa and Illinois state homeopathic state societies, and president of the AIH in 1888. Graduated Hahnemann (Phil.) in 1869.

Cranch, Edward (10-16-1851 • 5-20-1920) Prominent Erie, PA homeopath. An 1875 graduate of NY Med. Coll., Flower and Fifth Avenue Hospital.

Croserio, Simon Felix (11-16-1786or1769 • 4-13-1855). Author of first homeopathic book on obstetrics, *Homeopathic Manual of Obstetrics* (1866). Friend of Hahnemann.

Cross, Jerome E. (8-10-1839 • 10-1-1882).

Curie, Paul Francis (1799 • 1853) Wrote *Clinical Lectures on Homeopathy* (c. 1840) and *Practice of Homeopathy* (1838).

Curtis, Harvey W. (2-22-1824 • 4-30-1902) Noted abolitionist and Lt. Governor of Ohio.

Dake, Jabez Philander (4-22-1827 • 10-28-1894). Born Johnstown, NY, died Nashville, TN. Co-author of the *Cyclopedia of Drug Pathogenesy* with Hughes. Graduated HMC of PA 1851. Also penned *Therapeutic Methods: An outline of principles...* (1886). He was AIH president in 1857. He helped edit the *Phila. Journal of Hom., U.S. Journal of Hom.*, and *North American Journal of Hom.* He practiced most of his life in Pittsburgh, where he had the largest practice of any physician in that city.

Dayfoot, Herbert M. (•) An 1867 graduate of Cleve. Homeo. Med. Coll. and author of *Homeopathy for the People* (1868).

Dearborn, Frederick Myers (7-13-1876 • 1-25-1960) He wrote *American Homeopathy in the World War* (1923) and *Diseases of the Skin with Illustrations* as well as ten other books. He served in the Spanish-American War and WWI as a lieutenant colonel. He was prof. of dermatology at the NY Hom. Med. Coll., his alma mater (grad. 1900). He lectured widely on his specialty at the homeopathic medical colleges and was on the staff of many of the NYC hospitals. He is the son of H.M. His son F.M.Jr. (c. 1913 • 2-27-1958) rose to a high level in the U.S. government, serving as a special assistant to Pres. Eisenhower for security operations coordination.

Dearborn, Henry Martin (11-19-1846 • 2-16-1904). Author, teacher and physician. He soon developed an enormous reputation as a clinician and served on many clinical posts: visiting physician to the Metropolitan Hospital (formerly Ward's Island Homeo. Hospital, 1881), state examiner in lunacy (1882), etc. He was professor of the theory and practice of medicine to the NY Med. Coll. and Hospital for Women, professor of dermatology at the NY Homeo. Med. Coll. and Hospital, etc. He was assoc. editor of the *North American J. of Homeopathy,* wrote many papers and belonged to many homeopathic societies. Father of F.M. Dearborn.

Deschere, Martin (6-8-1848 • 7-21-1902). Graduated NY Hom. 1875. Associate editor of *North American Journal of Homeopathy.* Developer of a potentizer.

Detweiler, A.C. (• 7-6-1883). Died in a boating accident with W.A. Detweiler.

Detweiler, W.A. (• 7-6-1883). Died in a boating accident with A.C. Detweiler.

Detwiller, Henry (12-13-1795 • 4-21-1887). Came to the US from Switzerland in 1817. The pioneer of homeopathy in PA, having given the first homeopathic dose *(Puls.,* for a difficult case of retarded menstruation and severe colic) in that state on 7-23/8-1828 and the first to successfully practice it in the United States. He was co-founder of the Allentown Academy in 1835 and also of the AIH in 1844. "His Herbarium contained the most complete samples of fauna *(sic)* in the state..." *The Layman Speaks,* 28:8, p. 190 (1975).

Detwiller, John Jacob (4-26-1834 • 2-28-1916) Son of Henry, he developed a very successful surgical practice. He was a member of the first homeopathic examining board established by the state of Pennsylvania.

Dewey, Willis Alonzo (10-25-1858 • 4-1-1938). Author. Teacher. Graduate of NY Hom. 1880. Taught at Hahnemann Med. Coll. (San Francisco), and the U. of Mich. Homeopathic Med. Dept. He wrote *Practical Homoeopathic Therapeutics* (1901, 3rd ed. 1933) and *Essentials of Ho-*

meopathic Materia Medica (1894, 5th ed 1926) and with Wm. Boericke wrote *The Twelve Tissue Remedies of Schuessler* (1888, 6th ed in 1928). He was editor of the *California Homoeopathic Journal* and the *Medical Century*, and assoc. editor of the *Universal Homoeopathic Observer* and the *JAIH*.

Dhawale, M.L. (1927 • 1987) Famous Indian homeopath and author of *Principles and Practice of Homeopathy*.

Dickinson, Wilmot Horton (9-19-1829 • 10-x-1889). Prof. at U. of Iowa Homeopathic Dept. Author of *Homeopathic Principles and Practice of Medicine* (1883). 1858 graduate of Cleveland Homeo. Med. Coll.

Dieffenbach, Wm. Hermann (1865 •)

Dixon, Charles A. (1870 • 10-1-1959, Akron, OH) He was one of the great homeopaths of the generation after J.T. Kent. "I am thoroughly convinced that if all of our homeopathic doctors were practicing pure homeopathy that our school would be the dominant school of medicine throughout the whole civilized world before many years."—*HT* 2/1996, p. 28.

Dodge, Lewis (~1815 • ~1897) Upon graduation from Hahnemann (Phil.) in 1850, he was enlisted to teach materia medica and obstetrics at Cleve. Homeo. Med. Coll.

Douglas, James S. (7-4-1801 • 1878) Professor at Cleveland and St. Louis Hom. Med. Colleges. Helped prove *Gelsemium* and did partial provings of *Cimicifuga racemosa*. Pres. of the AIH in 1866. Author of *Practical Homeopathy, for the people...* (1875).

Douglass, Melford Eugene (•) Homeopath and author of *Characteristics of the Homeopathic Materia Medica* (1905) and *Pearls of Homeopathy* (1903).

Drysdale, John James (1817 • 8-20-1892). English homeopath. Developer of *Pyrogenium*. Author of *An Introduction to the study of homeopathy...* (1845).

Dubs, Samuel Richard (11-8-1811 • 12-26-1889). Founder of Philadelphia Provers Union and helped prove *Oxalic ac., Cucumis colocynthis, Lobelia cardinalis,* and the first to prove *Cimicfuga race.* Developed the decimal scale of potencies in the US. He adopted homeopathy when he was cured of a persistent cough and gastromalacia. He was one of the founders of the AIH and of the Homeo. Med. Coll. of PA.

Dudgeon, Robert Ellis (3-17-1820 • 9-8 or 9-1904). English. Translator of many of Hahnemann's works. Author of *Lectures on the Theory and Practice of Homeopathy* (1854). Developed a sphygmograph.

Dudley, Pemberton (10-17-1837 • 3-25-1907) An 1861 graduate of Hahnemann Medical College (Phil.) and served some 40 years as Professor and Dean of Faculty. Editor of the *Hahnemannian Monthly* for seven years and wrote an article on 'homeopathy' for the *Encyclopedia Ameri-*

cana. He was a voluminous writer. Served twelve years on the Pennsylvania State Board of Health and was Secretary of the AIH for seven years and its President in 1896. He was intimately involved in virtually every aspect of homeopathy in Philadelphia during his life.

Duncan, Thomas Cation (1840 Scotland • 6 or 7-16-1902). Author of *How to be Plump, Diseases of Children*, and others.

Dunham, Carroll (10-29-1828 • 2-18-1887) Author. Educator. Pupil of Boenninghausen. Developer of Dunham potencies, teacher at N.Y. Hom. Med. College. Co-editor *Amer. Hom. Review*. He was president of the AIH.

Dunsford, Harris F. (1808 • 1847) Wrote *The Practical Advantage of Homeopathy ...* (1842).

Dutt, Babu Rajendra (•) The first real popularizer of homeopathy in India.

Eaton, Morton Monroe (•) Wrote *Domestic Practice for Parents and Nurses* (1882). Had a son, Jr., who graduated from Pulte Med. Coll. in 1888.

Edson, Susan Ann(1-24-1823 • 11-12-1897) Graduate of Cleveland 1854. Physician to President James A. Garfield. Founder of Washington Homeopathic Free Dispensary. She served in the Army for two years during the Civil War.

Ehrhart, Urban J. (• 6-12-1877) Physician who turned pharmacist and founded Ehrhart and Karl Pharmacy in Chicago in 1912. His son Roger became a pharmacist and continued in the business.

Ehrmann, Ben (3-3-1812 • 3-15-1886).

Ehrmann,Francis (•) Practiced in the Carlisle, PA area.

Eisfelder, Henry W. (• 7-17-1975) an active proponent of homeopathy. He founded and edited the homeopathic journal, *The Annals of International Therapeutics*. He graduated from NY Homeo. Med. Coll.

Ellis, Sarah M. (1828 •) an 1859 graduate of the Western Homeo. Coll. (Cleve.). She was the first woman professor of anatomy in America when for two years she taught the subject at the NY Homeo. Med. Coll. for Women (1862-4). She practiced in Florida in an itinerant fashion.

Ellis, John (11-26-1815 • 12-3-1895 or 6) He wrote a homeopathic domestic book and was one of the pioneers of homeopathy in Detroit. He was president of the Michigan Institute of Homeopathy. In 1868 he gave up homeopathic practice and went into manufacturing. Continued to write on morality, temperance and other related subjects. He wrote *The Avoidable Causes of Disease*. Professor at Western Coll. of Homeopathy for 6 years. He invented a new process of refining petroleum, securing patents on that invention. Valvoline was the name of his product!

Epps, John (2-15-1805 Kent, England • 2-12-1869) Wrote *Domestic Homeopathy.*

Espanet, Alexis (1811 • 1886) Eminent French homeopath and author. Wrote *Traite Methodique et Pratique de Matiere Medicale et de Therapeutique base sur la loi des semblables* (1860).

Everest, Thomas Roupell (• 1855). Homeopath and author of *A Popular View of Homeopathy* (2nd, 1842).

Farley, W.B. (1868 • 5-25-1899).

Farrington, Ernest Albert (1-1-1847 • 12-15/7-1885). Graduate of Hahnemann Med. Coll (1868) and was professor of materia medica at his alma mater for over 11 years. Author. Died at age 38. A devout follower of Swedenborg, he refused allopathic help saying, "If I must die, I want to die a Christian." He wrote *Clinical Materia Medica* (1887).

Farrington, Harvey (6-12-1872 • 6-9-1957). Son of E. A. Farrington. Pupil of Kent. Taught at the AFH post graduate school. President IHA 1922 and author of *Homoeopathy and Homoeopathic Prescribing.*

Fellger, Adolphus (6-14-1821 • -19-1888) Noted homeopathic surgeon.

Feveile, Crik Nisson (1819 • 3-x-1873) Early Danish homeopathic pioneer who founded, in 1860, the *Popular Homoeopathic Review*. He translated Hering's *Homoeopathic Family Doctor*. He had a large practice and influenced many young homeopaths.

Fincke, Bernhardt (1-7-1821 • 10-21-1906). Was born in Saxony (Germany). Creator of the Fincke potencies (high potencies). President of the IHA in 1896. Graduated NYU School of Medicine in 1854. He possessed a superior musical ability, mastering the piano, violin, cello, and horn. He wrote voluminously and had a large and worldwide correspondence.

Fisher, Charles E. (3-7-1853 •) Homeopathic surgeon, author. An 1872 grad. of Detroit Hom. Med. Coll. He edited many homeopathic journals, most notably the *Southern J. of Hom.* (1885-1893) and *Medical Century.* He served as prof. of obstetrics to Hering and Hahnemann in Chicago for a number of years. He authored two comprehensive volumes, *Diseases of Children* (1895) and *Homeopathic Textbook of Surgery* (1895).

Flagg, Josiah Foster (1-11-1789 • 12-30-1853). An early homeopath in Boston. Co-founder of the AIH.

Flasschoen, Charles Isidore (1842 •) French homeopath and author of *Le Triomphe de l'homoeopathie...* (1908).

Fleury, Rudolph (1916 Swiss •) Distinguished Swiss homeopath.

Foote, George F. (3-13-1817 • 5-8-1889). Founder of Middletown State Hospital.

Fortier-Bernoville, Maurice (1896 • 1939) French homeopath and author. He was the founder and editor of the journal *L'Homoeopathie Moderne* (1932). He was active in LIGA affairs and published a number of books:

Une etude sur Phosphorus (1930), *L'Homoeopathie en medecine infantile* (1931), his best known *Comment guerir par l'Homoeopathie* (1929, 1937), and an interesting work on iridology, *Introduction a l'etude de l'Iridologie* (1932), etc. He was a proponent of artificial phylectenular autotherapy.

Foubister, Donald MacDonald (10-31-1902 Scotland • 1-31-1988). Worked at the London Homeopathic Hospital for a number of years and was a Fellow of the Faculty of Homoeopathy for many years in addition to being its president and dean. He wrote an excellent book, *Tutorials on Homoeopathy* (1989).

Fowler, Ada A. (11-11-1858 •) an 1889 grad. of Hahnemann (Chic.). She became house physician to the Chicago Nose and Throat Hospital

Freligh, Martin (1-23-1813 • 8-31-1889). Wrote *Homeopathic Practice of Medicine*, a domestic book for the layperson.

Freytag, Eberhard (c. 1764 • 3-14-1846). One of the first homeopaths in the USA (Bethlehem, PA).

Frost, James (5-24-1825 • 1-21-1875). Author of Obstetrics. Co-editor and founder of *Hahnemannian Monthly* 1865-8. He studied under H.N. Guernsey and graduated in 1850 from the Homeo. Med. Coll. of PA (Phil.)

Furr, E.B. (6-30-1922 • 7-26-1993). Homeopathic pharmacist. With his father (W.B.), ran Washington Homeopathic Pharmacy, Bethesda, MD for many years. Now it is owned and operated by J. Lillard.

Gallavardin, Jean-Pierre (1825 • 1-22-1898). French homeopath. Author of *Homeopathic Treatment of Alcoholism* (1890). His son, Jules (1848-1917) was also an influential French homeopath.

Gatchell, Horatio P. (~1814 • 1885) An 1842 graduate of the Eclectic Med Institute and soon became a professor at the Western Homeo. College, becoming a popular doctor in that city as well. He was also professor at Hahnemann College (Chic).

Gause, Owen B (6-x-1825 •) An 1857 graduate of the Homoe. Med. Coll. of Pa. and was professor of obstetrics and diseases of women and children for some twenty years. He was co-founder of the Homeo. Med. Soc. of Pa. and its president in 1869.

Geary, John Fitzgibbon (•) Compiled reviews and articles from the works of Hering (1858).

Geddes, Annie Lowe (6-4-1855 • 7-1903) Author and graduate of the NY College and Hospital for Women (1890). "A woman of strong character, of impressive presence, a good homeopathist and a brilliant operator, who would have made her mark as a gynecologist if she had lived. She joined the Institute in 1895."—*AIH Transactions,* 1904.

Gentry, William Daniel (9-8-1836 • 1-27-1922). Author of the six volume, 5500-page *The Concordance Repertory* (1890), which took 15 years to write. Two years after, he became a charismatic healer, claiming that "I alone can speak for you in the name of Jesus Christ." An 1880 graduate of Homeo. Med. Coll. of St. Louis, Missouri.

Getman, Volkert (8-11-1865 • 7-20-1950). Born Johnstown, NY. NY Hom. 1904. Prover of *Adrenalinum.*

Getsinger, Edward Christopher (1-9-1866 •) was supposedly a homeopath but retired from medical practice after just three years. He then devoted himself to uncovering the mysteries of life and lecturing on popular science. He traveled extensively and claims to have discovered the astronomical source of alphabets and chronology of the ancient proper names. He was associated with the Baha'i faith.

Gibson, D. M. (3-22-1888 • 3-8-1977). English author and homeopath. Retired to Toronto, Canada where he died at the age of 89.

Gladish, Donald (1900 • 6-30-1967) A 1933 grad. of Hahnemann (Phila.). He practiced homeopathy in Glenville, IL and was very active in organizational work and wrote many articles. He helped to establish the AFH's *The Layman Speaks.*

Gladwin, Frederica E. (2-18-1856 • 5-7-1931). Pupil of Kent in St. Louis. Came with him to Philadelphia. Taught at the AFH post graduate school which was the forerunner of the NCH Summer School. She taught Pierre Schmidt and E. Wright-Hubbard. She was one of the founders of the American Foundation of Homeopathy. She authored many articles.

Glassburn, John R. (8-11-1908 •) a 1934 graduate of Hahnemann (Phil.) and worked for many years at the Pittsburgh Homeo. Hospital (Shadyside). President of the Allegheny County Homeo. Soc. and the 1951 president of the Homeo. Med. Soc. of the State of PA.

Goldenberg, John (1810 • 1-1-1888) an early pioneering Russian homeopath who was the first homeopathic doctor to practice homeopathy in Moscow (for 45 years!).

Goldberg, Benjamin (1897 • 1978) a graduate of OSU when it was still homeopathic. He practiced for some 55 years in the Cincinnati area. He was a three term president of the Southern Homoeopathic Med. Assoc., and a former president of the Ohio State Homeopathic Med. Assoc.

Goodno, Wm. Colby (•) An 1870 graduate of Hahnemann (Phila.) who became associated with his alma mater in varying capacities. He was professor of the practice of medicine and lecturer on microscopy, histology and pathological anatomy. It was in this latter position that he gained his reputation as he coupled his knowledge of photography with microscopy to create very interesting classes. His lectures were the epitome of clarity and directness and indicated his mastery of the subject. He was a successful surgeon and practitioner of homeopathy.

Goullon, H. (•) German homeopath and author of *Scrofulous Affections* *and the Advantages of their Treatment According to ...* (1872, trans. by Emil Tietze).

Gram, Hans Burch (1786 • 2-26-1840). The first homeopath in the US - 1825. He was born in Boston, yet in 1808 his father died and he returned to Copenhagen to attend to his father's estate. He stayed there for some 15 or so years and received his medical degree from the Academy of Surgery in Copenhagen becoming a very skilled anatomist and surgeon. In 1825, he returned to NYC and set up practice and taught many budding homeopaths.

Gramm, Edward M. (7-28-1858 •) Son of G.E. Gramm who was also a Philadelphia homeopath. Edward studied under Hering and graduated from Hahnemann (Phila.) in 1880. His specialties as lecturer at his alma mater were dermatology and syphilology.

Grauvogl, Eduard von (2-18-1811 German • 8-31-1877). When Hering read Grauvogl's *Textbook on Homeopathy* (1870, *Lehrbuch der Homoopathie*) he said, "At last we have got a thinker." He also wrote *Homoopathisches Aehnlich-keitsgesetz*. Grauvogl proposed the three constitutions: hydrogenoid, oxygenoid, and carbo-nitrogenoid. See also dictionary entries for the three constitutions.

Gray, John Franklin (9-24-1804 • 6-6-1882). The second homeopath in the US. Pupil of Gram. Co-editor of the *American Journal of Homoeopathia* 1835 and *Homeopathic Examiner* 1843-5. Author of *Homeopathy in NY and the Late Abraham D. Wilson* (1865).

Green, Arthur Brooks (11-7-1884 • 5-12-1977) Brother of J.M. Green and active lay homeopath. He edited *The Layman Speaks* for many years. "It is more essential for a homeopathic physician to know thoroughly the remedies he has than to wait for new ones. In the pioneering days, the early homeopaths had something like 80 remedies all told, and did so much with them that they scared the traditionalists for their medical lives."—*The Layman Speaks,* Nov. 1970, p. 345. Wrote an impressive article on homeopathy published in the *Atlantic Monthly* (March, 1925).

Green, Julia Minerva (1871 • 12-11-1963) practiced homeopathy for over sixty years. Ms. Green was cured of a serious case of pneumonia by homeopathy and thus was her homeopathic introduction. She made house calls on a bicycle and later in a car. Until her eighties she made night house calls. She was an inspiration to many a homeopath. "Until shortly before her death, she slept outdoors six months a year, exercised for 15 minutes a day and ate only two meals 'of well selected food' daily."—*The Washington Post,* Dec. 12, 1963. She helped found the American Foundation of Homeopathy, which created the Post-graduate course in homeotherapeutics for physicians. It trained homeopaths (Dixon, Spalding, Shupis, Neiswander, Wright-Hubbard, etc before WWII and Williams, Panos, Clark, etc. after WWII). Dr. Maesimund Panos preceptored with Dr. Green in 1959, eventually taking over her practice.

Gregg, Rollin R. (8-19-1828 • 8-4-1886). Author of *An Illustrated Repertory of Pains in the Chest, Sides and Back.* President IHA 1885. Editor *Homoeopathic Quarterly* 1869-70.

Gregg, Samuel (7-1-1799 • 10-25-1872) pioneer of homeopathy in New England.

Griesselich, P.W.L. (1804 • 1848) Influential German homeopath and editor of the homeopathic journal *Hygea.*

Griggs, Wm. R. (• 6-15-1970) an 1894 graduate of Hahnemann (Phila.). "In May 1896 he established the Pediatric Dept. in the Women's Homeo. Hosp. of Phila. and was continuously connected with it as Chief until this year when the hospital passed into other hands. He studied pediatrics in Berlin in 1900. In 1912 he began as lecturer on the Organon in the Hahnemann College. In 1915 he was elected Assoc. Professor in Therapeutics, which post he held until 1950. In 1916 he assumed the directorship of the Constantine Hering Laboratory of Homeopathic Research and carefully proved 19 basic elements [indol, skatol, sarco-lactic acid, butric acid, hippuric acid, menthol, thymol, malic acid, and glycerine and partial provings on amylum, inulin, glycogen, blood albumen, gallic acid, lime, oenanthic acid, oelic acid, propionic acid, stearic acid, amorphous sulphur, tannic acid, and valerianic acid]." -*The Hahnemannian,* July/Sept. 1951, p. 164.

For years he had a free day in his office during which he never charged any of the patients that came to see him, but told them that during such time he'd use experimental methods of treatment.

He supposedly received a telegram from Rome - Pope Pius XII needed help with a recalcitrant case of hiccups. Griggs telegraphed the answer, *Hyos.,* which cured!

Grimmer, Arthur (8-29-1874 • 3-5-1967). "Together with Kent, Roberts, and Boger he belongs among the homeopath immortals."—E. Wright-Hubbard. 1906 graduate of Hering Med. Coll. (Chic.). He was a close pupil of Kent. President of the AIH in 1953. Recently, A. Currim, M.D. compiled and published *The Collected Works of A.H. Grimmer* (1996).

Gross, Gustav Wilhelm (9-6-1794 • 9-16 or 18-1847). One of the original Provers' Union. Prover of *Chamomilla* and other remedies. Bradford reported that when Gross' child died, he told Hahnemann that 'homeopathy cannot cure everything,' and that Hahnemann was 'displeased'.

Grosvenor, Lemuel Conant (3-22-1833 •) An 1864 graduate of Cleveland Homeopathic Medical College. An expert obstetrician, he was associated with the Chicago Homeo. Med. Coll. and the Hahnemann Medical College (Chic.). During the great Chicago fire of 1871 his home was spared and he tirelessly attended to the victims of that conflagration. He was a three-time president of the Chicago Academy of Homeopathic Physicians and Surgeons.

Guernsey, Egbert (7-8-1823 • 9-19-1903). President of the Medical Board, Metropolitan Hospital (NY) 1875-1903. Professor of materia medica at the NY Hom. Med. Coll. for six years. A founder of the State Hospital for the Insane (Middletown, NY). He authored *Domestic Practice* (1855). He edited the *Medical Union* in 1872, which later became the *Medical Times*. He was instrumental in converting the Inebriates Asylum (Wards Isl., NY) into a homeopathic hospital in 1877. Wrote *The Gentleman's Handbook of Homeopathy Especially for Travelers and for Domestic Practice* (1857).

Guernsey, Henry Newell (2-10-1817 • 6-27-1885). Author of many works including *Obstetrics* (1867) and an advocate of homeopathic keynotes, i.e., *The Key-Note System* (1868). Prof. and Dean of Hahnemann Med. College of Philadelphia. He studied under Alvin E. Small and practiced and was a great popularizer of homeopathy throughout the suburbs of Philadelphia. J.C. was his son. His brother, W.F. studied under him.

Guernsey, Joseph C. (3-25-1849 •   ) Graduate and valedictorian of Hahnemann Med. Coll. of Pa., 1872. Like his father, H.N., he was very active in homeopathy and with the affairs of his alma mater. He edited his father's works as well as Trans. of the World's Congress in 1876, etc. He was president of the Homeo. Med. Soc. of Pa. in 1893.

Guernsey, William Fuller (12-12-1814 •) completed his homeopathic education under his brother H.N. and graduated in 1852 from the Homeo. Med. Coll. of PA (Phila.) and practiced in Philadelphia for many years.

Guernsey, William Jefferson (2-15-1854 • 3-27-1935). Authored several works, namely *Guernsey's Boenninghausen* (1889), *The Card Repertory* (1885), *Desires and Aversions* (1883), *Hemorrhoids* (1882).

Gutman, William (•   ) 1965 AIH President. Prominent NY homeopath.

Haass, Friedrich Joseph (1780 • 1853) British homeopath and author of *A Guide to the Practice of Homeopathy...* (1844).

Haehl, Richard (12-15-1873 German • 2-7-1923). Wrote the definitive biography of Hahnemann, *Samuel Hahnemann: His Life and Work,* Vol. I & II (1922). Degree from Hahnemann Phila in 1898. Was responsible for saving many of Hahnemann's valuable artifacts, retrieving the 6th edition of the *Organon* and publishing it in 1921.

Hahnemann, Marie Melanie d'Hervilly Gohier (2-2-1800 • 5-27-1878) Second wife of Samuel (married on Jan. 18, 1835 and in 1836 they moved to Paris). She was an accomplished poet and painter. Hahnemann called her one of the finest homeopaths in Europe. Hahnemann's first wife was Johanna L.H. Kuchler (1764-1830).

Hahnemann, Samuel (4-10-1755 • 7-2-1843). See entry in dictionary proper.

Haines, Oliver S. (8-12-1860 •) 1882 grad of Hahnemann (Phila.). He was lecturer on clinical medicine and obstetrics at his alma mater.

Hale, Edwin Moses (2-2-1830 • 1-15-1899). Author of *Materia Medica of New Remedies* (1864) and other books. He introduced *Hydrastis can., Iberis amara, Phytolacca dec.,* etc. into practice. He graduated from Cleveland Hom. Med Coll. in 1859 and taught materia medica at Hahnemann (Chic.) for some 18 years. One of the 12 pioneers of homeopathy in Michigan.

Hall, Edwin Cesar Malan (7-16-1858 • 2-4-1939) An 1883 graduate of the New York Hom. Med. Coll. He was an esteemed physician in New Haven, CT for many years. He authored *Remedies in Pertussis* (1936).

Hallock, Lewis (6-30-1803 • 3-3-1897). Organized the "Medical and Philosophical Society" in N.Y.C., of which Gray, Gram, Kirby, and Hull were members. Practiced 75 years! He made many contributions to homeopathic journals.

Hamer, James H. (10-1-1847 •) Studied under Adolphus Fellger and graduated from Hahnemann (Phila.) in 1875. He served as professor of chemistry at his alma mater.

Hamilton, Edward (1824 • 1899) Author of *The Flora Homoeopathica* (1852,3).

Harding, George T. (6-12-1844 • 11-19-28). Father of President Harding. 1873 graduate of Cleveland Homeo. Med. Coll.

Harris, W. John (6-17-1852 •) He graduated in 1875 as valedictorian of his class, Homeo. Med. Coll. of Missouri (St. Louis) and continued on at his alma mater teaching clinical medicine anatomy, genito-urinary surgery, and sanitary science.

Hartlaub, Carl George Christian (•) Homeopathic physician and author of *Katechismus der Homoopathie* (1824).

Hartmann, Franz (5-18-1796 • 10-10-1853) A personal disciple of Hahnemann and one of his provers. Editor and founder of *Allgemeine Homoeopathic Zeitung.* He wrote a number of books, e.g., *Practical Observations of Some Chief Homoeopathic Remedies* (1841).

Hart, C. P. (1827 •). Co-editor of the *American Homeopathic Observer,* 1875-82.

Hastings, Caroline Elizabeth (4-21-1841 • 7-10-1922) an 1868 graduate of the NE Female Med. Coll. She was physician to the NE Moral Reform Society.

Hawkes, Alfred E. (1849 Scotland • 1919) Scottish homeopathic gynecologist and author.

Hawley, Wm. A. (• 5-15-1891).

Hay, William Howard (8-14-1866 • 10-29-1940). IHA member and founder of the "Hay System of Diet." His anti-vaccination speech was read into the Congressional Record in the late 1930s.

Hayes, Royal Elmore Swift (10-21-1871 • 8-3-1952). Member of the IHA. Author. Graduate of the Eclectic Med. Coll. of New York (1898), converted to homeopathy in 1900.

Heinigke, Carl (• 1889) German homeopath and author of *Handbuch der Homoopathischen...* (1880).

Heinroth, Johann Christian August (1773 • 1842) German homeopath and author.

Helmuth, William Tod (10-30-1833 • 5-15-1902). Was the main speaker at the dedication of the Hahnemann Monument in Washington, D.C. where he offered salutory comments entitled 'Ode to Hahnemann'. Graduate of the Homeopathic College of Pennsylvania in 1853. He held professorships at several homeopathic medical schools and was Chief Surgeon at the New York Homeopathic Medical College and Hospital for some thirty years and its Dean from 1893-1902. President of the Collins State Homeopathic Hospital. Poet and homeopathic surgeon. President of the AIH in 1867. He had a son, W.T.H. II, who also took up homeopathy and served as a homeopath in WWI.

Hempel, Charles Julius (9-5-1811 Germany • 9-24-1879). Settled in America in 1835. He translated many important books into English, enabling the struggling American homeopaths to get educated. Dean of Materia Medica at Ann Arbor, MI. Co-editor of the *Homeopathic Examiner* 1843-45. Professor at Hahnemann (Phil.) and Chair of Materia Medica (1857). He went blind as a result of all his translating/writing. Despite this misfortune and with the help of his wife he wrote *Materia Medica and Therapeutics*. He was primarily a low-potency advocate.

Henshaw, George Russell (1896 •3-29-1985) Born in Uniontown, PA. Creator of the flocculation test. As a young lad he was mechanically inclined but decided on a medical career graduating from the OSU homeopathic medical dept. He interned at Shadyside Hospital (Pgh., PA) and was a resident for two years at Middletown Insane Asylum and Hospital. He served as assistant director of pharmacology at the NY Homeo. Med. Coll. and later, in 1929, moved to Montclair, NJ where he practiced until his death. He wrote *A Scientific Approach to Homeopathy* (1980). See HENSHAW FLOCCULATION TEST.

Hering, Carl (•) Son of Constantine and owner of Globe Printing in Philadelphia. He wrote 'Chronology of Events Concerning the Life of C. Hering of Phil. PA, the father of homeopathy in America' (trans. *IHA*, 6-1919, 29 p.)

Hering, Constantine (1-1-1800 • 7-23-1880). Father of American Homeopathy and first president of the AIH. He was the first to prove *Lachesis* (the bushmaster snake, *Trigonocephalus*) in 1828 and the first to use *Nitroglycerin*. In 1835, with W. Wesselhoeft, Detwiller, Bute and Romig established the North American Academy of Homoeopathic Healing, the

Allentown Academy, and later, Hahnemann Med. Coll. (Phil). He was intimately involved with that institution until his death. He wrote *Domestic Physician* (1835) and *The Guiding Symptoms of Our Materia Medica* (1879-1891) as well as other works. He said: "If our school ever gives up the strict inductive method of Hahnemann, we are lost and deserve only to be mentioned as a caricature in the history of medicine."

Hering, Gottlieb (c. 1815 • 10-10-1888) Early Russian homeopath who practiced for many years in St. Petersurg. Was president of the Russian Society of Homoeopathic Physicians.

Hill, B.L. (12-18-1813 • 5-13-1871) was a surgeon of national reputation. Along with J.C. Douglas he conducted provings of Black cohosh *(Cimicifuga/Actaea racemosa)* with forty students, male and female, and published the results in *J. of Homeopathy* (1858, p. 256). He taught at Cleve. Hom. Med. College. In 1863 he was appointed U.S. Consul at San Juan, Puerto Rico. Wrote a book with Hunt entitled *Hill and Hunt's Homeopathic Surgery.*

Hirschel, Bernhard (1815 • 1874). German homeopath and author of *Die Homoopathie...* (1851). He studied medicine at the Academie Medico-chirurgicale of Dresden and the U. of Leipzig. Practiced in Dresden.

Holcombe, William Henry (5-29-1825 • 11-28 or 29-1893). Author.

Holland, George Calvert (1801 • 1865) British homeopath who wrote *A Domestic Practice of Homeopathy* (1859).

Holt, Daniel (1810 • 1883) Author of *Views of Homeopathy* (1845).

Honigberger, John Martin (1794 • 1869) Introduced homeopathy into India in 1835 and to Pakistan (Lahore) one year later. See TONNERE and DUTT.

Hooker, Worthington (1806 • 1867) Author of *Homeopathy: An Examination of Its Doctrines...* (1851).

Hooper, Joseph (• 2-28-1876) Taught for a short period of time at Cleve. Homeo. Med. Coll.

Houghton, Henry Clark (1-22-1837 • 12-1-1901). Author of *Lectures on Clinical Otology.* Student of H.C. Allen. Prof. at N.Y. Ophthalmic Hospital, N.Y. Hom. Med. College, and N.Y. Med. College for Women.

Houghton, Henry Lincoln (7-3-1869 • 6-17-1948). Pupil of Kent. Taught at the AFH post graduate school. IHA President 1917.

Howard, Erving M. (9-11-1848 •) Received his medical degree from Hahnemann (Phila.) in 1877. He served as lecturer on pharmacy, toxicology, and materia medica at his alma mater.

Hoyle, E. Petrie (8-15-1861 • 8-17-1955). Graduate of Hahnemann in Calif. 1900. Editor of many international proceedings. Practiced in Kittery, Maine.

Hoyne, Temple S. (10-16-1841 • 2-3-1899). Author. Dean of Dunham Medical College in Chicago. Wrote *Clinical Therapeutics* (1878-80).

Hrdlicka, Ales (3-29-1869 • 9-5-1943). Born in Bohemia/Moravia and died in Wash. D.C. Graduated N.Y. Homeopathic Medical College in 1894. Interned at the Middletown Homeopathic Hospital in 1896. Curator of the U.S. National Museum (a division of the Smithsonian). Anthropologist, espoused the theory of trans-siberian migration. Wrote *Tuberculosis Among the Indians*, as well as other books.

Hughes, Elizabeth C. (•) she studied medicine under her Baltimore, MD brother Alfred Hughes before graduating from the non-homeopathic Penn Med. Coll. (Phil.) in 1860. She was the first woman to practice medicine in VA.

Hughes, Richard (1836 • 4-9-1902). Very influential British homeopath. Author of *Manual of Pharmacodyamics* (1st-1867, 2nd-1868) and *Encyclopedia of Drug Pathogenesy*, as well as *The Principles and Practice of Homoeopathy* (1902). President of the International Congress in London, 1881. The dominant force in homeopathy in the U.K. He practiced in Brighton and at the Royal London Homoeo. Hosp. He considered modalities and pathological symptoms to be of upmost importance, and advocated the use of low potency remedies (below 30C).

Hull, Amos Gerald (1810 • 4-25-1859). Translator and editor of Jahr's works and editor of several homeopathic journals. Son-in-law of John Gray, MD. He was taught by Gram.

Humphreys, Erastus (• 1848) Father of Frederick, he was first an allopath and in 1840 converted to the homeopathic system. He worked hard though unsuccessfully to establish a homeopathic medical college in western New York.

Humphreys, Frederick (3-11-1816 • 7-7-1900). An 1850 graduate of the Homeo. Med. Coll. of Pa. Founder of Humphreys' Specifics, a line of combination products. First prover of *Apis* (1852) and *Plantago* (1871). He was expelled from the AIH in 1855 because of his viewpoints on combination homeopathy! His company, Humphreys' Homoeopathic Medicine Co., still exists today as Humphreys' Pharmacal. He wrote papers, a repertory on the diseases of the sexual system, and his domestic guide (in part a vehicle to sell his 'Specifics'). *Humphreys' Manual of Specific Homeopathy* (1st ed. 1858, last ed. in 1925) went through ten editions. Millions of copies were sold or distributed free of charge. He also wrote *Manual of Veterinary Specific Homoeopathy* (in 1860) and manufactured veterinary homeopathic remedies. He was an ordained Methodist minister.

Hunt, James G. (6-12-1821 •) An 1848 grad. from Eclectic Med. Inst. and Professor of Surgery at Cleve. Hom. Med. Coll. See HILL.

Hurndall, John Sutcliffe (•) Homeopathic veterinarian who wrote *Veterinary Homeopathy in its application to the horse* (1896).

Ivins, Horace Fremont (10-20-1856 •) An 1879 grad of Hahnemann (Phila.). He was a specialist on laryngology, otology, and ophthalmology and lectured on those subjects at his alma mater. He wrote *Diseases of the Nose and Throat* (1893).

Jackson, Mercy B. (9-17-1802 •   ) Despite her eleven children (two sets of twins, boys and girls) she managed to become interested in medicine studying with Dr. Capen, an allopath, in Plymouth, MA. One day she was introduced to homeopathy via 'the powders' and talked to Dr. Capen of her enthusiasm. So interested, he drove to Boston to find a homeopathist (1841), found none, but "...procured her both books and medicne, in the use of which he liberally participated." Finally in 1860, at the age of 58, she graduated from the NE Female Med. Coll. She declined a professorship at Lozier's school, but did become active in the Boston University School of Medicine as professor of diseases of children.

Jahr, George Heinrich Gottleib (1-30-1800 • 7-11-1875). Author of *40 years of Practice, Jahr's Symptomen Codex, Manual of Homoeopathic Medicine, A New Homoeopathic Pharmacopoeia (Handbuch der Haupt=Anzeigen fur die richtige Wahl der Homoopathischen Heilmittel* -Dusseldorf, JE Schaub, 1834, one of the earliest and most important homeopathic pharamcopoeias it is divided into two parts, materia medica and a therapeutical and symptomatological repertory. Along with the works of Joseph Benedict Buchner and Carl Ernst Gruner it formed the basis of C.J. Hempel's *New Homeoeopathic Pharmacopoeia* published in NYC in 1850), etc. He believed that all potencies worked but felt that the difference between the high and low potencies was not necessarily due to their dynamis but due to the development of remedy idiosyncrasies as dependent upon the potency. He was born in Saxony and graduated from the University of Bonn in 1828. He practiced in Paris for over 40 years and enjoyed a friendship with Hahnemann during that time. Toward the end of his life he became an itinerant, being virtually homeless. He practiced in Paris for 35 years and was a great popularizer of homeopathy, as he wrote tirelessly. He was also a poet.

James, Bushrod Washington (8-25-1836 •) An 1857 graduate of the Homeo. Med. Coll. of Pa. He was quite active in the organizational aspect of homeopathy and was the president of the Homeo. Med. Soc. of Pa. in 1873 and president of the AIH in 1883.

James, John Edwin (1-18-1844 •) 1876 saw the beginning of his involvement with Hahnemann Med. Coll. as adjunct professor of surgery, later becoming dept. head. He remained active for many years at Hahnemann and deserves the credit for developing its high level of clinical instruction.

Jeager, Gustav (1832 • 1917) German homeopath who wrote a number of pamphlets on homeopathy (1888-1891).

Jeanes, Jacob B. (10-4-1800 • 12-18-1877). Wrote the first book on homeopathy in the English language, *Practice of Medicine* (1838). Co-founder of the Hom. Med. Coll. of Pa. in 1848 and co-founder of the AIH in 1844. He was professor of the practice of medicine at the school he helped found.

Jenichen, Julius Caspar (1787 • Feb, 1849). Maker of high potencies in Germany and the first to make high potencies such as 2500C, 6000C, etc. Developed the idea of "potency". Believed it was the succussion and not the dilution which was important. Hahnemann denounced him. He eventually committed suicide.

Jensen, Soren (1811 • 7-5-1887) Early Danish homeopath who practiced in Copenhagen and was a pupil of Feveile.

Jimenez, Marcos (1902 • 1994) Mexican homeopath.

Johnson, Isaac D. (8-10-1827 • 1-20-1911). Author of *Johnson's Domestic Guide*, a very popular homeopathic domestic treatise.

Jones, Eli (1850 • 1933). Wrote *Definite Medication.*

Jones, Gaius J. (2-27-1840 • 2-7-1914) He was a graduate of Homoeo. Med. Coll. (Cleve.) in 1872 and intimately involved in Cleveland homeopathy in all respects for some 40 years. Dean of the Cleveland Homeopathic Med. Coll., 1890-97. He was on the staff of the Huron Street Hospital. President of AIH 1911. Wrote *Notes on Practice of Medicine, 1895-1903*.

Jones, Samuel Arthur (1834 • 3-9-1912). Author of *The Grounds of a Homeopath's Faith.* Teacher at Ann Arbor. His personal papers are in the library at the University of Illinois in Champaign-Urbana. An 1860 graduate of Homeo. Med Coll. of PA and Homeo. Med Coll of Missouri, St. Louis.

Jones, Stacy (1828 • 1906) Author of *The Medical Genius: A guide to the cure* ... (1887). Graduated in 1853 from Hahnemann (Phil.).

Joslin, Benjamin Franklin (11-25-1796 • 12-31-1885). Worked in NYC with P. P. Wells. Author of *Principles of Homeopathy* (1850). His son B.F., Jr. became a homeopath.

Jousset, Pierre (12-x-1818 • 12-23-1910). French homeopath and author and, along with Jean-Paul Tessier, leader in French homeopathy. He wrote *Elements de Medecine Pratique, Elements de matiere medicale experimentale et de therapeutique positive,* etc., and numerous journal articles particularly for *L'Art Medical.* He was involved in the formation of La Societe Francaise d'Homeopathie in December of 1889.

Julian, Othon Andre (6-18-1910 • 3-14-1984). Influential French homeopath. Wrote *Materia Medica of the New Remedies* (1960) and *Treatise of Dynamized Micro-Immunotherapy.*

Kahlke, Charles Edwin (1-13-1870 •) An 1894 graduate of Hahnemann (Chic.), where he became professor of surgery and was associated with Cook County Hospital for many years. He served in WWI, attaining the rank of major.

Kanjilal, J.N. (•) Noted Indian homeopath.

Kapadia, Sarabhai (10-20-1928 • 7-2-1987) Prominent Indian homeopath who wrote *Homeopathic Reminiscences.* He was active in society affairs and noted for his work with the Indian government in spreading homeopathy.

Keatinge, Harriette Charlotte (4-10-1837 • 11-11-1909) She studied medicine under her aunt, Clemence S. Lozier, who was also the founder of the NY Medical Coll. and Hospital for Women. After graduating she moved to New Orleans and was regarded as the pioneer woman physician of the Gulf states. Later she moved back to New York City.

Keim, Wm. H. (3-15-1843 •) He graduated from Hahnemann (Phila.) in 1871 and stayed on to lend his services in many capacities, primarily as demonstrator of surgery and anatomy. As a physician he had a large practice primarily devoted to the disease of women and children.

Kellogg, E. M. (9-20-1826 • 6-6-1905). First homeopath to advocate graded course study in medicine. NY Homeopathic was the second school in U.S. to do it.

Kent, James Tyler (3-31-1849 • 6-6-1916). Wrote several very important classics, including *Repertory of the Homoeopathic Materia Medica* (1877), *Lectures on Homoeopathic Philosophy* (1900), and *Lectures on Homoeopathic Materia Medica* (1905). Prof. materia medica, Homoeo. Med. Coll., St. Louis, 1881-88. Prof. materia medica and dean of the Post-Grad. Sch. of Homeopathy, Phila., 1890-99. Prof. of materia medica, Hahnemann Med. Coll. and Hosp., Chicago, 1903-09. Hering Med. Coll. and Hosp., 1909. Co-editor of *Homeopathic Courier* St. Louis 1881-82. Founded Postgraduate School in 1890 in Philadelphia. Graduate of the Eclectic Med. Inst. (1871, Cinc., OH). IHA President in 1887. He said,

"The physician who is the most successful is he who will first heal for the love of healing, who will practice first for the purpose of verifying his knowledge and performing his use for the love of it." Married to Clara L. Kent (1856 • 1943).

King, John B. S. (2-12-1855 • 8-28-1929). President IHA 1913. Teacher at Hering College. Took over editorship of the *Medical Advance.*

King, William Harvey (2-21-1861 • 7-24-1942, Scarsdale, NY). Author of the 4 volume *History of Homeopathy in America.* Professor of electrotherapeutics at New York Homeopathic College and later Dean from 1903-8. Performed first demonstration of x-rays in a US school. He was an 1882 graduate of the New York Homeopathic Med. College. He received a gold diploma from his alma mater in 1932. In his acceptance speech he commented, "(a) good joke will often prove a better remedy in the sick-room than any pills." He urged his fellow doctors to cultivate a sense of humor.

Kinne, Theodore Young (1839 • 3-4-1904). Worked on the HPUS. Also served on the Auxiliary Committee for the Hahnemann Monument in Washington, D.C.

Kirby, Stephen (5-21-1801 • 3-6-1876). Opened first homeopathic dispensary in NYC on Oct. 1845.

Kirch, Ruth Beckwith (•) Wife of D. Beckwith. 1892 grad. of Cleveland Med. College.

Kishore, Jugal (•) Noted Indian homeopath who created *The Kishore Cards* (repertory).

Kitchen, James (3-8-1800 • 8-19-1894). One of the first teachers at Hom. Med. Coll. of PA, and as one can see was long-lived, practicing homeopathy into his nineties. He translated Boullard's *Treatise on Rheumatism* and Jahr's *Homoeopathic Pharmacy*.

Knerr, Calvin Probst (12-27-1847 • 9-30-1940). An 1869 graduate of Hahnemann (Phila.). Son-in-law of Hering. Co-editor along with C.G. Raue, C. Mohr and Walter Hering (Hering's son) of the massive *Hering's Guiding Symptoms of our Materia Medica* (Vol. 1-10). Author of *Life of Hering* (1940) and *Knerr's Repertory* He was a member of the Church of the New Jerusalem (Swedenborgian).

Koerndoerfer, Augustus (10-27-1843 • 6-10-1923). Pupil of Hering. Co-editor of *Hering's Condensed Materia Medica*. 1868 Graduate of Hahnemann (Phil.) and Chair of Clinical Medicine there from 1876-81. He was president of the Homo. Med. Soc. of Pa. in 1890. See POTENCY in the dictionary.

Korsakoff, Iseman von (• 1853). Russian nobleman and homeopath. Developed the Korsakoff potencies in c. 1829.

Kozowski, Jerzy (1909 • 1987) Polish homeopath who trained in Germany with Kurt Hermann, M.D. He gave the first regular lectures on classical homeopathy in Poland. He wrote *First Steps in Homeopathy*.

Kraft, Frank (1-8-1851 • 7-19-1908, June 6 also, but July in most journals). Pupil of Kent (St. Louis 1884). Editor *St. Louis Periscope, American Homeopathist*.

Krichbaum, Philip Echel (• 7-17-1928). Member of the IHA. Hering Med. Coll., Chic. 1896.

Kunzli, Jost (full name Jost Kunzli von Fimmelsberg) (1915 • 1992). Author of *The General Repertory* or *Kent's Repertorium Generale*. This massive and important repertory is based on Kent's Repertory but includes referenced updates from 71 other important sources. This important Swiss homeopath verified remedies from his own practice, indicated in his repertory by 'black points' (bullets).

Laird, Frank Foster (4-15-1856 •) An 1880 graduate of Hahnemann (Phila.), he had the second highest grade point average ever (Van Lennep was first). He was medical director of the Utica Homeo. Hospital. He was an author and advocated the low potencies.

Lamasson, Francois (4-22-1907 • 5-30-1975) French homeopath and author. He was a professional associate of the Vannier family (Henry, Edward, and Leon) and Henry and Jean Boiron. He was very active in organizational work. He was Secretary General (the principal executive officer) and President of the Societe d'Homeopathie Francaise (created in 1952), and with Couturier, Bernard, Demarque and Rousson founded l'Institut National Homeopathique Francais. He penned many articles on isotherapy, materia medica, general homeopathy, and clinical homeopathy. Issue #4 (1976) of *Les Annales Homeopathiques Francaises* is entirely devoted to his work.

Laurie, Joseph (• 12-9-1865). Translated the works of Jahr. A graduate of the Homoeopathic Med. Coll. of Pa., he lived in England and was the senior physician to the Westminster and Lambeth Homoeopathic Med. Inst. and Dispensary. The 10th American Ed. (B & T, 1871) of his *Domestic Medicine* work was the most comprehensive and clearly written treatise on the homeopathic domestic medicine. It was written in six parts.

Lavelle, James I. (• 5-31-1976) though not a physician he was active in organizational affairs particularly of the American Foundation for Homoeopathy (AFH) where he served as treasurer for 30 years (1942-1972).

Lawler, James P. (1894 • 1978) a 1929 graduate of Hahnemann (Phil.) and a member of the AIH for many years.

Leavitt, Sheldon (4-9-1848 • 1-1-1933) An 1877 graduate of Hahnemann Med. Coll. (Chic.) where he served as professor of obstetrics and professor of gynecology at the Chicago Homeo. Med. Coll. He authored several books: *The Science and Art of Obstetrics* (1882), *Psycho-Therapy* (1903), *Volo-therapy* (1917), *Living a Century* (1928), etc. See VOLO-THERAPY in the dictionary.

Lee, Donald S. (8-9-1916 • 3-3-1990). Intimately involved with Boericke and Tafel (Phila.) for over 30 years (1958-1989).

Lee, Edmund James (1854 • 5-25-1922) The major editor of the classical homeopathic journal, *The Homoeopathic Physician.* 1877 graduate of NY Homeo. Med. College.

Leeser, Otto (1-7-1888 • 11-9-1964). Re-established the Robert Bosch Homeopathic Hospital in Germany. Spent WWII in England. Wrote *Textbook of Homeopathic Mat. Med.* (trans. by Linn Boyd) and *Grundlagen der Heilkunde.* "He was one of those rare human beings—fortunately not too rare among homeopaths—who devoted his whole life enthusiastically to homeopathy."—Wm. Gutman, *JAIH* 1/2, 1965.

Leggett, Sarah L. Guild (1846 • 5-27-1928). A 1888 graduate of Homeo. Med. Coll. of Missouri, St. Louis. Pupil of Kent.

Lilienthal, Samuel (12-5-1815 • 10-2 or 3-1891). Author; *Homoeopathic Therapeutics* (1878) was his opus. Taught at N.Y. Homeopathic College and then Hahnemann Medical College of the Pacific, sometimes just referred to as San Francisco. He was editor of the *North American Journal of Homoeopathy* and held professorships at the NY Hom. Med., Coll., and NY Coll Hosp. for Women. Birthdate may have been 11-5-1815 according to *Homoeopathic Physician.*

Lippe, Adolph (5-11-1812 • 1-28-1888). His full name was Adolphus Graf zur Lippe-Weissenfeld. His major literary work was *Lippe's Materia Medica.* One of the first graduates of Allentown. With Hering and Raue taught at Hahnemann Med. Coll. (Phila). One of the founders of the IHA. He was one of the finest homeopaths. Constantine Lippe was his son.

Lippe, Constantine (7-1-1840 • 1-1-1885). Son of Adolph Lippe. Author of *Lippe's Repertory to the more Characteristic Symptoms*, which he dedicated to Constantine Hering.

Lodge, Edwin A. (5-6-1822 • 1-25-1887). Pharmacist and founder (1864) and editor of *The American Observer.* Detroit, MI.

Loomis, Joseph G. (• 10-25-1853). Professor of Obstetrics and Diseases of Women and Children at the Homeopathic Med. Coll. of Pa.

Loos, Julia C. (5-28-1869 • 8-28-1929). Editor, *The Homeopathician.* Pupil of Kent in Philadelphia. Co-founder of the AFH.

Lozier, Clemence Sophia (12-11-1813 • 1 or 4-26-1888) Founded the New York Homeopathic Women's Medical College in 1863 and was intimately associated with that institution until her death, serving as dean for 25 years. She was a cousin of C. Dunham and aunt of Harriette Keatinge.

Lozier, Jennie de la Montaigne (~1850 •) She was a graduate of her mother-in-law's school and later taught physiology there. See CLEMENCE LOZIER.

Ludlam, Reuben (10-7-1831 • 4-29-1899). U. of Pennsylvania, 1851. Author of *Diseases of Women.* General Secretary of AIH 1870-1. Co-editor of the following journals: *N. Amer. Jrn. of Homeo., Chicago Homeopath, Medical Investigator, U.S. Med. and Surg. Jrn., The Clinique.*

Lund, Hans C. (• 4-17-1846). First homeopath in Denmark and teacher of Gram, the first homeopath in the U.S.A. C.L. Lund was his son (1818-1875) who also practiced homeopathy. See next entry, HENRICH C. LUND.

Lund, Henrich C. (c 1800 • 2-26-1889) A lay homeopath who practiced avidly in Denmark for some time. He wrote a monograph on *Arnica.* See PABST and THOMSEN and FEVEILE.

Lutze, Ernest Arthur (6-1-1813 • 1870) Wrote *Lehrbuch der Homoeopathy*

(1867). He created controversy when he attempted to publish an unautho-rized/falsified 6th Ed. of the *Organon*, in 1865.

Lutze, Frederick H. (8-19-1838 • 11-30-1924). Wrote a very good book on neuralgia as well as many journal articles. An 1882 graduate of NY Homeo. Med. College.

Lux, Wilhelm J.J. (4-6-1776 • 1-29-1849). First homeopathic veterinarian and first to coin the term 'isopathy'. This term first appeared in his book *Zooiasis or Homoeopathy in its Application to the Diseases of Animals* (1837).

Luyties, Carl Johann (9-15-1860 • 12-23-1917) an 1884 graduate of the Homeo. Med. Coll of Missouri (St. Louis). He taught diseases of children and chemistry at his alma mater. He was the son of Diedrich Reinhard Luyties (• 1-10-1879) who was a homeopathic physician and founder of Luyties Pharmacal in the 1850s. Carl also received a degree in pharmacy from the St. Louis College of Pharmacy in 1881. Walter Augst was his son.

Macfarlan, Donald (1885 •) Homeopath and author of *Concise Pictures of Dynamized Drugs Personally Proven* (1936).

Macfarlan, Malcom (6-8-1841 Elderslie, Scotland • 12-8-1921). Did a series of high potency provings by giving them frequently in water until they produced unmistakable and violent effects. He served as a surgeon during the Civil War and while stationed at Fort Morgan read Hahnemann's *Organon* and became convinced of the superiority of the homeopathic system. After his discharge from the military he was appointed professor of Clinical Surgery at Hahnemann (Phil.) in 1869.

Mack, Charles Samuel (1856 •) Author of *Philosophy in Homeopathy* (1890).

MacKenzie, George W. (• 8-5-1945)

MacLeod, George (• 9-5-1995). Leading homeopathic veterinarian from Scotland. Author.

Majundar, J.N. (•) Noted Indian homeopath.

Malcolm, John Gilmore (•) 1866 graduate of NY Hom. Med. Coll. and author of *A Regional and Comparative Materia Medica* (1895, with O.B. Moss).

Marcy, Erastus Edgerton (1822 • 1901) Author of *Homeopathy and Allopathy: Reply to an examination of the docrines...* (1852). Editor for 15 years of the *North American Homoeopathic Journal*.

Martin, George Henry (3-31-1859 •) An 1881 graduate of Boston Univer-sity School of Medicine. He accumulated a wealth of clinical experience and later became chair of clinical medicine at Hahnemann (San Fran-cisco). Later he took over the chair of mental and nervous diseases when Samuel Lilienthal retired. He was very active in California homeopathic organizations. He was assoc. editor of the *Pacific Coast J. of*

Homoeopathy.

Martin, Henry Noah (10-20-1829 • 10-1-1889). Co-editor, with Hering, of *American Journal of Homeopathic Materia Medica.* Professor at Hahnemann in Phila.

Mathur, K.N. (1906 • 1977) Noted Indian homeopathy who wrote *Principles of Prescribing* and *Systematic Materia Medica.*

Matthes, G. Felix (12-31-1809 • 3-17-1889).

Mazumdar, P.C. (•) Noted Indian homeopath who, along with B.N. Banerjee, struggled to popularize homeopathy in India around the turn of the 20th century. The two edited for a time the *India Homeopathic Review.*

McClatchey, Robert (4-6-1836 • 1-15-1883) 1856 graduate of the Homeo. Med. Coll. of PA (Phila.) and later a professor there. Editor, *Hahnemannian Monthly* 1868-78. 1856 grad. of and teacher at Homeo. Medical College of Pa. Served for 12 years as president of the Hahnemann Club of Philadelphia. Was president of the Homeo. Med. Soc. of Pa in 1874. He originated the movement to found the Children's Hospital of Philadelphia. For a time he studied under W.T. Helmuth.

McClelland, James Henderson (5-20-1845 • 1913) AIH president in 1893-4. He did a preceptorship with JP Dake and JC Burgher finally graduating from the Homeo. Med. Coll. of PA (Phila) in 1867. He helped found the Homeo. Med. and Surgical Hospital and Dispensatory of Pgh., PA.

McCoy, Louis (4-3-1929 • 8-19-1980) Converted to homeopathy late in life after being cured of blindnesss by high potency *Arnica.* He and his wife, Faye, studied with Vithoulkas in Greece. Faye studied with Ray Seidel. Louis was also a magician and entertained at NCH meetings and in Greece at Vithoulkas' school. His dying words to his wife were "Please project homeopathy," which she has done tirelessly.

McDowell, Charles (9-30-1857 • 8-31-1945) An 1878 graduate of the NY Homeo. Med. Coll., he later became demonstrator and professor of physiology and hygiene there for some 40 years. The Homeo. Med. Coll. of the State of New York was founded in 1860 and changed its name several times. In 1869 it became the NY Homeo. Med. Coll., in 1887 the New York Homeo. Med. Coll and Hospital, in 1908 the NY Homeo. Med. Coll. and Flower Hospital, and in 1935, the New York Medical College.

McKinnell, Henry (1805 • 1893) the first homeopath who came to Oregon-in 1853 (Bradford says it was L.J. Coombs). He organized and became the first president of the Portland Homeo. Med. Soc. (in 1876), which became the Oregon State Homeo. Soc. in 1893. The last decade of the 1890s saw 20 physicians practicing medicine in Portland, 5 of them were homeopaths. The first woman to practice in Oregon was Callie Brown Charlton. "...homeopathy had become something of a fad among the well-to-do in Portland in the late 1880s." -Olof Larsell, *The Doctor in Oregon* (1947, p. 417).

McManus, Felix R. (5-30-1807 • 3-3-1885). Pioneer of homeopathy in Maryland. In 1837, while at the funeral of one of his patients, the clergyman convinced him to investigate homeopathy. He spoke with Dr. Matlack of Phila. who convinced him to study homeopathy. Even though there were no works in English available Felix hired a German tutor so that he could read the German homeopathic texts. He helped found the AIH and was its president in 1847. His son Frederick A. was a homeopath

Meuller, Clotar (• 1877) German homeopath and author.

Middleton, Melbourne F. (1-21-1842 •) 1868 graduate of Hahnemann (Phila.).

Miller, R. Gibson (1862 • 5-10-1919). Came from Glasgow to study with Kent in 1884. Author of many articles.

Millspaugh, Charles Frederick (6-20-1854 • 9-15-1923). A graduate of the New York Hom. Med. Coll. in 1881 after studing at Cornell U. from 1871-73. Born in Ithaca, NY, he was a friend of Louis Agassiz from childhood. Edited the *Homoepathic Recorder* (1888-90) and wrote *American Medicinal Plants* (1884) and *Repertory to Eczema* (1885). He published many botanical papers from 1890-1915. He was curator of botany at the Field Museum of Natural History in Chicago, Professor of Botany at the U. of Chicago and Professor of Medical Botany at the Chicago Hom. Med. College.

Minton, Henry (3-4-1831 • 6-1-1895). Author of *Uterine Therapeutics*. Editor of *Homoeopathic Journal of Obstetrics*. He helped found the Brooklyn Homeopathic Lying-In Asylum. He declined a professorship at the New York Homeo. Med. Coll and a clinical position at the Homeo. Hosp. of New York because of the weight of his private practice and other activities. He was an 1853 graduate of the Homeo. Med. Coll. of PA (Phila.). "He paid his college fees by serving as the janitor's assistant, working far into the night, sweeping the halls, sawing the wood, and attending the furnaces." -Cleave, p. 472.

Mitchell, John N. (4-10-1847 •) A 1873 graduate of Hahnemann (Phila.) who stayed on to become demonstrator and later professor of obstetrics.

Moffit, Eliz. (6-23-1815 •) Born on a farm in Chillicothe, OH she studied general subjects under her stepfather a graduate of Harvard. Later she had an "...opportunity of enlarging her knowledge of the world she made a visit to Chicago which lasted about a year." -Cleave, p. 226. While there she studied some homeopathy. Later when the financial crisis of 1857 overtook the country, she was widowed and needed someway to support her family. She took up the domestic study of homeopathy eventually opening a shop to sell books and remedies and counsel people.

Mohr, Charles (5-2-1844 • 10-31-1907). Pupil of Hering. Co-editor of Hering's *Guiding Symptoms.* Graduated in 1873 or '75 from Hahnemann (Phila.).

He was professor of materia medica, clinical medicine and physical diagnosis, and lecturer on pharmacy at his alma mater. He proved a great many substances, including *Indium met., Nat. phos., Zincum pic., Lilium tig., Chininum ars., Zincum phos.,* and *Stannum met.*

Moore, Charles L. (1873 • 1-7-1944) 1899 graduate of Cleve. Med. Coll. He served as faculty member of his alma mater. Born in Orangeville, OH.

Moore, George (1803 • 1880) British homeopath and author of *Popular Guide to Homeopathy...* (1866).

Moore, Thomas (7-2-1827 • 3-25-1882). Author of works on homeopathic veterinary medicine. He converted to homeopathy after being treated by Hering.

Morales, Leonardo Jaramillo (• 1967) Mexican homeopath, wrote *Homeopathic Doctrine: The Reform of Medicine.*

Moss, Oscar Burnham (1845 •) Graduate of Cleve. Homeo. Med. Coll in 1870 and co-author of *A Regional and Comparative Materia Medica* (1895, with M.J. Gilmore).

Mure, Benoit-Jules (5-15-1809 • 3-14-1858). Author of *Materia Medica of the Drugs of the Brazilian Empire.* First to suggest that lower potencies be used for acute conditions and higher potencies be used for chronic conditions.

Murphy, Forrest J., Sr. (• 12-10-1974) Owner and president of Luyties Pharmacal Co. Actively involved in organizational work, e.g. AFH, AIH, and the AAHP. His son, F.J., took over the helm of Luyties when his father passed away.

Nash, Eugene Beauharnais (3-8-1838 Hillsdale, NY • 11-6-1917). Graduated Cleveland Homeopathic in 1874. Taught at NY Hom. Med. College. IHA President, 1903. Had 'a fine tenor voice' that led the choir at Methodist meetings. He wrote the excellent book *Leaders in Homoeopathic Therapeutics* (1898) as well as *Leaders for the Use of Sulphur.*

Neatby, Edwin Awdas (11-16-1858 British • 12-1-1933). Along with Stoneham he wrote *Manual of Homeotherapeutics.* Founded the Missionary School of Homeopathy.

Nebel, Antoine (1870 • 7-17-1954) Great French homeopath, researcher, author, and proponent of the high dilutions and advocate of drainage homeopathy and typology. Issue #1 (1955) of *Actes de la Societe Rhodanienne d'Homeopathie* is devoted entirely to his work. He conducted a proving of *Tuberculinum* (Koch) in 1901 and entered it into the materia medica as *Tuberculinum residuum.*

Neidhard, Charles S. (4-19-1809 • 4-17-1895). Author. While in medical school he was cured of an illness with homeopathy and thus enrolled in and graduated from the Allentown Academy in 1837. Co-founder of the

AIH. He was a prolific author and co-editor of the *American Journal of Homoeopathia* 1838, and the *North American Journal of Homoeopathy* 1862-68.

Neiswander, Harry (c. 1880 • 1960) A 1912 graduate of Cleve. Hom. Med. Coll. His wife, Rosella, studied medicine with her husband and did most of the repertory work for him. Clifford-Arthur Neiswander (1-31-1914 •), their son, practiced homeopathy for many years after graduating from the Ohio State U. Med. Sch. in 1942. Clifford-Arthur's wife Georgiana edited the *JAIH* for many years during the 1970s and 1980s.

Norton, Arthur Brigham (9-15-1856 • 6-18-1919). Teacher at NY Ophthalmic and author. 1881 graduate of NY Homeo. Med. College. Author of *Ophthalmic Diseases and Therapeutics.*

Norton, George S. (12-8-1851 • 1-31-1891). Teacher at NY Ophthalmic and author. Brother of A. B.

Ockford, George M. (1845 • 6-25-1921) 1872 graduate of Cleve. Homeo. Med. Coll. and author of *A Handbook of Homeopathic Practice* (1882).

Okie, Abraham Howard (• 9-21-1882). Translated Boenninghausen's *Therapeutic Pocket Book*. Practiced in RI. "It is a great pity that a man of such talents, and even genius, is as good as lost to the profession, having taken for the last decade, no interest whatever either in society meetings or in other enterprises concerning homeopathy."—Bradford's Scrapbooks.

Orme, Francis Hodgson (• 1-28-1913) Homeopathy no doubt spread in the south because of his successes treating yellow fever epidemics in Savannah, GA.

Ortega, Proceso Sanchez (1919 •) Noted Mexican homeopath and expert on miasms. He wrote *Notes on the Miasms or Hahnemann's Chronic Diseases* (1980).

Pabst, Johan C.L. (1795 • 5-18-1861) A popular early Danish homeopath.

Palmer, Alonzo Benjamin (1815 • 1887) Wrote *Four Lectures on Homeopathy* (1869), and *Homeopathy, What is It?* (1880).

Paschero, Tomas Pablo (1904 • 1986) Prominent Argentinian homeopath and pioneer in elucidating miasmatic theory especially as it relates to environmental factors as opposed to congenital ones.

Paterson, John (1890 • 1954 or 5) A British homeopath and associate of Bach and Wheeler who worked extensively on the therapeutic use of bowel nosodes. He wrote several books including *Sycosis and Sycotic Co. (Paterson)* and *The Role of the Bowel Flora in Chronic Disease.*

Patch, Frank Wallace (3-22-1862 • 9-7-1923). Pupil of Kent. President of IHA 1907.

Payne, William E. (11-25-1815 • 3-9-1877). First homeopathic practitioner in

Maine after convincing himself by reading Hahnemann's *Organon* at the age of 25. He abandoned allopathy after curing a patient of pneumonia with homeopathy. He delivered an oration at the celebration of the centennial birthday of homeopathy in Boston, 1855. AIH President, 1851.

Pease, Giles M. (5-3-1839 • 12-14-1891) practiced in Cambridgeport, MA. His son, Jr., saw first hand during the war the successes which homeopathy had treating yellow fever. He practiced in Boston and gained a great reputation as a surgeon.

Perez, Higinio G. (•) the foremost apostle of homeopathy in Mexico during the turn of the 20th century.

Peters, John Charles (1819 • 1893) Author of *The Science and Art or the principles and practice of medicine* (1859) and *A Complete Treatise on Headaches ... based on T.J. Reuckert's clinical experiences...* (1859).

Petersen, Fred Julius (1863 •) Author of *Materia Medica and Clinical Therapeutics* (1905).

Pettingill, Sarah Brooks (5-16-1810 •) she was an circa 1859 graduate of Penn Medical University (Phila.) and later desirous of studying homeopathy yet unable to prevail upon the Hom. Med. Coll. of PA to allow her to matriculate she did manage to sit in on materia medica lectures, "...if she would sit like a 'veiled nun' behind a partition, screened from the students." This she did and for two sessions. She was the woman pioneer practitioner in Phila. In 1871, the first year women were accepted into the AIH, she was duly admitted.

Phatak, S.R. (• 1981) Important Indian homeopath and author of *Materia Medica of Homeopathic Medicines* and *A Concise Repertory of Homeopathic Medicines.*

Phelan, Richard (Ireland, 1836 • 11-14-1902). Successfully treated Kent's wife in St. Louis and thus converted Kent, an allopathic physician, to homeopathy. Taught Kent. Organized Hering Medical College of St. Louis in 1880 which merged with Hom. Med. Coll. of St. Louis in 1882. He graduated from the Homeopathic Coll. of Phil (1867) and fought in the Civil War.

Pierce, Willard Ide (1857 • 1-8-1913). Professor at N.Y. Homeo. Med. College and author of *Plain Talks on Materia Medica...* (1911).

Pomeroy, T.F. (5-11-1816 • 4-2-1892) 1853 grad. of Cleveland Homeo. Med. Coll. He served as vice president and president of the Homeo. Med. Soc. of the State of Michigan.

Pope, Alfred C. (9-11-1830 • 3-26-1908). British.

Porter, Eugene Hoffman (8-7-1856 • 8-11-1929) Graduated from N.Y. Homeopathic Med. College in 1885 and was a professor of physiological materia medica there in 1902. Received his Doctor of Public Health degree from Syracuse U. Was a lecturer at Cornell U. and became N.Y. Commisioner of Foods and Markets from 1917-1923. Editor of the *N.A. Journal of Homeopathy* (1892-1927). From 1905-1914 he was N.Y. State Commissioner of Health. He was an officer of the AIH in 1900.

Powelson, Harvey (c. 1920 • 3-26-1991) Early on suggested to Drs. S. Messer and S. King to form a homeopathic naturopathic organization. This humble suggestion resulted in the formation of the Homeopathic Academy of Naturopathic Physicians (HANP). He said, "There's not much difference between good medicine and no medicine, but there's a lot of difference between good medicine and bad."—*JAIH,* 84:2, p. 32.

Preston, M. (1-22-1839 • 10-2-1895).

Pruzzo, Neil (c. 1942 • 9-9-1991) Texas homeopath who also practiced cranial osteopathy. His wife, Judy, also practiced homeopathy. "Dr. Pruzzo treated 8 cases of heat exhaustion successfully with *Carbo veg.*"—*JAIH,* 84:4, p. 119.

Pulford, Alfred (5-4-1863 • 8-4-1948)

Pulford, Charles H. (12-18-1859 • 6-12-1925) 1888 graduate of Hahnemann (Chicago).

Pulford, Dayton (1899 • 5-25-1964). Son of Alfred. He authored two books, *Key to the Materia Medica* and *Pneumonia.* He studied under Royal E.S. Hayes. A 32nd degree Mason, he was nicknamed 'G.G.', short for 'Galloping Gondola', "because he was long and lean and fast and quaint."— Eliz. W.-Hubbard, *JAIH,* 5/6, 1964.

Pulford, Wm. Henry (1831 • 1-16-1919) 1894 graduate of Cleveland Homeopathic Medical College.

Pulte, Joseph Hypolyte (10-6-1811 • 2-24-1874). Graduated with a degree in medicine from the U. of Hamburg, Germany. Emigrated to America in the mid-1830s. Author of *Pulte's Domestic Physician* (1850). Teacher at Allentown. Settled in Cincinnati and founded the Pulte Homoeopathic Medical College (1872). He was a co-founder of the AIH. He lectured at the Homeopathic College of Cleveland and was chair of the Dept. of Obstetrics and Diseases of Children.

Quin, Frederick Foster Hervey (1799 • 11-24-1878). First homeopath in England (1932) and often considered its Father. Pupil of Hahnemann, spending time with him in Leipzig. He himself was cured of cholera which convinced him without a doubt of the supremacy of homeopathy. He was a man of charm and a raconteur par excellence. He was sought in high circles and his influence in establishing homeopathy in Britain was unquestioned. He co-founded the British Homoeopathic Society in 1844 and was elected its president

Rabe, Rudolph Frederick (1-18-1872 • 3-18-1952). Professor at NY Homeopathic Medical College and Dean from 1920-1. IHA President 1923. Wrote *Medical Therapeutics for Daily Reference* (1920).

Radde, William (1800 • 5-19-1884). Founder of a pharmacy and publishing company in NY.

Radde, William Jr. (• 3-15-1862). Bought pharmacy of Jacob Sheek in Philadelphia. Then F. E. Boericke bought it when Radde died.

Rademacher, Charles L. (• 1861)

Rademacher, Johann Gottfried (1772 • 1850). Author of *Rademacher's Universal and Organ Remedies* (2 vol., 1st ed. 1841, trans. by A.A. Ramseyer) which was based on Paracelsian organopathy. He practiced medicine in Goch, Germany. It is questionable whether or not he was considered a homeopath in the true definition of the word.

Rae, Malcolm (1-18-1913 • 3-31-1979). British homeopath. Expert and pioneer in the field of homeopathic radionics. He carried out research on energy patterns and developed many instruments, the most famous being the Rae Magnetic Homeopathic Potency Simulator, which made homeopathic remedies by using geometric patterns—rates or templates—which he developed. "The Magneto-Geometric pattern from a simulator card is received by the water molecule in distilled water or blank pills as soon as they are placed in the simulator well." Rae developed many instruments, perfecting and expanding the scope of each. It was his intent to write a book but by his death he never had. See RADIONICS in the dictionary.

Raeside, John R. (1926 • 6-26-1972) Scottish homeopath and assistant to M. Blackie at the Royal London Hom. Hospital. A great researcher, he proved many remedies. He was killed in the 1972 plane crash (see end of this section).

Raievsky, Nicolas (1811 • 6-10-1889) An erudite, pioneering Russian homeopath. He authored works which were never published except for his 1886 pamphlet which popularized homeopathy.

Raue, Charles Gottleib (5-11-1820 • 8-21-1896). Associate and longtime friend of Hering. Co-editor of Hering's *Guiding Symptoms*. He wrote *Special Pathology and Diagnostics with Therapeutic Hints* (1868). He was professor at Hahnemann Med. Coll. of Phil. He also had a great love of psychology and wrote monographs on that subject, e.g., *Mental Symptoms* (1870), *Psychology as a Natural Science* (1889), etc., and would probably align himself with the Gestalt school of psychotherapy. Gottleib translates as 'Godlove'.

Rau, Gottlieb Ludwig (1779 • 1840) Homeopathic practitioner and author.

Raue, C. Sigmund (1873 •). He was Clinical Professor of Paediatrics at Hahnemann (Phil.) and author of *Diseases of Children: A text-book for the use of students and practitioners of medicine.*

Reckeweg, Hans Heinrich (5-20-1905 • 6-13-1985). Founder of BHI (Albuquerque, NM) and chief exponent of homotoxicology. See HOMO-TOXICOLOGY in the dictionary.

Reid, Bill (3-8-1936 • 11-10-1993) A California homeopathic physician who was active in teaching, healing and organizational work with the Ca. Hom. Med. Soc. and the HPCUS.

Reid, Fidelia Rachel Harris (4-19-1826 • 1-x-1903) an 1857 graduate of the Eclectic Med. Coll. (Cinn.) and after her marriage to a Unitarian minister (H.A. Reid) the two began to study homeopathy.

Remarkevitsch, Anthony (1824 • 4-x-1891) Early pioneering homeopath who practiced in Poland and Russia. Very popular physician who had a huge practice in Warsaw.

Renner, John (8-1-1890 • 6-27-1989). Like Cookinham, helped to keep homeopathy alive during its dark years (the middle of the 20th century). See *Brass Tacks: Oral Biography of a 20th Century Physician* (Adelaide Suits, 1985).

Reuckert, Ernst Ferdinand (1795 • 1843) Homeopath and author of *Therapeutics of Homeopathy* (1846).

Reuckert, Theodor Johann (c.1800 • 1885) German homeopath and author of *Klinische Erfahrungen in der Homoopathie* (1854).

Reynolds, L.S. (1814 • 1890).

Roberts, Herbert Alfred (5-7-1868 • 10-13-1950). Pupil of Close. Practiced in CT. Taught at the AFH post graduate school.

Rodman, Wm. Woodbridge (1817 • 1900) Author. Gave the 1865 AIH address.

Romig, John (1-3-1804 •   ) a graduate of the U. of Penn in 1825, he became interested in homeopathy in 1833 and was one of the original members of the Northampton Homeo. Med. Faculty and along with Hering, Wesselhoeft, Detwiller, Freytag, etc. established the first homeopathic school in the world, North American Academy der Homoeopathische Heikunst at Allentown, PA. In 1838 he moved to Baltimore but returned to Allentown two years later.

Romig, William H. (1-3-1804 • 2-10-1885) an 1871 graduate of Hahnemann (Phila.) and son of John Romig. Wm. and his brother Geo. M. (1845 • 12-6-1925, 1870 grad. of Hahnemann, Phila.) became associated with their father in the practice of medicine.

Rood, Marion Belle (8-11-1898 • 12-22-1995) Graduate of New York Medical College (formerly Homeopathic) in 1932 and practiced in Lapeer, MI for over 50 years. She was a colleague of Grimmer and a student of Harvey Farrington. She donated vast sums of her personal savings to the legal effort to keep the HPUS an official compendium.

Rosenstein, I.G. (•) Pioneer of homeopathy in Louisville, KY. Author of

Theory and Practice of Homeopathy (1840).

Rosa, Storm (7-18-1791or4 • 5-3-1864) Pioneer of homeopathy in Ohio and the mid-west. "When the Eclectic Medical College of Cincinnati was organized, it was understood by the legislature that chartered it and the original faculty that it was to be organized upon the broadest basis of true eclecticism. Drs. Morrow, Hill, Gatchell and other able men were members of the faculty, and Dr. Rosa was selected by the homoeopathists of Ohio as a suitable person to occupy the chair of theory and practice of homoeopathy. His labors in that college mark an era of homoeopathy in the west. They gave an impetus to the system that is felt even to this day. He began one course of lectures, which had the effect of converting not only one-third of the class, but two of his most prominent eclectic colleagues in the faculty, Drs. Hill and Gatchell. This was a result not relished by the eclectic school and Dr. Rosa was deposed from his postition." King, *(History of Homoeopathy, Vol. 1,* p. 182,3).

Rose, Roger A. (9-11-1925 • 6-14-1997) pioneer of resonance homeopathy.

Ross, A. C. Gordon (1904 • 1982) He was an author and popular homeopath in Scotland. He wrote *Homoeopathic Green Medicine* (1978).

Ross, T. Douglas (3-30-1932 • 9-8-1964) Noted Scottish homeopath. He served for two years as head of the Faculty of Homeopathy at the Royal London Hom. Hosp. before his untimely death at 32. "Life is a valley we inhabit lying between the peaks of two eternities—unscalable to us—but we do not lose the influence of a man like Douglas Ross by his death." - R.G. Laing, *(JAIH,* 11/12-1964, p. 340)

Royal, George (7-15-1853 • was still writing in 1931). Author. Prof. of materia medica and therapeutics at the Homeo. Med. Dept. State U. of Iowa. He wrote *Text-Book of Homoeopathic Theory and Practice of Medicine* (1923) and *Text-Book of Materia Medica* (1918).

Ruckert, Theodor Johann (1800 • 8-6-1885) A direct disciple of Hahnemann who took part in Hahnemann's provings. He wrote an extensive essay, 'On Epilepsy' as published in the *Allgemeine Homoeopathische Zeitung.*

Ruddock, Edward Harris (1822 • 12-23-1875). Author of *Vade Mecum, The Disease of Infants and Children, The Lady's Manual of Homoeopathic Treatment, Stepping Stones of Homoeopathy and Health,* and many other texts. A British homeopath, he was a member of the Royal College of Physicians and consulting physician to the Reading and Berkshire Homoeopathic Dispensary.

Runnels, Orange Scott (6-11-1847 • 8-15-1929) An 1871 grad. of Cleve. Hom. Hosp. Coll. and Pres. of AIH in 1886. He was surgeon general of Indiana in 1897.

Ruoff, A. Jos. Friedrich (•) German homeopath and author of *Ruoff's Repertory Nosologically Arranged* (2nd ed., 1845).

Rushmore, Edward (5-18-1845 • 11-24-1925). President of IHA in 1893.

Russell, John Rutherford (1816 • 1866) British homeopath and author, writing essays published in the *British Journal of Homeopathy* (1858-1866) and editor of *Homeopathy in 1851* (1852).

Sampson, Marmaduke Blake (• 1876) British author of *Homeopathy: Its Principles, Theory and Practice* (3rd ed., 1850).

Sanders, John C. (7-2-1825 •) Intimately involved with the Cleve. Homeo. Medical College. He was president of the AIH in 1883.

Sankaran, P. (1922 • 1979) Noted Indian homeopath and teacher of homeopathy at the Homeopathic College (Bombay). First editor of the *Indian Journal of Homeopathic Medicine*, and a founder of the All India Homeopathic Association. A personal associate of Eliz. Wright-Hubbard. Father of Rajan Sankaran, author of *The Spirit of Homeopathy* and *The Substance of Homeopathy.*

Santee, E. M. (•). Author of *Repertory of Convulsions.* Developed Santee potentizer.

Sawyer, Albert I. (10-31-1828 • 5-7-1891). A graduate of Western Coll. of Homeopathy and later the Cleveland Homeo. Hosp. Coll. He was instrumental in getting the homeopathic medical department established on the University of Michigan campus. He was mentor and preceptor of J.C. Wood, M.D.

Sawyer, Brig. Gen. Charles E. (1-24-1860 • 9-23-1924). Physician to President Harding. Pres. of AIH.

Schley, James Montfort (4-1-1852 • 10-22-1924) He became an esteemed physician in New York City and gained a reputation as a diagnostician *par excellence.* He was professor of physical diagnosis at the New York Med. Coll. and Women's Hospital. His father, James Montfort, was a noted homeopath in the South.

Schmid, Franz (3-13-1920 • 1-5-1997) German homeopath, author and renowned expert on pediatrics. He was also an expert on cell therapy and congenital diseases, especially Down's syndrome. He wrote *Biological Medicine* and the massive, 13,429-page *Handbook of Pediatrics.*

"For him, a fulfilling life meant work, meant leadership by example. He put up with countless hostilities and disadvantages on behalf of 'his' children with Down's syndrome but found fulfillment in the shining eyes of those whom he rescued from the semi-darkness of a life of disability and (in many case) set on the road to a near-normal daily life."—*Biomedical Therapy,* 15:2, 1997, p. 39.

Schmid, F.W. (1918 • 5-15-1984). Practiced in San Francisco. Was a president of the AIH.

Schmidt, Pierre (7-22-1894 • 10-15-1987). The great Swiss homeopath, he was responsible for reintroducing classical homeopathy into Europe. He studied under Frederica E. Gladwin, who had been a pupil of Kent's. He was associated with J.H. Clarke and Sir John Weir of England. A co-founder of the LIGA and active participant in that organization for many years. He wrote *Defective Illnesses* (1980) and *Hidden Treasures of the Last Organon*, which brought public attention to Hahnemann's changes in the 6th edition (such as the Q potencies) which had otherwise gone unnoticed in the homeopathic community since the 1920-21 publication of the 6th edition.

"His death is no cause for vain mourning on the part of his pupils and those whom he influenced. Now is the time for them to show their appreciation for all that Pierre Schmidt meant to them, and to bear witness by their actions. Many owe him more than their professional orientation; they owe him the quality of their lives. To them belongs the honor to ascertain the survival of their master's work.

"Let us hope that the seed so liberally sewn by Dr. Pierre Schmidt's generosity throughout the world will ripen to a bountiful harvest." -Jacques Baur, M.D., *(CHQ,* 1/1988, p. 38).

Schmidt, Roger (• 10-19-1975). The brother of Pierre Schmidt and a fine homeopath in his own right. He practiced for some fifty years in the San Francisco area. President of the AIH in 1958.

Schmidt-Nagel, Dora (1-6-1898 • 3-21-1986). Operated and founded the Laboratoire Homeopathique in Geneva, Switz. She produced remedies of unquestioned reliability.

Schneider, Nathaniel C. (1839 • 1895) An 1864 graduate of Cleveland Homeo. Med. College. Later he taught at his alma mater and worked diligently at the Huron Street Hospital. He was a partner with D.H. Beckwith, too.

Schuessler, Wilhelm Heinrich (8-21-1821 • 3-30-1897) Founder of the Biochemic system of medicine in which twelve cell salts are employed to cure illness by balancing and revitalizing cellular activity. He wrote *Twelve Tissue Remedies* (1880). Obituary in *Homeopathic Recorder* (Vol 13, p. 499). See dictionary entry. Whether or not he can be called a homeopath is questionable.

Schwabe, Willmar (•) Founder of the German homeopathic company Schwabe & Co. in 1865. Author of *Lehrbuch der Homoopathischen...* (1887).

Schwartz, F. Adele (• 1-26-1945)

Scudder, J. M. (9-8-1829 • 2-17-1894). Prominent eclectic physician, author, and educator.

Seidel, Ray E. (• 5-29-1980) Homeopathic physician who practiced in south Philadelphia for over forty years. He introduced Julian Winston to homeopathy. He was a 1935 graduate of Hahnemann (Phil.). Served as president of the Pan American Homeopathic Medical Congress.

Selfride, James M. (• 3-4-1906) California homeopath.

Senn, Dominique (1912 • 1992) Noted Swiss homeopath who did seminal work in bioenergetics and its relationship to homeopathy, and conducted research in nosodal therapy and nosode theories.

Seward, S.A. (9-3-1810 • 2-8-1897).

Shadman, Alonzo Jay (7-20-1877 • 3-6 or 4-6-1960). Homeopathic surgeon who practiced in Boston and owned Emerson Hospital, which he purchased from its founder, Nathaniel Emerson. Graduated from Boston University Medical School in 1905. Honorary V.P. of the British Homeopathic Association. Author of *Who is Your Doctor and Why?* (1958).

Sharp, William (1805 • 1896) Author of *Tracts on Homoeopathy* (1853,4), a popular and important text. It consists of 12 tracts or essays which educate the reader and defend homeopathy. See TRACT in the dictionary.

Shedd, Percy William (1870 • 1-9-1911). Developed Shedd potentizer. Author, teacher, bacteriologist. Wrote *The Clinic Repertory* (1908).

Sheek, Jacob (• 1-1-1858). Co-owner, along with Charles Radermacher, of Radermacher and Sheek Pharmacy, which was purchased by Boericke in 1858.

Shepherd, Dorothy (1885 • 11-15-1952). Author of *The Magic of the Minimum Dose, A Physician's Posy, Homoeopathy in Epidemic Diseases*, etc. Studied at the Hering College in Chicago, ca. 1910. Born in Britain.

Sherman, Lewis (1843 • 7-20-1915) Noted Wisconsin homeopath and author of *Therapeutics and Materia Medica* (3rd, 1887).

Shipman, George Elias (1820 • 1893) Homeopath and author of *Homeopathy, Allopathy and the City Hospital* (1857) and *The Homeopathic Family Guide...* (8th Ed., 1873).

Simmons, George H. (1852 England • 1937) 1882 graduate of Hahnemann Med. (Chicago).

Simon, Leon (11-27-1798 • 5-13-1867). Writer, lecturer, and disciple of Hahnemann. Publisher along with Jahr and Croserio of *Annales de la Medicine Homoeopathique* in 1842.

Simpson, Stephen (1792 •) British homeopath and author of *A Practical View of Homeopathy...* (1836).

Sircar, Mahendra Lal (•) Noted Calcutta homeopath who started the *Calcutta J. of Medicine*, a homeopathic journal, in 1868.

Skinner, Thomas (8-11-1825 Scotland • 10-11-1906). Homeopathic author and developer of the Skinner potentizer. He was cured of hypochondria by E.W. Berridge, who prescribed *Sulphur*. He wrote *Homoeopathy and Gynaecology* (1878). Co-editor of *The Organon*.

Small, Alvan Edmond (3-4-1811 • 12-28 or 31-1886). Teacher of H. N. Guernsey. He was a professor at the Homeo. Med. Coll. of Pa and later was one of the chief founders of Hahnemann (Chic.). He wrote *Diseases of the Nervous System, Practice of Medicine, Diseases of the Chest,* and *Domestic Practice.* He was a popular lecturer and indeed a popular personage and was associated with the school he helped found for over 30 years. In 1873 he was president of the AIH.

Small, Herbert Elwyn (• 1911) Wrote *The Story of Homeopathy* (1889).

Small, Standley G. (1874 • 6-19-1915). 1898 grad of Cleveland Hom. Med. Coll.

Smith, A. Dwight (1885 • 3-2-1980) Homeopath in Glendale, CA for some 60 years. 1912 graduate of Hahnemann (Chic.), studied under Kent. He was very active in homeopathic organizations. Past president of the IHA and editor of the *Homeopathic Recorder* for many years. He edited the *Pacific Coast Homeopathic Bulletin* for 25 years.

Smith, David S. (4-28-1816 • 4-29-1891). Founder of Hahnemann (Chicago). "Father of Western homeopathy".

Smith, Henry M. (4-24-1835 • 3-16-1901) An 1876 grad. of the NY Hom. Med. Coll.. Secretary of the Monument Committee (1892-1902), which coordinated the erection of the monument to Hahnemann at Scott Circle in Washington, D.C. Co-editor with Dunham of *American Homeopathic Review*. His father (John T.S. Smith) founded Smith's Pharmacy in 1844.

Smith, J.Heber (12-5-1842 • 10-23-1898) an 1866 graduate of the Homeo. Med. Coll. of PA. Edited the *New England Medical Gazette.*

Snader, Edward Roland (1-10-1855 •) An 1884 graduate of Hahnemann (Phila.) and lecturer on physical diagnosis with a speciality in heart and lungs.

Snelling, Frederick Greenwood (1831 • 1878) Author of *Hull's Jahr: A New Manual of Homeopathic Practice* (1864).

Sparhawk, George E. (2-2-1830 • 3-16-1906). Member of the IHA. Practiced in VT. He preceptored with W.F. Guernsey and graduated in 1853 from the Homeo. Med. Coll. of PA. "His ministry of healing is twice blessed; it blesses him that gives and him that takes." - Cleave, p. 183.

Spork, Emily von Vegesach (3-x-1835 •) the daughter of Baron and Baroness Emil von Vegesach of Sweden. She had a great interest in medicine but the Swedish schools did not admit women so she studied massage-Swedish Movement Cure-and became very successful in Bergen, Norway. Still dissatisfied and unfulfilled she ventured to America and attended Hahnemann (Chic.) graduating in 1873. She became "...the first Scandinavian lady who has studied homeopathy and received the full diploma of Doctor of Medicine." -Cleave, p. 429.

Stapf, Johann Ernst (9.-9-1788 • 7-11-1860). Hahnemann's pupil, intimate friend, and prover of many remedies. He established the journal *Archiv fur die homoopathische Heilkunst* in 1822 and edited it with G.W. Gross.

He is considered the first in a long line of homeopathic physicians to treat the British royal family.

Staples, Henry Franklin (3-29-1870 • 5-26-1938) An 1896 graduate of Cleve. U. School of Medicine and professor of hygiene at Cleve.-Pulte, 1905-1914. President of the Ohio State Homeo. Med. Society in 1911 and honorary president of the AIH in 1936.

Stauffer, Abraham Kar (1870 • c.1930) German author of *Clinische Homoopathische arzneimittellehre* (1926).

Stearns, Guy Beckly (9-16-1870 • 3-21-1947) Author of *The Physical Basis of Homeopathy and a New Synthesis.*

Steiner, Rudolf (2-27-1861 • 1925) Though not a homeopath in the strict sense, his homeopathic legacy lives on in the anthroposophical practitioners of today who do use the homeopathic principle. He created/researched/ intuited an enormous amount of work which cannot be dealt with here. "There are in reality no allopaths because what is described as an allopathic remedy is subjected within the organism to a homeopathic process ... and heals only through, and by virtue of, this process. The homeopathic dosage has really, up to a point, been very carefully copied from Nature herself."—R. Steiner (*Lilipoh*, 32, p. 13). Steiner also said, "A real medicine can only exist when it penetrates into a knowledge which embraces the human being in respect to body, soul and spirit." See ANTHROSOPHY in the dictionary.

Stebbins, Nathaniel B. (1802 • 1888) Wrote *A Treatise of Biblical Medical Practice and homeopathy* (1857).

Stephens, Philetus J. (•) Eclectic and homeopathic physician, he was an 1875 graduate of Ecl. Med. Coll. of the City of NY. He wrote *A Record of the Surgical Clinics of W.T. Helmuth* (1875).

Stephenson, James Hawley (3-29-1919 • 3-20-1985). Author of *Homeopathic Provings, 1924-1959*. He was introduced to homeopathy when Elizabeth W.-Hubbard cured him of longstanding 'right lower quadrant pain'. He continued to study homeopathy under her tutelage. He had wide ranging interests: astrology, yoga, rolfing, cranial-sacral massage work. He was a prisoner of war after being shot down over Germany during WWII. He was active in organizational work and edited the *JAIH* from 1958 to 1968 and was the U.S. editor of *Acta Homeopathica* in 1968. He also authored *Index Medicus Homeopathicus Cumulativus 1963-65, A Doctor's Guide to Helping Yourself with Homeopathic Remedies* (1976), *Poetry in Vega, A Vision in Verse,* and *Lyrical Voices.* "A prodigious worker, an excellent teacher, James H. Stephenson was also a prince among men and will be missed by many."—H.N. Williams.

Stubler, Martin (1915 • 1989) Influential Austrian homeopath who "...managed to combine the clinical and scientific facts abut the remedies with the archetypal pictures of mythology, fairy tales and poetry, seemingly without any effort." - *Homoeopathic Links,* (1997, 10:2, p. 94)

Sturm, W. (6-x-1796 •   ) earliest practitioner of homeopathy in Cinncinati, in 1839 (Pulte started in 1840).

Sutherland, Allan D. (1897 • 1-31-1980) Author and pupil of H.A. Roberts. Dean of the AIH Post-Graduate School of Homeopathy, 1943-1979. 1925 grad of Hahnemann (Phil.).

Swan, Samuel (7-4-1814 • 10-17 or 18-1893; *Homoeopathic Physician* gives birth date as Oct. 18, 1815). Developer of *Lac caninum* as well as nosodes such as *Medorrhinum* and *Syphilinum.* Author of *A Materia Medica: Containing Provings and Clinical Verifications* (1888).

Tafel, Adolph J. (9-15-1839 • 3-9-1895). Founder of B&T along with F.E. Boericke in 1853. Obituary in *Homeopathic Recorder* (10:4, p. 145).

Taft, Mary Florence (6-19-1853 • 9-8-1927)

Talbot, Israel Tisdale (10-29-1829 • 7-2-1899). Founded the New England Female Medical College. Dean of Boston U. 1869-99. He studied medicine under the first physician in New England to adopt the homeopathic method, Samuel Gregg. He graduated from the Homeo. Med. Coll of Pa. in 1853. He performed the first successful tracheotomy in America on June 5, 1855. In 1866 he established the *New England Medical Gazette.* He was president of the AIH in 1872. His wife, Emily Fairbanks Talbot (2-22-1834 • 1902), was quite active in homeopathic affairs, not just assisting her husband but through numerous duties on her own, such as serving on the Board of Trustees of the Westborough Insane Hospital.

Talcott, Selden Haines (7-7-1842 • 6-15-1902). Medical superintendant of Middletown Homeopathic Hospital for the Insane for some 25 years. 1872 graduate of New York Homeopathic Medical College. He wrote many journal articles and a book entitled *Mental Diseases and Their Modern Treatment.* As a public speaker he had few equals.

Tarbell, Jonathan Adams (3-31-1810 • 1-21-1864). Author of *Homeopathy Simplified* (c.1856).

Tessier, Jean-Paul (1811 • 1862) Initially an allopath, his book *Recherches Cliniques* documents his conversion to homeopathy as it came about from his use of homeopathy in the treatment of cholera and pneumonia. He did much experimentation on pneumonia using homeopathic remedies. He was founder and editor of *L'Art Medical,* the major French homeopathic journal during that time. A large figure in the history of French homeopathy and a proponent of pathological homeopathy.

Teste, Alphonse (1814 • 1898). French homeopath and author. He wrote a very popular materia medica, *Systematisation Pratique de la Matiere*

Medicale Homoeopathique (1st ed., 1853), and *A Homoeopathic Treatise of Diseases of Children* (1862).

Thomas, Jean (1902 • 1977) French homeopath who developed serocytotherapy.

Thomas, Amos R. (10-3-1826 •) Dean of Hahnemann Med. Coll. (Phila.) for some 20 years as well as professor of anatomy. He edited the *American Journal of Homoeopathic Materia Medica*.

Thomas, Charles M. (5-3-1849 •) An 1871 graduate of Hahnemann (Phila.) and professor of ophthalmology and otology and operative surgery for many years.

Thomsen, Hans (1802 • 1864) Early Danish homeopath who was very popular with the poor. Along with Pabst they worked side by side in the cholera epidemic of 1853. Only 5 percent of their patients died compared to the allopaths' rate of 50-70 percent.

Thurston, R. L. (c.1851 • May, 1911). HMC Chicago 1882. Author.

Ticknor, Calbe B. (1805 • 1840) Author.

Tietze, C.D. (7-29-1799 • 6-23-1847)

Tonnere, C. Fabre (•) The first qualified physician to practice homeopathy in India.

Tooker, Robert (3-28-1841 • 11-8-1902). Co-editor, *Medica Era* 1883-85. Author, *Diseases of Children*.

Trinks, Carl Friedrich Gottfried (1800 • 1868) German homeopath and author of *Handbuch der Homoopathischen...* (1848).

Troup, Ronald M. (c. 1886 • 8-19-1973) A Berkeley, CA homeopathic physician who was very involved with the Cal. State Hom. Assoc. for many years during the 1960s and 1970s. He taught at the AFH postgraduate school. He studied homeopathy under Dr. Denman and was president of the AIH in 1962.

Turrill, Geo. R. (9-4-1829 • 6-21-1891) Taught anatomy at Cleve. Hom. Med Coll.

Tyler, Margaret Lucy (1857 British • 6-21-1943). She was a protege of Kent, although never studied with him. With money she inherited from her father she set up the Sir Henry James Tyler Scholarship Fund which sent several physicians, including D. Borland, and John Weir, to study with Kent between the years of 1908 to 1913. She worked in the London Homeopathic Hospital for over 40 years. Edited *Homoeopathy* for some eleven years. She wrote several books and pamphlets but her major works were, *Homoeopathic Drug Pictures* and *How Not To Do It* (1958). She created a correspondence course on homeopathy. Her father Sir H.J. Tyler (1849 • 1910), was a homeopath.

Underhill, Albert Edward (1895 •) Graduate of NY Homeo. Med. College.

Underwood, Benoni F. (12-12-1843 •) Author of *A Materia Medica of differential potency* (1884). An 1868 graduate of Hahnemann (Phila.). He proved iodiform.

Upham, Roy (•) President of AIH in 1921.

Van Baun, Wm. Weed (8-20-1858 •) An 1880 graduate of Hahnemann (Phila.) He was for many years a devoted editor of the *Hahnemannian Monthly*.

Van Denburg, Marvin W. (1843 • 12-8-1921) Wrote *A Homeopathic Materia Medica on a new and orginal plan, a sample fascicle containing the arsenic group* (1895).

Van Lennep, William Bird (12-1-1853 • 1-9-1919) A 1880 graduate of Hahnemann (Phila.), where he had the highest grade point average ever. He lectured at his alma mater on pathology and surgery. He was very active in homeopathic organizations and in clinical work. Co-editor of the *Hahnemannian Monthly*.

Vanderburgh, Federal (5-11-1788 • 1-23-1868). Pupil of Gram in NY. He wrote many pamphlets dealing with homeopathy and wrote *The Geometry of the Vital Forces*.

Vannier, Edouard (1869 • 11-23-1943) Pioneer French homeopath and elder brother of Leon. He had two sons who were also involved in French homeopathy: Henri Vannier and Pierre-Edouard Vannier.

Vannier, Henri (• 7-29-1990)

Vannier, Leon (10-30-1880 • 9-9-1963) Leader of French homeopathy, researcher, and author. Wrote a fine little introductory text, *Introduction a L'Etude de L'Homoeopathie* (1919). For a time he was editor of the journal he helped found, in 1912, *L'Homoeopathie Francaise*. In 1930 he founded le Dispensaire Hahnemann and le Centre Homoeopathique de France. In 1950 he founded la Maison de l'Homoeopathie. He did seminal research on nosodes, isotherapy, typology, sanguineous autotherapy, and drainage homeopathy.

Vannier, Pierre-Edouard (1899 • 1986)

Verdi, Tullio S. (1829 • 11-26-1902). Doctor to Secretary of State William Seward and prominent Washington, D.C. homeopath. In 1866 he suggested that an International Homeopathic Congress be organized, which was held 10 years later in 1876 in Philadelphia. An 1856 graduate of the Homeo. Med. Coll. of PA (Phila.).

Voegeli, Adolphe (1898 • 2-2-1993) A Swiss homeopathic doctor who in his mid 40s converted to homeopathy after reading L. Vannier's *Materia Medica*. He wrote 14 books on homeopathy, most published by Haug-

Verlag and traveled widely in his motor home through Germany and Switzerland teaching and consulting. "Don't study the remedies, but study the difference between the remedies . . . then think! Make your own opinion! *Esprit critique!"* and "Modern medicine doesn't want to cure people, but to prolong their lives" are a couple of his aphorisms. Obituary gleaned from *Homeopathic Links* (3/93, p. 11).

Vogel, Alfred (1902 • 1996) Esteemed naturopath who wrote several books, *The Nature Doctor* being his most popular. It was translated into 12 languages and went through fifty English language editions. He was instrumental in making echinacea a popular herbal remedy worldwide. He founded Bioforce, an herbal and homeopathic company, in 1963. His philosophy was "Be moderate and live in tune with nature."

Voll, Reinhold (2-17-1909 • 2-12-1989) German homeopath who was a leader in EAV. See dictionary entries for VOLL, VEGATEST, EAV.

Voorhoeve, Johannes (•) Wrote *Homeopathy in Practice* (1925).

Waffle, Willella H. (10-25-1854 • 11-12-1924) an 1886 graduate of Hahnemann (Chic.) and was the first woman physician to practice medicine in Los Angeles County, CA.

Wagner, Phillippina (4-12-1842 • 2-17-1915). Graduate of Hahnemann Med. Coll. of the Pacific in 1889.

Wait, Phoebe Jane Babcock (9-30-1838 • 1-30-1904) A graduate of the NY Med Coll and Hospital for Women in 1871, later serving that institution in various capacities (professor, dean) for many years.

Walsh, James Joseph (1865 • 1942) Homeopath and author.

Ward, Florence Nightingale (7-10-1860 •) Graduated from Hahnemann Med. Coll. (Chic.) in 1883. She practiced in San Francisco where she had the largest practice of any woman physician west of Chicago. In 1895, she married James William Ward.

Ward, Isaac Moreau (10-23-1806 • 2-24-1895). First homeopath in NJ. He converted to homeopathy after seeing its effectiveness in the 1832 cholera epidemic. He helped found the AIH in 1844, and in 1849, when the NY State Homeo. Med. Soc. was established, he served as its first president. He was associated with the two homeopathic medical colleges in NYC as well as Hahnemann in Philadelphia. His son, Joseph, became a homeopath (1858 grad of Homeo. Med. Coll. of PA) and served as a professor at the Homeo. Med. Coll. of Missouri (St. Louis) for 15 years.

Ward, James William (3-14-1861 • 7-12-1939). An 1883 graduate of New York Homeo. Med. Coll. He served as medical director of San Francisco in the earthquake of 1906. Surgeon, teacher, author. AIH president in 1910. He wrote *The Principles and Scope of Homeopathy* (1929) and *Unabridged Dictionary of Sensations "As If"*.

Weaver, Charles E. (2-25-1903 •) an 1930 graduate of Hahnemann (Phila.) and 1953 president of the Homeo. Med. Soc. of the State of PA. His uncle, Daniel W. Weaver, was an 1896 graduate of Hahnemann (Phila.)

Weaver, Rufus B. (1-10-1841 •) A longtime lecturer and professor at Hahnemann (Phila.). He was very skilled in anatomy and dissection. He made a complete dissection of the nervous system, working 10 hours a day for 6 months, and mounted it—the entire cerbro-spinal nervous system of a human being—in a single specimen.

Weaver, Wm. A., Jr. (9-15-1909 • 6-16-1974) a 1933 graduate of Hahnemann (Phil.) and was an assistant medical instructor there. He was active in AIH and AFH organizational affairs and was a fellow of the American Board of Homoeotherapeutics.

Wederkinch (1799 • 9-x-1876) Early Danish homeopath who, for a time, was assistant to Feveile.

Weir, Sir John (10-1879 Scotland • 4-17-1971) Physician to the British royal family for many years. He was first convinced of the merits of homeopathy by Dr. R. Gibson-Miller. He studied under J.H. Allen and Kent when he visited America. He was President of the Faculty of Homoeopathy in 1923. He wrote *Homeopathic Philosophy, Its Importance in the Treatment of Chronic Disease* (1915) as well as other references.

"Largely on Sir John's initiative, Parliament passed the Faculty of Homeopathy Act in 1947 *(The Times)*. His pharmacists were staggered on the occasion of the funeral of King George V to receive from Sir John prescriptions for three Kings and four Queens the same day *(The Daily Telegraph)*; for his practice in Royalty extended outside Great Britain to Norway."- *The Layman Speaks*, 24:6, 1971, p. 187.

Wells, Lucien B. (10-8-1810 • 3-23-1894)

Wells, Phineus Parkhurst (7-8-1808 • 11-23-1891 Brooklyn, NY). First President of the IHA (1881). 1862-6 co-editor of *American Homoe. Review.*

Weniavsky, Thaddeus (1817 • 6-20-1887) An early pioneering homeopathic physician who practiced in Poland and Russia.

Wenz, Eugen (1856 • 1945)

Wesselhoeft, Conrad (3-23-1834 • 12-17-1904) 1856 graduate of Harvard Medical School. His uncle, Wm. Wesselhoeft, interested him in homeopathy. He helped found the Boston University School of Medicine and was Professor of Pathology and Materia Medica there for some 30 years. He was president of the AIH in 1879. He was co-editor with Hughes and Dake of the *Cyclopaedia of Drug-Pathogenesy* and the AIH Pharmacopoeia. He translated Hahnemann's 5th edition of *The Organon* into English in 1876. Walter was his brother. Conrad was his nephew.

Wesselhoeft, Conrad (6-23-1884 • 12-2-1962) Son of Walter. He was a graduate of Harvard Medical School, 1911, but practiced homeopathy. He was considered an international authority on contagious and infectious diseases and wrote prolifically on those subjects. He held many medical appointments in the Boston area and at the time of his death was professor emeritus of clinical medicine at Boston University School of Medicine.

Wesselhoeft, J.G. (•) Owned German/English bookstores in Philadelphia, New York City, and Baltimore.

Wesselhoeft, Robert (1795 •) A hydrotherapist who joined his brother,Wm., in the United States. Wm. helped to teach him homeopathy and later the two founded the first hydrotherapeutic institution in the United States in Brattleboro, VT in 1846. Robert had two sons, Walter and Conrad Wesselhoeft.

Wesselhoeft, Walter (8-29-1838 • 8-17-1920) Walter, brother of Conrad, was also a homeopathic physician and held professorships of clinical medicine, anatomy, and obstetrics at Boston U. Sch. of Medicine from 1873 to 1909. He had a son, Conrad, who became a homeopathic physician and served with the 26th division during WWI.

Wesselhoeft, William (1794 • 9-1-1858) Prominent homeopath and companion of Detwiller during the early days of homeopathy in Pennsylvania. He was educated by Goethe and was a friend of Stapf. Along with brother Robert they established a water-cure establishment in VT.

Wesselhoeft, William Fessenden (3-4-1862 • 6-27-1943) grandson of Wm. He was the father of Mrs. L. Saltonstall (wife of Gov. Saltonstall of Mass.) He was chief surgeon at the Mass. Memorial Hospital and Clinical Professor of Surgery at the Boston U. School of Medicine. He served in WWI as the commanding officer of Base Hospital #44, which was organized by the Mass. Memorial Hospital.

Wheeler, Charles Edwin (1868 Australia • 2-2-1947). He moved to England. Author of *Bowel Nosodes* and *Introduction to the Principles and Practice of Homoeopathy* (1920, with Bodman and Kenyon). Associate of John Paterson and T.M. Dishington. He edited *Homoeopathic World* for a number of years and was President of the LIGA in 1936.

Wheeler, John (~1795 • 2-10-1876) Was a professor at Cleve. Hom. Med. College and served as President of the Board of Trustees and advised and directed the college during the first 10 years of its existence. He was a much-loved physician in that city.

White, Sarah Jane (1840 •) an 1873 graduate of the Womens Homeo. Med. Coll. of New York. She preceptored with E. Bayard. She qualified to receive her diploma after her first course of lectures but according to the by-laws had to attend the full course. She carried out the establishment of a Women's Free Medical College in NY opening in 1871.

Wilcox, De Witt Gilbert (1-15-1858 • 9-26-1951) An 1880 graduate of the Homeopathic Hospital College in Cleveland. Later he traveled to London where he worked under Joseph Lister and Lawson Tait (the leading abdominal surgeon and ovariotomist). He was attending surgeon at Buffalo Homeo. Hospital and later was attending gynecologist at Westborough State Hospital (Mass.). He was professor of gynecology at Boston University Medical School and 1914 president of the AIH. He was the first American surgeon to publish a record of an operation for a floating kidney and one of the first to perform an operation for ectopic pregnancy. He did pioneer work in brain surgery and was the first to operate on a criminal's skull in hopes of changing character where a head injury was believed to be the cause of criminal tendencies. He wrote *Health, Hygiene, Happiness* (1910) and *The Physical Awakening of the Boy* (1911).

Wilkinson, Garth J.J. (1812 • 1899) First to make the remedy *Hekla lava* from potentized lava from Mount Hecla (Iceland), based on the observation that sheep grazing on the mountain developed bony exostoses on their jaws. He was the first to translate Swedenborg's *Arcana Coelestia, Regnum Animale*, and *Oeconomia Regni Animalis* from Latin into English. Wilkinson, educated at Hahnemann Medical College, 1853 (Phil.), was a Swedenborgian. He authored *The Human Body and Its Relation to Man* (1851). About homeopathic remedies he had this to say: "[They] are more like ideas than material bodies."

Williams, Carl Alonzo (2-1-1872 • 12-24-1956) an 1895 graduate of Hahnemann (Phila.). Past-president and for 15 years was member of the Florida State Board of Medical Examiners. He lived in New London, CT, Worcester, MA and St. Pete. FL. He translated into English *Diseases of the Respiratory Tract* by F. Cartier. He was a heart specialist and wrote several papers on that as well as other subjects.

Williams, Nancy T. (• 1903) Noted homeopathic physician and largest individual donor to the erection of the Hanemann Monument in Washington, DC. She contributed $4,510.

Williams, Savina L. (10-27-1825 •) was a graduate of the Eclectic Med. Coll. (Cinn.) and along with her husband, Isaiah, converted to homeopathy and practiced for many years.

Williamson, Walter (1-4-1811 • 12-19-1870). Founder, with Hering and Jeanes, of the Hom. Med. Coll. of PA. Co-editor, *North American Journal of Homeopathy* 1862-69. Helped organize the AIH in 1844 and the NY Hom. Med. Coll. in 1848. An 1833 graduate of U. of Pennsylvania, he converted to homeopathy in 1836. President of the AIH in 1848. He had three sons who all became homeopathic physicians: Walter M. (1857 grad of Homeo. Med Coll. of Pa.), Matthew S. (1872 grad of Hahnemann-Phila.), and Alonzo P. (1876 grad of Hahnemann, Phila.)

Wilsey, Ferdinand Little (6-23-1797 • 5-11-1860). He was first a merchant, then a graduate of medical school. He was the first homeopathic patient in

America. By 1828 he was seeing many patients himself. A pupil of Gram. His doctor, John Gray, became Gram's first pupil in NYC.

Wilson, Thomas P. (11-9-1832 •) Professor at Cleveland and Pulte Homeo. Med. Colleges. An 1857 graduate of Western College of Homeopathy (Cleve.), later professor and Dean, too. He was editor of the journal, *Medical Advance*. His specialty was ophthalmology. He was 1871 president of the Ohio State Medical Society.

Winslow, Caroline Brown (11-19-1822 •) a graduate with honors from the Eclectic Med. Coll. in 1853. She was the first female graduate in medicine west of the Allegheny Mountains. She, in 1856, graduated from the Western Coll. of Homeopathy (Cleve.). She became a skillful surgeon in Utica, NY before moving to D.C. to become intimately involved in homeopathy in the nation's capital.

Winterburn, George William (9-19-1845 • 11.11.1911). Editor, *American Homeopathist* 1883-6. Graduated Eclectic College in 1875. Authored a repertory entitled *A Repertory of the Most Characteristic Symptoms of the Materia Medica* (1886).

Wolf, M.A.A. (1828 • 9-30-1891). Wrote a number of scholarly journal articles.

Wood, James Craven (1-11-1858 • 8-29-1948). President of the AIH in 1902. Surgeon, author. Wrote *Textbook of Gynecology (1st-1894, 2nd-1898)* and *An Old Doctor of the New School* (1942). An 1879 graduate of the U. of Michigan Homeopathic Medical Dept. President of the Michigan and Ohio Homeopathic Societies.

Woodbury, Benjamin Collins Sr. (1836 • 6-8-1915). Graduate of Hahnemann in Phil. in 1866.

Woodbury, Benjamin Collins Jr. (8-13-1882 • 1-22-1948). Author of *Homeopathic Materia Medica for Nurses*, a five-act play about Hahnemann's life, and many journal articles. Pres. of IHA in 1948. His father was also a homeopath.

Woodbury, John Henry (8-8-1832 •) influential and prominent Boston homeopath who took an active role in homeopathy in that city and in New England for many years. An 1855 graduate of Cleveland Homeopathic Medical College.

Woods, Harold Fergie (1883 • 1-15-1961). Pupil of Kent (1908). Wrote *Herbal Simples*.

Woodward, A.W. (•) Author of *Constitutional Therapeutics* (1903).

Worcester Samuel H. (2-16-1824 •) Cured of a scrofulous affection of the eye by H.B. Gram in 1837. First a clergyman, he later studied medicine and graduated in 1861 from the NY Homeo. Medical College. He wrote the massive *Insanity and It's Treatment* (1882). His son Samuel (2-5-

1847 •) became a homeopath as well.

Wright, Ida M. (1872 • 6-30-1915, *JAMA* lists 8-5-1915). 1911 graduate of Hahnemann in Chicago.

Wright-Hubbard, Elizabeth (2-18-1896 • 5-22-1967). First woman president of the AIH (1959) and editor of the *JAIH* for many years. She studied for a year with Pierre Schmidt, MD in Geneva, Switzerland and later with Emil Schlegel. She practiced in New York City. She wrote *A Brief Study Course in Homeopathy* and taught at the AFH post graduate homeopathic school. IHA President 1945-46. She edited the *Homoeopathic Recorder*. President of the Anthroposophical Society in America. Dr. Rabe cured her of scarlet fever with *Amm. carb.* 10M.

Yeldham, Stephen (•) Homeopath and author of *Homeopathy in Venereal Disease* (1888).

Yingling, W. A. (1-12-1851 • 4-3-1933). Author and member of the IHA. William Augustus lived and practiced in Emporia, KS from 1896 until his death. He was educated for medical missionary work, but after receiving his appointment to go to Bombay, India he became ill and could not carry out that mission. He filled the pulpit at Findlay, OH for seven years, then moved to Dodge City where he engaged in the cattle business. He named the Ness county town of Nonchalanta in 1886. He reluctantly returned to the practice of medicine to relieve the suffering in the area north of Dodge City. His practice became extensive, extending to the neighboring states. He was quite religious and missed Methodist church services just once in 32 years.

Youlin, John J. (12-31-1821 •) an 1854 graduate of the Cleve. Homeo. Medical College. Though he attended homeopathic medical college he was an opponent of the system and it was not until he was cured of a fever that he took up a belief in homeopathy. He was such a bitter opponent of homeopathy voicing his opinions so loudly and for so long that once convinced of its merit it took him two years to tell his parents. He was president of the NJ State Homeo. Medical Society for 11 years and was president of the AIH in 1874!

Young, William W. (12-5-1900 • 4-4-1974) Pres. of AIN in 1970.

Zerns, William M. (• 9-20-1887). 1872 graduate of Homeopathic Med. Coll. of Pa.

TWELVE HOMEOPATHS PERISH IN AIRLINE DISASTER

In 1972, several homeopathic doctors and associates lost their lives in an airline crash. This is the notice of that tragic incident as published in the *JAIH*.

It is a most grievous and tragic loss to have to write 'finis' to the lives of so many splendid homoeopathic doctors, pharmacist and friends who lost their lives last June 26 in an airline crash while enroute to the International Homeopathic Congress in Brussels. The British European Airways supplied the following list of names of those doctors who were on board the ill-fated airplane: Doctors I. Campbell, Golomb, Kay Kadalla (27 years old who was applying for a license to practice in the U.S.), Kadleigh, Lanza, Ruben, Raeside, Stevenson, Slinger, E. Stewart, T. Fergus Stewart (a guest at the AIH convention several years ago), and Dr. and Mrs. D.W. Everitt (the pharmacist of the homeopathic firm of Nelson & Co). To all their bereaved families and friends the American Institute of Homeopathy and the American Foundation for Homoeopathy sent a cablegram on June 28 to the British Faculty of Homoeopathy in London expressing deepest sympathy at this unfortunate tragedy.

APPELLATIONS, JOURNALS and PROFESSIONAL ASSOCIATIONS

AAHP American Association of Homoeopathic Pharmacists

AAP American Academy of Pediatrics

AATA American Art Therapy Association

ABAI American Board of Allergy and Immunology

ABFP American Board of Family Practitioners

ABHT American Board of Homeotherapeutics

ABMP Associated Bodywork & Massage Professional

ABOM American Board of Oxidative Medicine

ABPN American Board of Psychiatry and Neurology

ACM alternative and complementary medicine

ACN American College of Nutrition

ACR Advanced Certified Rolfer

ACSW Academy of Certified Social Workers

AH *American Homeopath* (journal)

AHMA American Holistic Medical Association

AHNA American Holistic Nurses Association

AHPhA American Homeopathic Pharmaceutical Association

AIH American Institute of Homeopathy

AK Acupuncturist (Pennsylvania)

AMTA American Massage Therapy Association

ANMP Association of Natural Medicine Pharmacists

AOBTA American Oriental Bodywork Therapy Association

AP Acupuncture Physician

APMA American Preventive Medical Association

ARNP Advanced Registered Nurse Practitioner

ASG Affiliated Study Group of the National Center for Homeopathy

ATR Art Therapist-Registered

AHZ *Allgemeine Homoopathische Zeitung* (journal)

ATHA Alternative Therapies Health Association

ATMOA Alternative Therapies Medical Outcomes Association

AVMA American Veterinary Medical Association

BA Bachelor of Arts

BALCCH Bachelor London College of Classical Homeopathy

BAMS Bachelor of Ayurvedic Medicine and Surgery

BHJ *British Homeopathic Journal*

BHMS British Homeopathic Medical Society

BHMS Bachelor of Homeopathic Medicine and Surgery (India)

BKH Beroepsvereniging voor Klassieke Homoeopathie (The Netherlands)

BN Bionutritionist

BS or **BSc** Bachelor of Science

BSN Bachelor of Science, Nursing

CA Certified Acupuncturist

CAAPM Clinical Associate of the American Academy of Pain Management

CAC Certified Animal Chiropractor

CAc Certified Acupuncturist

CAH Chiropractic Academy of Homeopathy

CAMT Certified Acupressure Massage Therapist

CAR Certified Advanced Rolfer

CAT Certified Acupressure Therapist

CAT/CNAT Certified AMMA Therapist/Nurse *(emphasis on bodywork)*

CBPM Certified Bonnie Prudden Myotherapist

CCH Certified in Classical Homeopathy

CCH Certified Clinical Hypnotherapist

CCN Certified Clinical Nutritionist

CCRH Central Council for Research in Homeopathy (India)

CCSP Certified Chiropractic Sports Physician

CEU Continuing Education Unit(s)

CFNP Certified Family Nurse Practitioner

CFP Certified Feldenkrais Practitioner

CHE Council on Homeopathic Education

CHF Centre Homoeopathique de France

CHom Certificate of Homeopathy

CHt Certified Hynotherapist

CHC Council for Homeopathic Certification

CHE Council on Homeopathic Education

CHES Certified Health Education Specialist

CISW Certified Independent Social Worker

CMR Certified Medical Representative

CMT Certified Music Therapist

CMT/CMP Certified Massage Therapist/Practitioner

CNCB Clinical Nutrition Certification Board

CNM Certified Nurse Midwife

CNS Certified Nutrition Specialist

COI Certified Ohashiatsu Instructor

CPT Certified Polarity Therapist

CRNP Certified Registered Nurse Practitioner

CRRN Certified Rehabiliation Registered Nurse

CSPOMM Certified Specialty in Proficiency Osteopathic Manipulation Medicine

CUIM Capital University of Integrative Medicine

CVA Certified Veterinary Acupuncturist

CVO College of Veterinarians of Ontario

CvBGH Clemens von Bonninghausen Gesellschaft fur Homoopathik e.V. (Germany)

CWO Dutch Homeopathic Scientific Research Committee

DAAPM Diplomate of the American Academy of Pain Management

DABFP Diplomate of the American Board of Family Practice

DABIM Diplomate of the American Board of Internal Medicine

DAc Diplomate in Acupuncture

DACVD Diplomate of the American College of Veterinary Dermatology

DC Doctor of Chiropractic

DDS Doctor of Dentistry

DGKH Deutsch Gesellschaft fur Klassische Homoopathie

(Germany)

DHANP Diplomate of the Homeopathic Academy of Naturopathic Physicians

DHM Diploma in Holistic Medicine

DHM Diploma/Diplomate in Homeopathic Medicine

DHMS Diploma of Homeopathic Medicine and Surgery (India)

DHPh Diploma in Homeopathic Pharmacy

DHom(Med) Diplomate of Homeopathic Medicine

DHt Diplomate of Homeo-therapeutics

DHU Deutsche Homoopathie-Union

DIHom Diploma of the Institute of Homeopathy

DMD Doctor of Dental Medicine

DNBHE Diplomate of the National Board of Homeopathic Examiners

DO Doctor of Osteopathy

DOM Doctor of Oriental Medicine

DPM Doctor of Podiatric Medicine

DSH Diploma (from the) School of Homeopathy

DSKH Dansk Selskab for Klassisk Homoopati (Denmark)

DVM Doctor of Veterinary Medicine

DVetHom Diploma in Veterinary Homeopathy

ECCH European Council for Classical Homeopathy

ECH European Committee for Homeopathy

ESCOP European Scientific Cooperative on Phytotherapy

FAAEM Fellow of the American Academy of Environmental Medicine

FAAFP Fellow of the American Academy of Family Practitioners.

FAAN Fellow of the American Association of Nurses

FAAP Fellow of the Association of American Pediatrics

FAAPMR Fellow of the American Academy of Physical Medicine and Rehabilitation

FACA Fellow of the American College of Allergies

FACACN Fellow of the Council of Applied Clinical Nutriton

FACD Fellow of the American College of Dentists

FACGP Fellow of the American College of General Practitioners

FACHP Fellow of the American College of Homeopathic Physicians

FACOG Fellow of the American College of Obstetrics and Gynecology

FACP Fellow of the American College of Physicians

FACS Fellow of the American College of Surgeons

FAGD Fellow of the Academy of General Dentistry

FAIM Foundation for the Advancement of Medicine

FCAH Fellow of the Canadian Academy of Homeopathy

FDA Food and Drug Administration

FFHOM Fellow of the Faculty of Homeopathy

FHR Foundation for Homeopathic Research (India)

FIACA Fellow of the International Academy of Clinical Acupuncture

FIAOMT Fellow of the International Academy of Oral Medicine and Toxicology

FICCMO Fellow of the International College of Cranio-Mandibular Orthopedics

FICPA Fellow of the International Chiropractic Pediatrics Association

FNP Family Nurse Practitioner

FONMUNA Federation of Natural Medicine Users of North America

FRCP Fellow of the Royal College of Physicians

FRCS Fellow of the Royal College of Surgeons

FRSAHA Fellow of the Royal South African Homeopathic Association

FSHom Fellow of the Society of Homeopaths (U.K.)

GHP Good Homeopathic Practice *(see dictionary entry)*

GMP Good Manufacturing Practices

HANP Homeopathic Academy of Naturopathic Physicians (USA)

HAV Homoopathischer Arzte Verband (Switzerland)

HCC Homeopathic Community Council

HF Homoopathie Forum (Germany)

HH *Homoeopathic Heritage* (Indian journal)

HIIHD Hahnemann International Institute for Homeopathic Documentation

HL *Homoeopathic Links* (Swiss journal)

HMD Homeopathic Medical Doctor

HMO Health Maintenance Organization

HMRG Homeopathic Medicine Research Group

HNA Homeopathic Nurses Assoc.

HNC Certified Holistic Nurse

HOMINT Homeopathy International

Homeopatisk Tidskrift (homeopathic journal)

HPCUS Homoeopathic Pharmacopoeia Convention of the United States

HSF Homoeopaths sans [*without*] Frontieres

HSG Homeopathic Study Group

HT *Homeopathy Today* (USA journal)

IAACN International and American Associations of Clinical Nutritionists

IACH International Academy for Classical Homeopathy

ICCH International Council for Classical Homeopathy

ICHom International College of Homeopathy, or Institute of Classical Homeopathy

ICR Institute of Clinical Research (India)

IFH International Foundation for Homeopathy

IHA International Hahnemannian Association

IMD Doctor of Integrative Medicine

IOMA International Oxidative Medicine Association

IRHIS Institute for Research in Homeopathic Information

ISSSEEM International Society for the Study of Subtle Energies and Energy Medicine

ISH Irish Society of Homoeopaths

(Ireland)

JAIH *Journal of the American Institute of Homeopathy* (USA)

JAMA *Journal of the American Medical Association*

JD Juris Doctor (Doctor of Law)

KHA Kent Homeopathic Associates

KIKOM Kollegiale Instanz fur Komplementare Medizin (U. of Berne, Switz.)

LAc Licensed Acupuncturist

LCH Licentiate of the College of Homeopathy

LCCH London College of Classical Homeopathy

LCCHI London College of Classical Homeopathy International

LCCHOTP London College of Classical Homeopathy Overseas Training Programme

LCEH Licentiate of the Court of Examination in Homoeopathy and Biochemistry

LCSW Licensed Clinical Social Worker

LD Licensed Dietitian

LicAc Licensed Acupuncturist

LIGA refers to International Homeopathic Medical League

LL Laymen's League

LM Licensed Midwife

LMHI Liga Medicorum Homoeopathica Internationalis (International Homeopathic Medical League, LIGA)

LMHP Licensed Mental Health Practitioner

LMP/LMT Licensed Massage Practitioner/Therapist

LMPFH Licensed Medical Profes-

sionals for Homeopathy

LN Licensed Nutritionist

LNC Certified Licensed Nutritionist

LPN Licensed Practical Nurse

MA Master of Arts

MAc Master of Acupuncture

MASc Master of Ayurvedic Science

MBBS Bachelor of Medicine and Bachelor of Surgery (India)

MCH Member of the College of Homeopathy

MD Doctor of Medicine

MD(H) Homeopathic Medical Doctor (in Arizona)

MFCC Marriage, Family and Child Counselor

MH Master Herbalist

MFHom Member, Faculty of Homeopathy (U.K.)

MNIMH Member of the National Institutes of Medical Herbalists (UK)

MNNP Master of Nursing, Nurse Practitioner

MOM Master of Oriental Medicine

MRC Medical Research Council

MPH Master of Public Health

MRCGP Member of the Royal College of General Practitioners

MS/MSc Master of Science

MSD Master of Science in Dentistry

MSN Master of Science in Nursing

MSW Master of Social Work

MT/MsT Massage Therapist

NANHE North American Network of Homeopathic Educators

NASH North American Society of Homeopaths

NASTAT North American Society of Teachers of the Alexander Technique

NBHE National Board of Homeopathic Examiners

NC Nutritional Counselor

NCAHF National Council Against Health Fraud

NCCA National Commission for the Certification of Acupuncturists

NCH National Center for Homeopathy

ND Naturopathic Doctor

NEHA New England Homeopathic Academy

NEJH *New England Journal of Homeopathy*

NESH New England School of Homeopathy

NHL Norsk Homeopaters Landsforbund (Norway)

NIH National Institutes of Health

NJH *National Journal of Homoeopathy* (India)

NLP Neuro-Linguistic Programming

NMD Naturopathic Medical Doctor (in Arizona)

NP Nurse Practitioner

NWPVH NWP Vakgroep Homoeopathie (Netherlands)

NZICH New Zealand Institute of Classical Homoeopathy (NZ)

OAM Office of Alternative Medicine

OD Doctor of Optometry

OGHM Austrian Association for Homeopathic Medicine

OIRF Occidental Institute Research Foundation

OMD Oriental Medical Doctor

OSHMS Ohio State Homeopathic Medical Society

PA Physician Assistant

PA Professional Associate

PAC/PA-C Certified Physician Assistant

PharmD/PD Doctor of Pharmacy

PhD Doctor of Philosophy

PMD Doctor of Physiatric Medicine

PsyD Doctor of Psychology

PT Physical Therapist

RAc Registered Acupuncturist

RCCM Research Council for Complementary Medicine

RD Registered Dietitian

RM Reiki Master

RMT Registered Music Therapist

RMT Registered Massage Therapist

RN Registered Nurse

RN-C Certified Registered Nurse

RN, C/RNCS/RNC-S Registered Nurse Clinical Specialty

RNNP Registered Nurse, Nurse Practitioner

RPh Registered Pharmacist

RPP Registered Polarity Practitioner

RPT Registered Physical Therapist

RSHom(NA,UK) Registered with the Society of Homoeopaths (NA-North America; UK-United Kingdom)

SAKH Svenska Akademian for Klassisk Homoeopati (Sweden)

SH Suomen Homeopaatit (Finland)

SHMA Southern Homeopathic Medical Association

Simillimum (USA journal)

SHO Dutch Foundation for Homeopathic Education

SOH Society of Homeopaths (UK)

SVHA Swiss Association for Homeopathic Doctors

The Homeopath (UK journal)

TLfD&P *Townsend Letter for Doctors and Patients*

TT Therapy Technician

VBKH Vereniging ter Bevordering van Klassieke Homoeopathie (Belgium)

VHAN Society of Homeopathic Physicians in the Netherlands

VKH Vereniging ter Bevordering van Klassieke Homeopathen (Belgium)

VKH Verband Klassischer Homoopathen/Innen (Switzerland)

VMD Veterinary Medical Doctor

VSM the initials of a pharmacy in The Netherlands which manufactures homeopathics

ZDN Zentrum zur Dokumentation fur Naturheilverfahren (German)

ZKH *Zeitschrift fur Klassische Homoopathie* (German journal)

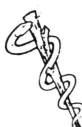

CADUCEUS
(L., 'heralds' staff/wand')

Two types of caduceus are confused in modern iconography. The symbol which uses a single snake entwined about a bough is the correct one when used in reference to the medical profession. It is the sole symbol of the AMA and other medical groups.

This single snake adorned the staff of Aesculapius (Roman) or Asklepios (Greek) who was a famous human physician circa 1200 BCE who was later worshipped as a god. (According to some versions he was the son of Apollo, tutored in surgery by a centaur, a 'monster' having the head, trunk and arms of a man and the body and legs of a horse). Whichever, there were temples erected to him in ancient Greece. This god or man of healing was often pictured/depicted with a rearing snake at his feet, and by 200 BCE his snake-laden wand represented medicine. Amongst the temples at Epidaurus the ancient Greek school of medicine grew. The sick came to sleep in the temples, hoping to be cured or granted a vision of the cure. Over the years the priests observed the ill people and learned the art of diagnosis.

Sir William Butts, physician to King Henry VIII, was granted the caduceus as his crest. This was permitted because it had also become "the symbol of military heralds seeking to negotiate peace with an enemy; the physician's enemy being disease. In 1856 the U.S. Marine Health Service, the predecessor of today's Public Health Service, made a two-snake caduceus its symbol. Accompanied by an anchor, it remains the PHS symbol today. In 1902, it was adopted by the Army Medical Corps."* The Army Medical Corps version consists of a staff with two formal wings at top in addition to the two entwined serpents. This staff is not regarded as a medical emblem but as an administrative emblem, implying neutrality.

The two-snake depiction is the symbol of Mercury (Roman) or Hermes (Greek), the winged messenger of the gods. It was originally an olive branch with green twigs (eventually becoming ribbons) wound around it. According to myth, Hermes once saw two snakes fighting. He hurled his staff between them, whereupon they wound about it and became friends. However, this myth may have evolved because of confusion with the staff's streamers. This versatile and busy god was also considered the god of commerce, protector of thieves and guide of departing souls to Hades.

Nevertheless, despite its shrouded and mysterious origin, the single-snake staff is, according to the American College of Surgeons, "the symbol of choice by scholars and those in the medical profession, representing 'the power and mystery of the healing art'."

---

*'Medicine's Symbol: An Age-Old Debate.' V. Cohn in the *Washington Post*, 1992.

VAN HOY PUBLISHERS

THE DUNHAM LECTURES by J. T. Kent, M.D.
Edited by Christopher Ellithorp and Jay Yasgur
The editors have brought together four of Dr. Kent's lectures, *Chamomilla, Anthracinum, Pulsatilla,* and *Phosphorus,* which he delivered in 1899 at Dunham Homeopathic Medical College in Chicago. These lectures are different than the ones in his materia medica and are especially interesting and vivid. The lecture on *Anthracinum* is a special treat.

35 pages / $8.00 ppd

SOME CLINICAL EXPERIENCES of Erastus E. Case, M.D.
with selected writings
Edited by Jay Yasgur
This volume is a reprint of Dr. Case's classic, S*ome Clinical Experiences* in which Dr. Case presents over 200 of his cases and 100 prescribing drills. One hundred pages of additional information is included to make this a more useful work. Discussions Case had with Kent, Boger, Stuart Close, the Allens, and Wesselhoeft are appendixed, as are ten of Dr. Case's published papers.
"A singularly fine volume that should be on the shelf (and in the mind) of everyone who loves homeopathy."—Homeopathy Today, April 1992.

330 pages / $28.50 +$3.00 s&h.

HOMŒOPATHIC MATERIA MEDICA for NURSES
Benjamin C. Woodbury, with selected writings
Edited by Jay Yasgur
The title of this book leads one to believe that it is just for nurses. However, this is not the case ... it is useful for all as it contains sections on homeopathic principles, homeopathic pharmacy and homeopathic nursing. Dr. Woodbury was an expert in the field of materia medica. This is a reprint of the second edition of his 1922 book. 114 remedies are succinctly discussed, yet all the essential points are covered. Approximately ninety pages of additional material is included ... a dozen published papers in all, including a repertory of cancer of the tongue, notes on *Kobaltum,* Hering's Law of Cure, materia medica study, outline of

Sulfadiazine and Succinimide of Mercury. This volume will assist your study of the remedies and help you understand the evolution and arrangement of the materia medica. *Foreword by Maesimund Panos, M.D.*

300 pages / $18.95 + $3.00 s&h.

CUMULATIVE INDEX TO
THE HOMOEOPATHIC PHYSICIAN
Edited and compiled by Jay Yasgur
Foreword by Julian Winston

The *Homoeopathic Physician* was a high quality, classically-oriented homeo-pathic journal published from 188 to 1899. *In toto* it ran nearly 10,000 pages and contained countless clinical articles, communications, book reviews, proving reports, editorials, and historical materials related to the homeopathic community. Now, one of the finest pieces of homeopathic literature can be searched easily and quickly. There are nine sections to the Index: 2 article title sections (one listed by volume, the other alphabetically), 2 author sections (one listed by volume, the other alphabetically), 2 book review sections (one listed by volume, the other alphabetically), an obituary section, and 2 remedy sections (one listed alphabetically, the other listed alphabetically as the remedy appeared in the article title). In addition to the Index, Mr. Yasgur has included about forty pages of clinical material and historical tidbits as gleaned from the journal.

330 pages / $ 75.00 ppd.

ANNUAL ANNOUNCEMENTS OF THE
HAHNEMANN MEDICAL COLLEGE AND HOSPITAL
(Philadelphia, 1885/1886)
and
RUSH MEDICAL COLLEGE
(Chicago, 1880-1881)

These reprinted medical college prospectuses were sent to prospective students who were interested in pursuing the career of medicine. They include information on the officers, faculty, administration, and hospital staff and describes the course of study, college fees, and curriculum, etc. Hahnemann (Phila.) was the oldest and first homeopathic college, while Rush is allopathic and included for comparative purposes. An interesting historical selection.

60 pages total / $ 10.00 ppd.

ABOUT THE AUTHOR

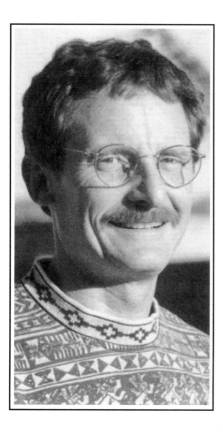

Jay Yasgur, R.PH., M.SC. is a licensed pharmacist, having received his pharmacy degree from Duquesne University and his M.Sc. in Allied Health from the University of North Florida. He became interested in the holistic health care field while studying massage in Florida. Later, while associated with a holistic health clinic, he pursued homeopathic studies under the direction of A.J. Trofe, a naturopath.

Jay has worked for Humphreys Pharmacal, the nation's second oldest manufacturer of homeopathic remedies, and Weleda, an anthroposophical firm, and currently works as an independent retail pharmacist blending homeopathy into his pharmacy practice. He is a member of several homeopathic organizations including the HPCUS (Homeopathic Pharmacopoeia Convention of the United States).

Mr. Yasgur has written homeopathic articles for *Pharmacy Times, American Druggist* and *American Pharmacy*, as well as *Resonance, Simillimum, Lilipoh, Homeopathic Links, Journal of the American Institute of Homeopathy, Alternative Therapies in Health and Medicine, Natural Pharmacy Newsletter, Natural Pharmacy, Lloydiana, Journal of Naturopathic Medicine,* and *Homeopathy Today.* His other books, which he edited, include *Some Clinical Experiences of E.E. Case, M.D.* and *Homoeopathic Materia Medica for Nurses* (by B.C. Woodbury, M.D.) Along with C. Ellithorp, he produced 'The Dunham Lectures of J.T. Kent.' He created a homeopathic calendar for 1995, and compiled the 300-page *Cumulative Index to the 'Homoeopathic Physician'.*

Mr. Yasgur was the first to offer certified continuing education credits on homeopathy to pharmacists when he presented his first talk and film to the Pinellas County Pharmaceutical Association, St. Petersburg, FL, in 1985.

While traveling in Nigeria in late 1992, Jay was invited to lecture on homeopathy. To recognize his publishing achievements and homeopathic expertise, he was honored by being made an Obong, or Chief, Obong Ikpaisong Ibibio and Annang A.K.S., Nigeria, of Traditional Medicine.

He is currently working on two books, the first dealing with the life of a homeopathic medical student at the turn of the century and the second blending the history of science with historical and clinical aspects of homeopathy. Mr. Yasgur may be contacted at Van Hoy Publishers, P.O. Box 636, Greenville, PA 16125

'Each time a [person] stands up for an ideal, or acts to improve the lot of others ... he sends forth a tiny ripple of hope, and crossing each other from a million different centers of energy and daring those ripples build a current that can sweep down the mightiest walls of oppression and resistance ...'

—Robert F. Kennedy

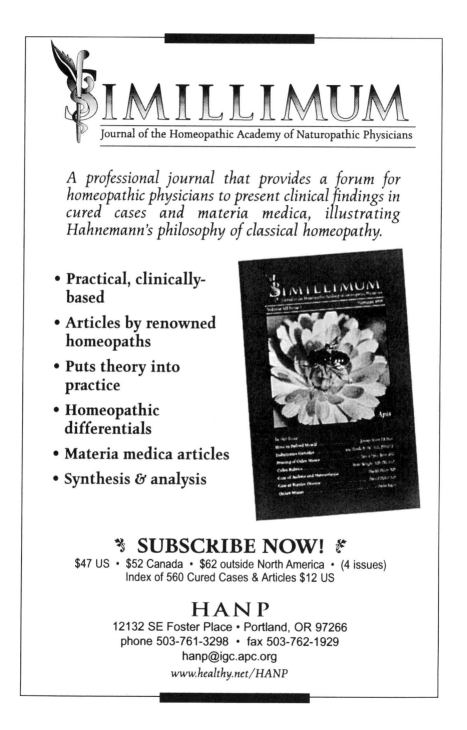

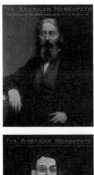

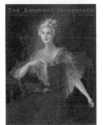
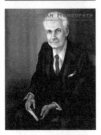
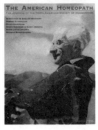
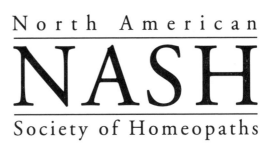

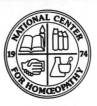